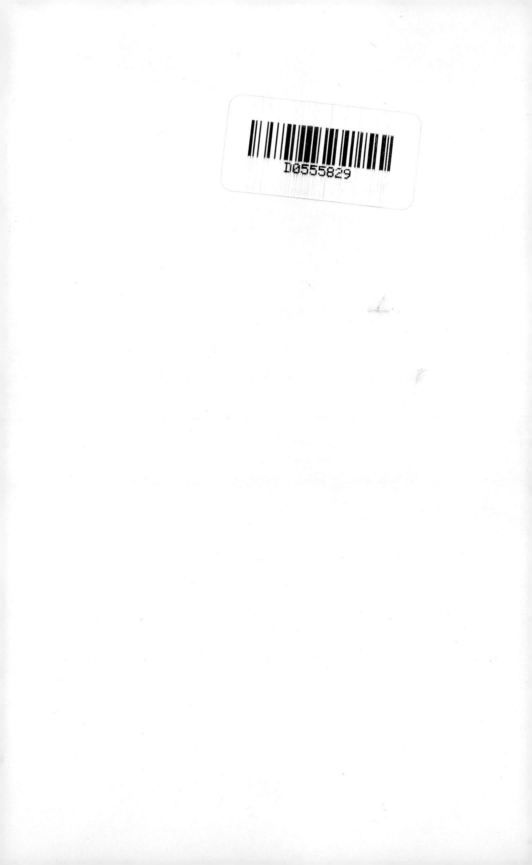

D0555829

The
Concept and Measurement
of
Quality of Life
in the
Frail Elderly

The
Concept and Measurement
of
Quality of Life
in the
Frail Elderly

Edited by

James E. Birren

Anna & Harry Borun Center for Gerontological Research
Multicampus Division of Geriatric Medicine and Gerontology
University of California, Los Angeles
Los Angeles, California

James E. Lubben

Department of Social Welfare
University of California, Los Angeles
Los Angeles, California

Janice Cichowlas Rowe

Multicampus Division of Geriatric Medicine and Gerontology
University of California, Los Angeles
Los Angeles, California

Donna E. Deutchman

Anna & Harry Borun Center for Gerontological Research
Multicampus Division of Geriatric Medicine and Gerontology
University of California, Los Angeles
Los Angeles, California

ACADEMIC PRESS, INC.

Harcourt Brace Jovanovich, Publishers

San Diego   New York   Boston   London   Sydney   Tokyo   Toronto

HV
1461
.C 658
1991

This book is printed on acid-free paper. ∞

Copyright © 1991 by ACADEMIC PRESS, INC.
All Rights Reserved.
No part of this publication may be reproduced or transmitted in any form or
by any means, electronic or mechanical, including photocopy, recording, or
any information storage and retrieval system, without permission in writing
from the publisher.

Academic Press, Inc.
San Diego, California 92101

United Kingdom Edition published by
Academic Press Limited
24–28 Oval Road, London NW1 7DX

Library of Congress Cataloging-in-Publication Data

The Concept and measurement of quality of life in the frail elderly /
    edited by James E. Birren ... [et al.].
        p.   cm.
    Based on a conference held Feb. 16–18, 1990 as a joint project of
UCLA's Multicampus Division of Geriatric Medicine and Gerontology
and the Jewish Homes for the Aging of Greater Los Angeles, sponsored
by the Anna and Harry Borun Center for Gerontological Research.
    Includes index.
    ISBN 0-12-101275-1
    1. Frail elderly--Services for--United States--Congresses.
2. Quality of life--United States--Congresses.   I. Birren, James E.
II. University of California, Los Angeles. Multicampus Division of
Geriatric Medicine and Gerontology.   III> Jewish Homes for the Aging
of Greater Los Angeles.   IV. Anna and Harry Borun Center for
Gerontological Research.
    [DNLM: 1. Aged, 80 and Over--congresses.   2. Frail Elderly-
-congresses.   3. Quality of Life--congresses.   WT 30 C744]
HV1461.C658   1991
362.6--dc20
DNLM/DLC
for Library of Congress   91-13951
                                                              CIP

PRINTED IN THE UNITED STATES OF AMERICA
91   92   93   94   9 8 7 6 5 4 3 2 1

Contents

CONCORDIA COLLEGE LIBRARY
2811 NE HOLMAN ST.
PORTLAND, OR   97211-6099

II *The Physical World and Quality of Life in the Frail Elderly*

III   *The Social World and Quality of Life
in the Frail Elderly*

IV   The World within Us and Quality of Life in the Frail Elderly

V

Autonomy as a Factor in Quality of Life in the Frail Elderly

13   Resident Decision Making and Quality of Life in the Frail Elderly
TERRIE WETLE

14   Sense of Control, Quality of Life, and Frail Older People
RONALD P. ABELES

Contributors

Numbers in parentheses indicate the pages on which the authors' contributions begin.

RONALD P. ABELES (**297**), Behavioral Sciences Research Program, National Institute on Aging, National Institutes of Health, Bethesda, Maryland 20892

SHARON B. ARNOLD (**50**), Prospective Payment Assessment Commission, Washington, District of Columbia 20024

ROBERT C. ATCHLEY (**207**), Scripps Foundation, Scripps Gerontology Center, Miami University, Oxford, Ohio 45056

JAMES E. BIRREN (**344**), Anna & Harry Borun Center for Gerontological Research, Multicampus Division of Geriatric Medicine and Gerontology, University of California, Los Angeles, Los Angeles, California 90024

NEENA L. CHAPPELL (**171**), Centre on Aging, University of Manitoba, Winnipeg R3T 2N2, Canada

JODI COHN (**28**), Department of Medicine, Anna & Harry Borun Center for Gerontological Research, Multicampus Division of Geriatric Medicine and Gerontology, University of California, Los Angeles, Los Angeles, California 90024

LISA DIECKMANN (**344**), Anna & Harry Borun Center for Gerontological Research, Multicampus Division of Geriatric Medicine and Gerontology, University of California, Los Angeles, Los Angeles, California 90024

GEOFF FERNIE (**142**), Centre for Studies on Aging, Sunnybrook Medical Center, University of Toronto, Toronto M4N 3M5, Canada

KATHLEEN M. GENTILE (**74**), School of Medicine, Anna & Harry Borun Center for Gerontological Research, Multicampus Division of Geriatric Medicine and Gerontology, University of California, Los Angeles, Los Angeles, California 90024

PRISCILLA GILLIAM-MACRAE (**226**), Department of Sports Medicine, Pepperdine University, Malibu, California 90265

BARRY J. GURLAND (**335**), Department of Clinical Psychiatry, Center for Geriatrics and Gerontology, Columbia University, New York, New York 10032

ROSALIE A. KANE (**315**), School of Public Health and School of Social Work, University of Minnesota, Minneapolis, Minnesota 55455

SIDNEY KATZ (**335**), Center for Geriatrics and Gerontology, Columbia University, New York, New York 10032

M. POWELL LAWTON (3), Philadelphia Geriatric Center, Philadelphia, Pennsylvania 19141

MORTON A. LIEBERMAN (120), Center for Social Sciences, University of California, San Francisco, San Francisco, California 94143

JON PYNOOS (91), Andrus Gerontology Center, University of Southern California, Los Angeles, California 90089

VICTOR REGNIER (91), Andrus Gerontology Center, University of Southern California, Los Angeles, California 90089

WANEEN W. SPIRDUSO (226), Department of Kinesiology and Health Education, Institute for Neurosciences, University of Texas, Austin, Austin, Texas 78712

E. PERCIL STANFORD (191), College of Health and Human Resources, San Diego State University, San Diego, California 92182

JUDITH A. SUGAR (28), Department of Psychology, Colorado State University, Fort Collins, Colorado 80523

TORBJÖRN SVENSSON (256), Gerontology Research Center, 222 20 Lund, Sweden

TERRIE WETLE (279), Institute of Living, Hartford, Connecticut 06106

Preface

As researchers begin to examine the issues of quality of life in the later years, they are faced with a fundamental stumbling block: The current literature base shows a weakness in research aimed at defining and measuring quality of life. No body of knowledge currently exists that can provide criteria to evaluate interventions to improve quality of life or to assess the relative values of the varied but interactive aspects of life quality. Obviously, the ability to assess quality of life in the later years is of paramount importance if older adults are to benefit meaningfully from health care and increased longevity. Factors influencing quality of life of the very elderly impact every level of health care and play a central role in the consequences of such care for the older individual, his or her family, and society.

This book brings together leading researchers in the field of aging to begin to define the concept of quality of life in the later years, to outline the issues of its measurement, and to evaluate existing interventions. It includes reviews of the literature; a report on a survey designed to assess and compare perceptions of quality of life among older adults, their families, and service providers; and discussions of current research and future research directions.

The roots of this volume are in the conduct of a national conference, sponsored by the Anna and Harry Borun Center for Gerontological Research, a joint project of UCLA's Multicampus Division of Geriatric Medicine and Gerontology and the Jewish Homes for the Aging of Greater Los Angeles. This conference provided a productive and critical forum for interaction among chapter authors and review of early drafts. The conference and the resulting publication are among the first efforts of the newly established Borun Center for Gerontological Research at UCLA, which is designed to expand the existing program of research on aging to include gerontological research and demonstration projects. The mission of the Borun Center is to create and test nonmedical interventions to improving the quality of life of the very elderly, especially the frail elderly receiving institutional and noninstitutional long-term care. The goal encompasses such objectives as identifying factors that affect the quality of life of frail older persons and elucidating the relative importance of and interactions among these factors. Research activities are truly interdisciplinary, conceived according to a model of frailty that addresses social, economic, environmental, and psychological problems, as well as deficits in health status. This book is based on the belief that to ensure a high quality of life in the later years it is necessary to address all aspects of the individual's internal life and his or her role in society.

We are grateful to the Anna and Harry Borun Foundation and to the ARCO Foundation for support of these efforts as well as to the Brookdale Foundation for its support of the senior editor. We also gratefully acknowledge the participation of the moderators, Barry Gurland, Rosalie Kane, Joseph Ouslander, and Victor Regnier, and that of the many attendees of the conference who asked critical questions and helped to enlighten the authors through interdisciplinary dialogue. Finally, we acknowledge the unfailing efforts of Alice M. Zeehandelaar and Georgina Ortega, without whose administrative expertise the conference and resulting book would not have been possible.

It is our hope that this book will provide the background and motivation to stimulate future research in this important area. Now that we are leading longer lives, we must turn our attention to making the increasing number of years of life meaningful and productive for all generations.

I

Background

1

A Multidimensional View of Quality of Life in Frail Elders

M. Powell Lawton

The phrase "quality of life" may well be established already as a marker concept of our own fin de siècle. In at least three arenas of scientific endeavor, sizable research enterprises have been built around quality of life: social accounting, medical treatment research, and social psychology. Since the social-accounting approach deals only in population aggregates, this chapter will focus on the individual aspects of quality of life typically studied by the medical and social sciences.

An index of the growth of interest in quality of life may be found by simply counting citations, for example, those in *Index Medicus,* which listed 77 articles in English in 1985 and was up to 149 in 1988. *Psychological Abstracts* first listed such an entry in 1985 (38 articles) and by 1988 the number was 80. MEDLINE and PSYCHINFO show even more citations. A surprising number of studies on quality of life make the media, including the Fickle Finger of Fate Award of a popular television show of the 1970s that was given to a group whose $300,000 grant concluded that healthier and wealthier people were happier than sick and poor people.

This chapter will not attempt a comprehensive review of the literature on quality of life (for such a review see Arnold, Chapter 3). The background literature on quality of life will be discussed selectively rather than exhaustively. Medical and nonmedical views will be contrasted and the need for a theoretically coherent conception discussed. A substantial portion of the chapter will be devoted to persistent issues in quality of life research: objective and subjective perspectives, positive and negative qualities, and the processes by which people regulate their preferred mix of qualities of life. It will be argued that a theoretical framework which subsumes all of what is meant by quality of life may be applied to people in every state of health. A major conclusion is that life qualities which depart in the positive direction from neutral have been relatively neglected in both theory and empirical research dealing with quality of life. Before laying out

Copyright © 1991 by Academic Press, Inc.
All rights of reproduction in any form reserved.

the general conceptual framework, the next section will consider the specific focus of the volume as a whole—frailty as it relates to quality of life.

Medical Quality of Life

As the number of indexed articles cited earlier implies, the volume of published material on quality of life seems almost twice as heavy in medical journals as in psychological and social-scientific journals. This surge of research activity in quality of life has been stimulated by several phenomena in contemporary health care. Chronic illness has become better recognized as the major social-medical problem of the day, portending the possibility of extended person-years of such illness as life expectancy is extended and the proportion of very old people increases. At the same time, aggressive surgical, pharmacological, and technological treatment possibilities have expanded, with frequent negative side effects for the persons receiving therapy. Ethical concerns surface over these phenomena in two ways. The obvious direction of such concern is for the comfort of the patient under both palliative and aggressive treatment: What intensity of negative side effects and symptom perseveration are justified by the gains of therapy or life extension? The second direction may best be characterized as a financial-ethical concern: To how great a proportion of society's resources is an individual entitled when therapy or life extension becomes highly expensive?

The ethical issues and their antecedent cause, the growing social importance of chronic illness and disability (hereafter referred to as *frailty*), appear to be the driving force behind much research on quality of life. There is much to cheer in such concerns that go beyond the physical aspects of medicine. It seems likely that concern for quality of life has resulted in greater perceived salience of the social and psychological implications of treatment of frailty in both the day-to-day practice of medicine and the teaching curricula of medical schools.

It is instructive to consider what is subsumed under the quality of life rubric in medical research. Treatment problems in clinical medicine have been the source of many of the measures of quality of life: hypertension (Wenger, 1988), stroke (Niemi, Laaksonen, Kotila, & Waltimo, 1988), and cancer (Habu, Saito, Sato, Takeshita, Sunagawa, & Endo, 1988). Clinical focus on specific diseases has led to attempts to scale the severity of symptoms characteristic of single diseases (Brook, Goldberg, Harris, Applegate, Rosenthal, & Lohr, 1979) as well as the symptoms and disabilities that may be occasioned by the treatment, for example, chemotherapy (Selby, 1985), intensive care (Patrick, Danis, Southerland, & Hong, 1988), or surgery (Mayou & Bryant, 1987).

Such a system of quality of life indicators based on disease symptoms and treatment consequences or side effects does constitute a structure consistent with clinical needs. Concurrently, however, there has been consistent recognition of the need to assess quality of life beyond the specific symptoms associated with any single disease and its treatment. Detailed accounting of the types of measures used across many studies may be found in literature reviews, some recent examples being those by Fowlie and Berkeley (1987), Hollandsworth (1988), Ochs, Mulhern, and Kun (1988), and Selby and Robertson (1987). A few examples of the domains that have been included in some research studies will suffice here. One of the earliest omnibus measures of quality of life was that of Spitzer *et al.* (1981), whose domains were activity, daily living, health, support, and outlook. Cassileth, Lusk, Miller, Brown, & Miller (1985) chose items measuring social ties, job satisfaction, use of psychotropic drugs, life satisfaction, subjective health, hopelessness, and amount of adjustment needed to cope with a new diagnosis. Ochs *et al.* (1988) grouped measures under the general categories of physical function, mental health, economic aspects, and satisfaction with function. Pearlman and Uhlmann (1988) used domains of physical function, intellectual function, social function, emotional function, and perceptions and health status in their research. Ware (1987) suggested physical health, mental health, social functioning, role functioning, and health perceptions. Some frequent single- or multiple-domain measures include the Sickness Impact Profile (Bergner, Bobbitt, Pollard, Martin, & Gilson, 1976), the Activities of Daily Living Index (Katz, Ford, Moskowitz, Jackson, & Jaffe, 1963), the Psychological General Well-being Index (National Center for Health Statistics, 1977), and the McGill Pain Index (Melzack, 1983).

Two conclusions emerge from the exhaustive reviews cited above and from this sampling of suggested components of quality of life. First, all components are plausible indicators of quality of life. Second, the components represent a jumble of content and levels of generality. Thus, there is a clear need to impose order on the quality of life construct. In fairness to some of the clusters of attributes already mentioned, some investigators have begun by searching for order. The Sickness Impact Profile for example, was derived from a content analysis of descriptive material from many different sources, which was generated by having people talk about how illness might affect a person's life. The 22-item Functional Living Index (Schipper, Clinck, McMurray, & Levitt, 1984) was distilled from 250 questions suggested by 11 experts to tap quality of life of cancer patients.

These latter two efforts exemplify one pole of a basic dichotomy in quality of life research: the health-specific, as opposed to generalized, conception of quality of life. Since virtually all of this stream of research emerged from the study of ill patients, it is not surprising that all are related to physical health. As Ware (1987, 474) notes: "The goal of the health care system is to maximize the health component of quality of life, namely health status. Measures of health outcomes should be defined accordingly." In contrast, "quality of life, as traditionally defined, is a much broader concept" (Ware, 1987, 474). If we accept the health-specific focus of quality of life, then the Sickness Impact Profile, which estimates the impairing behavioral effects of health on 12 domains (e.g., body care, emotions, work), is an excellent measure. An alternative approach begins with the theoretical perspective that health is only one of many related domains of quality of life.

A Conceptual Structure for Quality of Life

There are two requirements for a conceptual view of quality of life: designation of its structure and detailing of its content.

Structure of Quality of Life

A definition of quality of life may be offered here: Quality of life is the multidimensional evaluation, by both intrapersonal and social-normative criteria, of the person–environment system of an individual in time past, current, and anticipated. This definition is anchored within a conceptual framework whose earlier version the author has called "the good life" (Lawton, 1983). At that time, the intent was to not confuse the overall term "quality of life" with one of the component sectors of the good life, "perceived quality of life." At this point, accepted usage makes "quality of life" the preferable omnibus term.

This definition is structural and is meant to subsume the full spectrum of quality of life in its most inclusive meaning. Six terms used in the definition require elaboration: multidimensional, evaluation, intrapersonal, social-normative, person–environment system, and temporality.

A conceptual structure for quality of life is necessarily *multidimensional*, just as is life itself. Many arguments have been advanced in favor of a unidimensional measure of quality of life (Fanshel & Bush, 1970; Kaplan, 1988). A unidimensional measure may be produced directly or by combination of multiple attributes (see discussion later in this chapter). Research in both medical quality of life and classical treatments of this topic in the social sciences (Butt & Beiser, 1987; Campbell, Converse, & Rodgers, 1976; Flanagan, 1978; George & Bearon, 1980) has agreed that many domains are relevant to quality of life; the remaining problem is to identify which ones and how to combine them, questions to be discussed shortly. The World Health Organization definition of health (1948)—a state of complete physical, mental and social well-being—is totally consistent with the multidimensional view.

The *evaluation* aspect of the definition has the obvious meaning that the desirability versus undesirability of an aspect of life is implied (good versus bad, favorable versus unfavorable). A second, less obvious meaning subsumed under the term is that the evaluation may depart in either direction from a neutral point. Increments above the average, as well as decrements below it, are possible. This feature of the proposed structure for quality of life sets it apart most completely from medical quality of life, which typically is concerned with negative deviations from the average (symptoms, impairments, disabilities, side effects). A similar point was made by Rowe and Kahn (1987) when they distinguished "successful aging" from "usual aging." A complete conceptual framework for quality of life must give equal time to the facets of life that elevate people's evaluations, rather than assume a usual baseline from which only decrements occur (for example, the joy and benefits of physical activity [Spirduso & Gilliam-MacRae, Chapter 11]).

The *intrapersonal* aspects of quality of life express one essential ingredient of a comprehensive conception, that each individual has internal standards and evaluations of life that are idiosyncratic and not totally accountable to any external standard. A more usual term is *subjective,* or *perceptual,* used loosely. Many conceptions of quality of life depend solely upon subjective evaluations for the definition of quality.

The *social-normative* aspects of quality of life express the corollary assertion of the present view that objectively measurable or consensual evaluations of facets of life must also be considered in assessing quality of life. The whole story requires the use of both the intrapersonal and the social-normative perspectives.

The *person–environment system* expresses three important postulates. First, environment affects the person's well-being; and not all environments are equal in the life quality they afford. Second, people affect environment; they select their environments and shape them to their needs. Third, the relationship between person and environment is less often a matter of the person being either reactive or proactive, as in the first two postulates, as it is that of a transactional system in which the processes are dynamic and reciprocal.

The *temporal* aspect of quality of life emphasizes the dynamic, ongoing nature of the person–environment system. Specifically, remembered qualities of the past are present in the frames of reference by which qualities of the present and future are evaluated. For their own sake, qualities of the past remain active as memories and reminiscences. Expectations for the future clearly condition the present as well. In the context of chronic illness, the way a person construes the future course of illness and treatment—i.e., perceived prognosis—will condition his or her behavior and subjective state of the present and the way decisions are made regarding health care alternatives.

The structural concepts of multidimensionality, evaluation, intrapersonal versus social-normative frames of reference, person–environment transactions, and temporality lead to the second major conceptual issue, the content of quality of life.

The Content of Quality of Life

Specifying the content of quality of life demands, first, that every aspect of life be represented and that measures be provided. The dimensions of quality of life have been hypothesized earlier to include four large evaluative sectors: behavioral competence, perceived quality of life, objective environment, and psychological well-being, as denoted in Figure 1 (Lawton, 1983). Each of the four sectors may in turn be differentiated into as many dimensions as the details of one's attention demand.

Behavioral competence represents the social-normative evaluation of the person's functioning in the health, cognitive, time-use, and social dimensions. The details of the hierarchy of behavioral competence (Figure 2) have been described elsewhere (Lawton, 1982, 1983). The important feature for the present purpose is that this hierarchy and its categories are able to accommodate any externally observable facet of a person. Some, but not all, of the categories subsume *roles,* for example, paid employment, hobby, sport, spouse, family provider, or friend. Criteria for the social-normative evaluation of competence in these roles are a familiar component of social science. While there is no absolute criterion for biological health, objective indicators exist in the form of observable symptoms and measurable physiological function. Activities of daily living (ADL; Katz *et al.,* 1963) and cognition (e.g., the Mini-mental State Examination; Folstein, Folstein, & McHugh, 1975) are among the most ubiquitous measures of function. Virtually all conceptions of quality of life have included dimensions of these types, but there has been little consensus on which specific dimensions. The present conception adds, first, the specification that biological health, functional health, cognition, time use, and social behavior should all be included; and, second, that the appropriate indicators for measuring competence in each dimension are many, and must be chosen with regard to the individual being evaluated and the purpose of the evaluation.

Why these particular five categories of behavioral competence? They represent

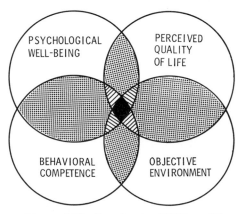

Figure 1 Four sectors of the good life. From Lawton (1983), p. 351, copyright Gerontological Society of America. Reprinted with permission.

COMPLEX

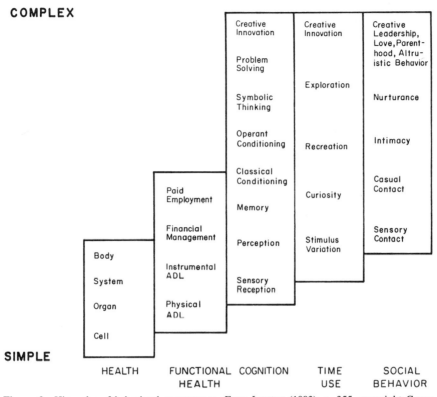

SIMPLE

| HEALTH | FUNCTIONAL HEALTH | COGNITION | TIME USE | SOCIAL BEHAVIOR |

Figure 2   Hierarchy of behavioral competence. From Lawton (1983), p. 355, copyright Gerontological Society of America. Reprinted with permission.

a hierarchy of complexity consistent with a system view of the person (see Seeman, 1989, for one of the more recent views of this type). Functioning within each level is relatively autonomous, yet each has reciprocal associations with both higher and lower levels of function, especially under threshold or stressful conditions. Each named category is capable of further differentiation, depending on the specificity of one's interest (for example, biological health may be specified in cellular, physiological, organ, or neural-organizational terms). As one moves up the hierarchy from biological to social complexity is also evidenced by the increasingly personal-preferential, social-normative, and environmental contribution to the evaluative criteria for competence. These particular five domains were chosen because they allow any facet of competence to be accommodated within one or another domain and because of their hypothesized hierarchy of complexity both within and across domains from the biological to the social.

Perceived quality of life has an internal structure that parallels directly the sector of behavioral competence. Whereas competence should be measured by performance or observation, perceived quality of life is by definition subjective. The person's subjective evaluation of function in any of the behavioral competence dimensions has formed the main content of perceived quality of life research (Andrews & Withey, 1976; Campbell *et al.*, 1976). Self-rated health (e.g., as measured by Mossey & Shapiro, 1982) is an operationalization of the health domain of perceived quality of life. Just as behavioral competence affords limitless detailing of specific dimensions for particular purposes, perceived quality of life has the same feature. For example, pain and discomfort have not constituted a usual component of assessment systems designed for the population at large (e.g., Campbell *et al.*, 1976). This dimension is central, however, to all approaches to health quality of life (Melzack, 1983). In much of the health research reviewed earlier, the excessively global term *perception* has been advanced as a component of quality of life, but without specification or conceptual rationale regarding which perceptual dimensions to evaluate. Pain and discomfort, being relevant to chronic illness, are in some health quality of life systems the only representatives of perceived quality of life. Here, it is suggested that the basic larger categories always be represented in quality of life assessment batteries, with the more specific dimensions being custom-selected to match the purpose of the inquiry. For example, pain, cognitive self-efficacy (Bandura, 1977), quality of spare time in general, and relationships with children and spouse might be appropriate perceived dimensions for quality of life assessment among frail people; whereas job satisfaction, sport efficacy, or sexual satisfaction would be less likely candidates as far as their relevance to the person's contemporary situation goes.

Behavioral competence and perceived quality of life are central sectors of quality of life. The other two sectors (environment and psychological well-being) are essential components of a loose causal model. The sector of *environment* is hypothesized to afford (i.e., be causally associated with) some forms of behavioral competence and not others and to constitute a subset of important conditions of the dimensions of perceived quality of life. Rather than having a dimension-to-dimension cognate relationship to behavioral competence and perceived quality of life, however, environment has a more diffuse relationship to dimensions within these sectors. Some objective environmental features are directly relevant to some dimensions of behavioral competence; for example, air and water quality is relevant to biological health, dwelling-unit physical access is relevant to mobility, and the richness of behavior settings (Barker, 1968) in one's environment is relevant to competence in time use. Other environmental attributes are best seen as "affordances" (Gibson, 1979), features inherent in the physical structure of the environment that allow, but do not elicit, behavior. For example, home and neighborhood are objective physical entities that afford, but do not guarantee, the enactment of behavioral competences in self-care, intellectual stimulation, and social behavior. Home, neighborhood, and social networks are examples of environmental objects that may also be evaluated subjectively. It is advantageous to search for objective facets of environmental objects that can be evaluated by physical or consensual criteria independent of the individual who experiences them. In this approach, deviations of the subjective from the objective evaluation themselves become objects for study and possible explanation. The causal nature of environment is not meant to imply a simplistic linear effect but, rather, to indicate that the relevance of all external environment to a particular person is limited and conditioned by its relevance to behavioral competences and perceived quality of life.

Psychological well-being is the ultimate outcome in a causal model of the open type. It may be defined as the weighted evaluated level of the person's competence and perceived quality in all domains of contemporary life. The "weighted" aspect of this definition implies that psychological well-being is more than a simple sum of competences and satisfactions. To explain the weighting process requires yet another conceptual superstructure, the self, which is a schema formed by proactive and reactive processes that provides a template for interpreting all aspects of past, present, and future experience. Typical indicators of psychological well-being include mental health (the Center for Epidemiological Studies Depression [CESD] Scale; Radloff, 1977), cognitive judgments of overall life satisfaction (the Life Satisfaction Index; Neugarten, Havighurst, & Tobin, 1961), and positive and negative emotion experienced as either states or traits (Watson, Clark, & Tellegen, 1988).

Atchley (Chapter 10) has detailed ways in which continuity of self is maintained in the face of normal aging and frailty. An essential aspect of psychological well-being is the ability of the person both to accommodate to loss and to assimilate positive information about the self. Frailty changes the dynamics of such continuity but not necessarily the strength of the self.

Objective and Subjective Quality of Life

Quality of life researchers have sometimes asserted that indicators of quality must be subjective. The four-sector view suggests that both perspectives are essential.

There are two reasons for insisting upon parallel objective and subjective evaluations of person and environment. The first reason is that social planning and the formulation of ethical and legal principles require us to make judgments about the objective qualities of people and environments. Without social norms as to what constitutes desirable, efficacious, or healthy behavior, there could be no process of individual socialization toward positive aggregate social goals. Similarly, without standards for architectural design, city planning, or the operation of social institutions we should have no way of aspiring to environments that benefit the greatest number of people or that are consonant with the needs of subgroups of people. Thus, social consensus, or sometimes even physical measurement (e.g., the soundness of the physical construction of a home), plays an important role in defining quality of life.

A second reason for giving objective measures of person and environment a major position in quality of life is that such measures provide an anchoring point from which individual perceptions may deviate. The nature of these deviations is itself a matter of interest. For example, a person may suffer from a disability and be unable to walk alone. This compromise in ADL competence is an important facet of quality of life. The same person's subjective view of his or her own competence is quite capable of having adapted to the objective disability and compensated so completely in both behavior (e.g., mastered the wheelchair) and psychological (e.g., no feeling of weakness) dimensions that the bottom-line meaning of the disabled status is negated.

Dependence and Independence among Aspects of Life Quality

Looking backward at these assertions regarding the content of quality of life, there is nothing new in suggesting any of the indicators of quality of life. What may be different from most conceptions is the assertion that the four sectors of the good life (as depicted in Figure 1)—behavioral competence, perceived quality of life, objective environment, and psychological well-being—encompass all possible indicators of quality of life, allowing for every individual's quality to be located within a theoretically determined structure. Conversely, quality of life cannot be fully represented without such a four-dimensional plotting of how the person stands.

This assertion means that well-being in one sector cannot be reduced to a combination of well-being in other sectors. The body of research in quality of life is full of demonstrations of dependencies among sectors. For example, social support seems to enhance mental health directly (Holahan & Holahan, 1987); neighborhood quality is associated with higher morale (Lawton, Nahemow, & Yeh, 1980); functional health and activity participation are correlated (Palmore, 1981); and physical health and mental health are almost always related to one another (Okun, Stock, Haring, & Witter, 1984). Yet we know that each marker of quality of life may be defined as a goal in its own right. The legitimacy of such autonomous goals does not depend on demonstrating that achievement of that goal leads in turn to better quality of life in all other domains.

Some examples from outside the scientific world help illustrate such "freestanding" aspects of quality of life. Many domains of behavioral competence are subsumed under the favorite psychological rubric of the day, self-efficacy (Bandura, 1977). History and the arts tell us even more about the lure of fame, power, ascendancy, and acquisition for their own sake. "Flow," the complete involvement of the actor with his activity (Csikszentmihaly, 1975, 36), has been creatively introduced into behavioral science, but literature and opera illustrate even better the place of thrill, novelty, and total engagement in human life. No psychological research has come close to operationalizing the romantic love domain of perceived quality of life (see Sternberg, 1987). Expertise (Glaser, 1981) driven by intrinsic motivation (Deci, 1975) as studied by the psychologist is a pale shadow of compulsive creativity. Autonomy is one of the needs that has had full play in the behavioral sciences recently (Baltes, Kinderman, Reisenzein, & Schmid, 1987; Hoflund, 1988; see Abeles, Chapter 14; Kane, Chapter 15; and Wetle, Chapter 13). Even more vivid are the moves toward autonomy in Eastern Europe and the astonishing new prevalence of smiling crowds in these countries. Environmental research has been hard put to demonstrate that housing has a major impact on mental health, yet note the consumer behavior that has led to a homeownership rate of 75% among the older population and their longitudinal history of successive upward approximations toward ideal housing (Lawton, 1978). Entertainment constitutes one of the main expenditures of people today, despite the fact that time budget categories of "recreation" and judged satisfaction with leisure activity have played relatively minor roles in quality of life research. One reason for choosing these examples is that the legitimacy of each of these goals is self-evident. We do not need to prove that they necessarily enhance mental health in order to accept them as human goals worthy of individual and social endorsement.

This chapter has digressed from behavioral science simply to concretize the power behind motivation to achieve different facets of quality of life. Such illustrations inevitably bring us to a multidimensional conception of quality of life. At best, correlations among the domains of life quality are imperfect. While it is not difficult to accept multidimensionality as a fact, it is not so easy to know how the dimensions add up. The usual outcome of quality of life research using the multidimensional perspective is a profile of domains of varying levels of quality. I shall provide a case study illustrating the problems of trying to integrate the disparate facets of quality of life into a coherent assessment of a whole life.

Quality of the Last Year of Life: A Multidimensional Research Study

Interviews were conducted with 200 surviving relatives of a group of recently deceased older people sampled from Philadelphia death records (Lawton, Moss, & Glicksman, 1990; Moss, Lawton, & Glicksman, in press). The purpose was to reconstruct a picture of the quality of that last year for people who spent most of the year in the community rather than in an institution. Quality was measured by having survivors rate the deceased person's month-by-month quality of life in a number of the domains named earlier: functional health, pain, mental clarity, interest in the world, visiting and being visited by family and friends, time use

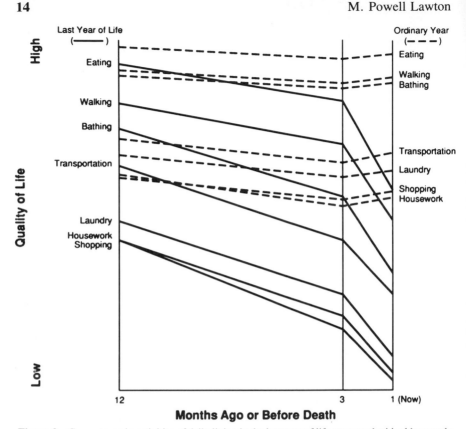

Figure 3 Competence in activities of daily living in the last year of life compared with older people in an ordinary year of life. From Lawton, Moss, and Glicksman (1990). Copyright, the Milbank Memorial Fund. Reprinted with permission.

(time spent doing nothing), satisfaction with time use, hope, and depression. Figures 3 and 4 show the trajectories of these indicators of life quality, compared with similar measures taken from an averagely healthy sample of living older people whose present life quality was rated by a close associate. The details of the research, including some information on the validity of the proxy reports, are in the cited reports.

The question at hand is: How can the overall quality of the last year be summarized quantitatively? Although one could do so by summing standard scores, such a summary would not be anchored in a scale with a meaningful metric or zero point. The researchers therefore arbitrarily established a point on each quality scale to designate the range of minimally acceptable quality. Since monthly ratings were obtained, it was possible to characterize each month of the

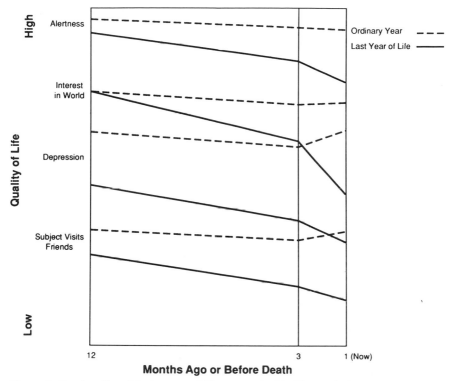

Figure 4 Rated quality of the last year of life compared with older people in an ordinary year of life. From Lawton, Moss, and Glicksman (1990). Copyright, the Milbank Memorial Fund. Reprinted with permission.

year as a good- or poor-quality month by each of the following nine quality rating indicators:

1. Pain: seldom or never
2. Mental clarity: clear all or most of the time
3. Functional health: no help at all or less than once a week
4. Social contact: an average of one to three contacts per month or more (family and friends)
5. Time use: five hours or less during the waking day spent doing nothing
6. Satisfaction with time use: satisfied always or most of the time
7. Depression: seldom or never depressed
8. Interest in the world: somewhat or very much interested
9. Hope: felt somewhat or very much that there was something to live for

Table 1 Percentages of Decedents Rated as Experiencing Positive Quality in Nine Domains across the Last 12 Months of Life

Month	Pain	Alert	ADL	Social	Satisfaction with time use	Null behavior	Depression	Interest	Hope	Total[a] +QQL%
12	63	91	71	74	82	84	73	79	89	84.7
11	62	90	67	74	81	84	73	78	89	83.7
10	60	88	66	74	81	83	73	78	89	83.7
9	60	88	67	74	81	82	74	76	87	81.2
8	60	86	68	73	80	83	73	75	86	81.6
7	60	86	67	73	79	82	72	75	86	81.7
6	58	85	65	71	79	81	72	73	85	81.2
5	57	83	64	71	77	81	71	71	84	80.1
4	50	81	59	70	73	79	69	69	81	78.5
3	49	79	55	67	72	76	65	66	80	74.9
2	45	74	50	67	69	67	62	60	77	68.1
1	42	73	42	67	64	60	62	57	74	64.9

[a]Percentage of subjects with positive quality in five or more domains.

From Lawton, Moss, and Glicksman (1990). Copyright, the Milbank Memorial Fund. Reprinted with permission.

Table 1 shows the percentages with high-quality ratings in each of the quality of life domains for each of the 12 months. The last column in Table 1 gives the percentages of persons each month who experienced a majority of high-quality indicators (i.e., five or more of the nine domains). Up to the end of life, almost two-thirds could be said to be living high-quality lives by these indicators.

The investigators believe that the result was not a bad description of the last year of life. However, consider the problems: The investigators' subjective decision determined both which dimensions to use and the point that divided good quality from poor quality on each; the rating scales themselves were not anchored in a true-zero scale; and the assumption was made that each of the quality indicators was equally important in determining overall quality.

Unidimensional Conceptions of Quality of Life

These problematic features are endemic to a multidimensional view of quality of life. Recognition of the problems of this approach led to a stream of research on quality of life designed to produce a single index of quality. This metric deals with the value assigned to life: the "utility" of, or preferences for, differing health states spread over differing periods of time (Fanshel & Bush, 1970; Patrick, Bush, & Chen, 1973; Torrance, Thomas, & Sackett, 1972). The utility approach deals explicitly with health-related quality of life, discounting the normal value of life by degradations associated with negative aspects of illness and its treatments. The proponents of this view argue that the lack of an absolute criterion of quality of life precludes any universal method of combining dimensions because each condition and each individual is so different. The way around this problem is to give people the opportunity to attach a value on life that can be expressed quantitatively as the wish to live y years under x conditions. The conditions represent different combinations of health quality of life indicators.

A number of methods have been proposed for arriving at such judgments. Notable among them is the "quality-adjusted life years" approach (QALYS; Bush, Fanshel, & Chen, 1972; Kaplan, 1982, 1988; Patrick et al., 1973), where the scaled quality of a functional health state is cumulated over time (remaining life span or a research-assigned time period in the future). Both health state and prognosis enter into the calculation of the QALYS. There are two major inputs into the determination of health state: function levels in the domains of social activity, mobility, and physical activity; and a limited set of physical "symptom/problem complexes," which a formula combines into a quality of well-being score, using weights determined by consensual ratings. The anchoring points used to establish the scale for consensus ratings were 0, representing death, and 1.00, representing optimum functioning, defined as "conformity to society's standards of physical and mental well-being, including the performance of activities usual for a person's age and social role" (Patrick et al., 1973, 8). We should note that "optimum" is clearly equated with "usual" in this conception.

The QALYS approach allows a value to be attached to a contemporary health state, which represents the reduced proportion of the normal life span that would be seen as equal in value to the longer reduced-quality life span, given the conditions of the illness. Any source of data (e.g., judgments of normal research subjects) may be used, data that are often independent of the judgment of the people with the condition.

Another frequently used method is the "time trade-off" (TTO) approach, which lends itself to determination of preferences either by the general public or by people who are experiencing the condition (Torrance, Thomas, & Sackett, 1972). As in the previous approach, anchoring points of 0 for death and 1.00 for optimal health are offered and the subject is asked to consider a scenario or vignette describing a chronic condition. Torrance (1982) has suggested a four-function scenario: physical function, health problems, activities of daily living, and social-emotional attributes. The subject is asked to choose between having the condition the rest of his or her life versus living a shorter life in good health. The length of shortened life is varied systematically. The length of life where the choice is equal between the longer chronic illness and the shortened life, the "indifference point," is the weighted measure of preference; the weight from 0 to 1.00 represents the proportion of normal life expectancy that would yield the same number of quality years as the longer but compromised quality life span.

In these and other approaches to single estimates of health, combining length of life with quality of life offers a metric with great appeal. Aggregation of quality years across people receiving different treatments allows treatments to be compared in terms of quality years added to life. The costs of quality years added may be compared among treatments, illnesses, and population groups.

Two major problems limit the usefulness of the health utility concept as a basis for planning treatment and health care policy. First is the limitation of concern to "health quality of life." Both the Kaplan and Bush (1982) and Torrance (1982) approaches do examine quality of life in four dimensions, yet the emphasis is always on whether physical illness or its treatment exerts a decrementing effect on the nonhealth dimensions. In fact, the World Health Organization (1948) definition of health is explicitly rejected by both Kaplan (1982) and Torrance (1987). Such a limitation of the quality of life to the health domain introduces a fundamental contradiction. The task in determining health preferences is always framed in terms of the value of life to the frail person. Yet, subjects making such value judgments from vignettes or function-problem combinations are given stimulus materials that are often lacking in social and psychological content. One doubts that the researcher's definition of health-related quality of life is as evident to them.

This physical health parochialism is matched by a second type of parochialism, a weighting system for determining quality years that allows only unidirectional decrement from the usual. Presumably, subjects are left on their own to define good health and their own "usual" functioning; the research task imposes on them the use of the familiar decremental view of aging and illness. The alternative view is that people weigh both increments and decrements to well-being in evaluating their present and expected quality of life.

Positive and Negative Aspects of Life

It is well established that affective experience is structured by most people into dimensions of positive affect and negative affect, that these two dimensions are at least partially independent of one another, and that both contribute to "happiness" (Bradburn, 1969; Diener & Emmons, 1984; Watson & Tellegen, 1985). Furthermore, research has shown that negative affect depends more on internal factors, including physical health, while positive affect is associated more strongly with stimulation from outside the person (Bradburn, 1969; Lawton, 1983). Zautra and Reich (1980) have shown that positive events have the capacity to elevate positive affect, while negative events increase negative affect but have a less-strong influence on positive affect. Other differential relationships to positive and negative affective states have been demonstrated for care-giving satisfactions and burdens (Lawton, Moss, Kleban, Glicksman, & Rovine, in press) and for social relationships (Lawton, Moss, & Kleban, 1986). In the latter research, social relationships based on shared feeling and communality (solidary relationships) were related to positive affect, but having more solidary relationships did not mitigate negative affect. A converse affect was seen in relationships based on status and competition. Of course there are crossover relationships as well; the research of Lewinsohn and colleagues has shown that producing positive experiences can sometimes mitigate depression (Lewinsohn, Sullivan, & Grosscup, 1980). Although the relationship of neural events to affective experience is far from clear, there appears to be substantial evidence in favor of differentiation between positive and negative affect at the neuropsychological level (Tucker & Williamson, 1984). The conclusion from research on the dimensions of affect is that mental health outcomes are strongly determined by the way people process both positive and negative experiences and the events associated with them.

The mental calculus that produces the feeling of satisfaction with one's life, hope, or the wish to live is very poorly understood at this juncture. The unidimensional utility approach to assessing quality of life certainly represents a laudable attempt to understand the process. On the other hand, research on positive affect as a neglected aspect of human experience is convincing enough to suggest that the decision-theoretic approach will also have to incorporate the positive aspects of human experience.

The present author's search of this literature has yielded no attempt to probe trade-offs between positive experiences and health-related decrements in life quality. Do frail people do better if they have a loved spouse, a fulfilling relationship with a child (see Chappell, Chapter 8), an area of expertise that can be applied despite the illness, a sphere of life where autonomy can still be exercised (Abeles, Chapter 14), or an ideology that organizes the meaning of pain, suffering, life, and death?

It is possible that one's hierarchy of values becomes rearranged in the face of frailty. Conceivably, heightened valuation of a family relationship, of one's remaining skills, or of religious conviction may occur *because* of the onset of illness. One remembers the classic finding of Turner, Tobin, and Lieberman (1972) that hostility in nursing home residents was associated with a better outcome. Did the sense of self-determination that accompanied hostile expression give them something to live for? (See also Abeles's discussion of personal control, this volume). Another study (Lawton, 1985) demonstrated how very impaired, homebound older people optimized their competence by establishing a control center in their living room chairs. From this vantage point they controlled their foreshortened life span and extended their span of control beyond the residence through television, telephone, reading matter, and mementos from the past. The angry residents' and the control center directors' lives certainly were diminished in quality by their frailty, but the increments in quality associated with their proactivity would be very difficult to capture in a health-utility preference game.

It is also probable that one's adaptation level for positive and negative experiences changes as one's life becomes more restricted. If frailty brings about a lessened prevalence of the types of high positive-affect experiences associated with a more vigorous earlier life, it may well be that one begins to savor smaller pleasures just as readily as the earlier ones. Conversely, the costs of frailty may engender some degree of adaptation to negative experience that blunts the pain, as illustrated neatly in the research that demonstrated lottery winners to be no happier than paraplegics (Brickman, Coates, & Janoff-Bulman, 1978).

This author has referred to increasing "density of differentiation" as an adaptive mechanism by which people whose physical life space has shrunk (i.e., the frail) come to perceive previously unrecognized distinctions among both positive and negative features of their psychological life space. We have little knowledge at present about how such newly differentiated pleasures and pains affect overall quality of life.

We need to expend as much effort deriving a weighted inventory of possible increments to overall life quality as was spent deriving the weighted decrements. It is possible that events of sufficiently positive impact occurring at a rate exceeding a particular individual's minimum requirement may reinforce the wish to live. This hypothesis seems quite possible to test. People may also vary in the extent to which avoidance of negative states, as compared with the proliferation of positive states, constitutes the most important life goal (see, for example,

Cloninger's [1987] tripartite view of personality as need orientations toward novelty seeking, harm avoidance, and reward dependence). Viewing life as a whole and expressing a judgment of the future value of life under x conditions absolutely demands the WHO-broadened view of health.

Quality of Life and Social Policy

The utility approach has emphasized universality, not individual differences. Two interesting sources of variation were reported, however, in one exploration of subgroup differences in health utilities (Sackett & Torrance, 1978). Age trends were found in the higher valuation of life under the hypothetical condition of dialysis or organ transplant conditions given by middle-aged (as contrasted with younger and older) people. The oldest group (ages 66–79) expressed a higher valuation of life under the condition that specified long-term hospitalization for an unnamed disease. Further, patients who themselves were actually experiencing renal failure expressed greater valuation of life extended by dialysis or transplant than did nonpatients making the same judgments in a hypothetical scenario. In another study where both older patients and their physicians rated patients' global quality of life, physicians consistently rated it more poorly than did patients (Pearlman & Uhlmann, 1988). The message is clear: Determining a gold standard for valuing life under different health conditions by obtaining the judgments of people not suffering from the condition—a "public consensus"—carries with it the heavy risk of misrepresenting the judgments of those who actually are in the health state.

A similar consideration is the question as to whether a person at one point in life is capable of assessing his or her preference at a future time. The environment will surely be different. Will even the self be different? (See Atchley, Chapter 10).

It is but a short step from the establishment of health utilities by consensus to the articulation of ethical principles for social aggregates to the neglect of the individual. The medicalization of quality of life enhances this danger. Although social policy inevitably must take account of utilitarian principles, a dialectic between the aggregate good and the individual right must be maintained. There is a strong political element implied in medical quality of life research, in that lowered quality often is used to justify withholding or reducing financial investment in health care for a group. A more balanced estimate of the quality of lives of frail people will come from two additional ingredients: equal time for positive experiences and the certainty that the criteria for quality established by consensus are always matched by those expressed by the affected people. We must learn how some frail people achieve a balance of decrements and increments to "usual" quality of life that enables them to go on by choice, living out their remaining quantity of years.

Research Needs

The multidimensional conception of quality of life specifies more domains than instruments now exist to measure. The conception also demands appropriate measurement at different levels of functioning within each domain. Therefore, a primary research need is for the creation of a better integrated set of assessment instruments. If successful, they will surely improve upon the existing ones, for example, the OARS (Duke University, 1978), the CARE (Gurland, Kuriansky, Sharpe, Simon, Stiller, & Berkett, 1977–1978), and the MAI (Lawton, Moss, Fulcomer, & Kleban, 1982).

Research is also needed to assess the overall valuation of life of frail people. The QALYS and TTO methods have great usefulness if properly seen as expressing one facet of valuation of life. Their methods are too cumbersome for the frail, and, above all, they are lacking in depth of representing quality of life.

This chapter has argued strongly for further attention to assessing the positive features of life. Psychological science now recognizes the significance of positive affect. We now need research to determine how people's environments can maximize opportunities for positive experiences.

Simultaneously, the intrapersonal processes of accommodation and assimilation as they are affected by frailty need to be better understood. Very little is known about how the perceptual, cognitive, and affective responses of people change in response to sources of enjoyment as they become older and more frail. The self as an object for research needs to have more attention.

The greatest need is to understand how some people maintain high quality of life despite the threat of illness and disability. Changes in expectations, adaptation level, choice of goals (e.g., "selective optimization with compensation"; Baltes, Dittmain-Kohli, & Dixon, 1984), and density of differentiation are mechanisms deserving more study.

Conclusion

It is therefore concluded that the breadth and depth of life as a whole, and maintenance of an appropriate focus on the individual rather than the aggregate, demand a multidimensional conception of quality of life. The searches for unidimensionality, for the single concept of medical quality of life, and for deviations expressed only as decrements are attempts at oversimplifications that a society concerned with individual differences cannot afford.

Although the majority of research on quality of life has adopted a multidimensional perspective, with varying inclusiveness of domains beyond health-related quality of life, few such endeavors have been based on a theoretical conception of quality of life. The four-sector structure suggested in this chapter is meant to ameliorate this situation. This conception will no doubt be superseded, in turn, by improved constructs. The one feature of the present conception that should be preserved in future theoretical structures is its claim to leave room for every facet of quality of life, including its provision for objective and subjective definitions of quality. Whatever else such a structure does, it must accommodate 100% of all possible attributes capable of being evaluated.

This structure is not meant to dictate operationalization of measurement of quality of life. The four sectors provide a way of accounting for the universe of domains of quality of life. Research application must continue to sample among all possible domains and ranges of functioning according to the purpose of each research endeavor. The meaning of the research will be much clearer if the portion of quality of life addressed in the research can be anchored within the four-sector framework.

References

Andrews, F. M., & Withey, S. B. (1976). *Social indicators of well-being.* New York: Plenum Press.

Baltes, M. M., Kinderman, T., Reisenzein, R., & Schmid, U. (1987). Further observational data on the behavioral and social world of institutions for the aged. *Psychology and Aging, 2,* 390–403.

Baltes, P. B., Dittmann-Kohli, F., & Dixon, R. A. (1984). New perspectives on the development of intelligence in adulthood. In P. B. Baltes & O. G. Brim, eds., *Life-span development and behavior,* vol. 6, pp. 33–76. New York: Academic Press.

Bandura, A. (1977). Self-efficacy: Toward a unifying theory of behavioral change. *Psychological Review, 84,* 190–215.

Barker, R. G. (1968). *Ecological psychology.* Stanford, Calif.: Stanford University Press.

Bergner, M., Bobbitt, R. A., Pollard, W. E., Martin, P., & Gilson, B. S. (1976). The Sickness Impact Profile: Validation of a health status measure. *Medical Care, 14,* 57–67.

Bradburn, N. M. (1969). *The structure of psychological well-being.* Chicago: Aldine.

Brickman, P., Coates, D., & Janoff-Bulman, R. (1978). Lottery winners and accident victims: Is happiness relative? *Journal of Personality and Social Psychology, 36,* 917–927.

Brook, R. H., Goldberg, G. A., Harris, L. J., Applegate, K., Rosenthal, M., & Lohr, K. N. (1979). Conceptualization in measurement of physiologic health in the Health Insurance Study. Santa Monica, California: Rand Corporation.

Bush, J. W., Fanshel, S., & Chen, M. M. (1972). Analysis of a tuberculin testing program using a health status index. *Social and Economic Planning Science, 6,* 49–68.

Butt, D. S., & Beiser, M. (1987). Successful aging: A theme for international psychology. *Psychology and Aging, 2,* 87–94.

Campbell, A., Converse, P., & Rodgers, W. (1976). *Quality of life in America.* New York: Russell Sage.

Cassileth, B. R., Lusk, E. J., Miller, D. S., Brown, L. L., & Miller, C. (1985). Psychosocial correlates of survival in advanced malignant disease? *New England Journal of Medicine, 312,* 1551–1555.

Cloninger, C. R. (1987). A systematic method for clinical description and classification of personality variants. *Archives of General Psychiatry, 44,* 573–588.

Csikszentmihaly, M. (1975). *Beyond boredom and anxiety.* San Francisco: Jossey-Bass.

Deci, E. L. (1975). *Intrinsic motivation.* New York: Plenum.

Diener, E., & Emmons, R. (1984). The independence of positive and negative affect. *Journal of Personality and Social Psychology, 47,* 1105–1117.

Duke University Center for the Study of Aging (1978). *Multidimensional functional assessment: The OARS methodology,* 2nd ed. Durham, N.C.: Duke University.

Fanshel, S., & Bush, J. W. (1970). A health-status index and its application to health-service outcomes. *Operations Research, 10,* 1021–1066.

Flanagan, J. C. (1978). A research approach to improving our quality of life. *American Psychologist, 33,* 138–147.

Folstein, M. F., Folstein, S. E., & McHugh, P. R. (1975). "Mini-mental state": A practical method for grading the cognitive state of patients for the clinician. *Journal of Psychiatric Research, 12,* 189–198.

Fowlie, M., & Berkeley, J. (1987). Quality of life—A review of the literature. *Family Practice, 4,* 226–234.

George, L. K., & Bearon, L. B. (1980). *Quality of life in older persons: Meaning and measurement.* New York: Human Sciences Press.

Gibson, J. J. (1979). *The ecological approach to visual perception.* Boston: Houghton-Mifflin.

Glaser, R. (1981). The future of testing: A research agenda for cognitive psychology and psychometrics. *American Psychologist, 36,* 923–936.

Gurland, B. J., Kuriansky, J., Sharpe, L., Simon, R., Stiller, P., & Berkett, P. (1977–1978). The comprehensive assessment and referral evaluation (CARE)—Rationale development, and reliability. *International Journal of Aging and Human Development, 8,* 9–41.

Habu, H., Saito, N., Sato, Y., Takeshita, K., Sunagawa, M., & Endo, M. (1988). Quality of postoperative life in gastric cancer patients seventy years of age and over. *Internal Surgery, 73,* 82–86.

Hoflund, B., ed. (1988). Autonomy in long term care. *The Gerontologist, 28,* (Suppl. 3) 1–96.

Holahan, C. K., & Holahan, C. J. (1987). Self-efficacy, social support, and depression in aging. *Journal of Gerontology, 42,* 65–68.

Hollandsworth, J. G. (1988). Evaluating the impact of medical treatment on the quality of life: A 5-year update. *Social Science in Medicine, 26,* 425–434.

Kaplan, R. M. (1982). Human preference measurement for health decisions and the evaluation of long-term care. In R. L. Kane & R. A. Kane, eds., *Values and longterm care,* pp. 157–188. Lexington, Mass.: Lexington Books.

Kaplan, R. M. (1988). Health-related quality of life in cardiovascular disease. *Journal of Consulting and Clinical Psychology, 56,* 382–392.

Kaplan, R. M., & Bush, J. W. (1982). Health-related quality of life measurement for evaluation research and policy analysis. *Health Psychology, 1,* 61–80.

Katz, S., Ford, A. B., Moskowitz, R. W., Jackson, B. A., & Jaffe, M. W. (1963). Studies of illness in the aged. The index of ADL: A standardized measure of biological and psychosocial function. *Journal of the American Medical Association, 185,* 914–919.

Lawton, M. P. (1978). Housing problems of the community resident elderly. *Occasional papers in housing and community affairs,* no. 1, pp. 39–74. Washington, D.C.: U.S. Government Printing Office.

Lawton, M. P. (1982). Competence, environmental press, and the adaptation of older people. In M. P. Lawton, P. G. Windley, & T. O. Byerts, eds., *Aging and the environment: Theoretical approaches,* pp. 33–59. New York: Springer.

Lawton, M. P. (1983). Environment and other determinants of well-being in older people. *The Gerontologist, 23,* 349–357.

Lawton, M. P. (1985). The elderly in context: Perspectives from environmental psychology and gerontology. *Environment and Behavior, 17,* 501–519.

Lawton, M. P., Nahemow, L., & Yeh, T.-M. (1980). Neighborhood environment and the wellbeing of older tenants in planned housing. *International Journal of Aging and Human Development, 11,* 211–227.

Lawton, M. P., Moss, M., Fulcomer, M., & Kleban, M. H. (1982). A research and service-oriented Multilevel Assessment Instrument. *Journal of Gerontology, 37,* 91–99.

Lawton, M. P., Moss, M., & Kleban, M. H. (1986). *Psychological well-being, mastery, and the social relationships of older people.* Philadelphia: Philadelphia Geriatric Center.

Lawton, M. P., Moss, M., & Glicksman, A. (1990). The quality of the last year of life of older persons. *Milbank Quarterly, 68,* 1–28.

Lawton, M. P., Moss, M., Kleban, M. H., Glicksman, A., & Rovine, M. (in press). A two-factor model of caregiving stress and psychological well-being. *Journals of Gerontology: Psychological Sciences.*

Lewinsohn, P. M., Sullivan, M., & Grosscup, S. J. (1980). Changing reinforcing events: An approach to the treatment of depression. *Psychotherapy: Theory, Research, and Practice, 17,* 322–334.

Mayou, R., & Bryant, B. (1987). Quality of life after coronary artery surgery. *Quarterly Journal of Medicine,* New Series, *62,* 239–248.

Melzack, R., ed. (1983). *Pain measurement and assessment.* New York: Raven Press.

Moss, M., Lawton, M. P., & Glicksman, A. (in press). The role of pain in the last year of life of older persons. *Journals of Gerontology: Psychological Sciences.*

Mossey, J. M., & Shapiro, E. (1982). Self-rated health: A predictor of mortality among the elderly. *American Journal of Public Health, 22,* 800–808.

National Center for Health Statistics (1977). A. F. Fazio, *A concurrent validation of the NCHS General Well-Being Schedule.* HHS NO.HE20.6208.2., September. Washington, D.C.: U.S. Government Printing Office.

Neugarten, B. L., Havighurst, R. J., & Tobin, S. S. (1961). The measurement of life satisfaction. *Journal of Gerontology, 16,* 134–143.

Niemi, M.-L., Laaksonen, R., Kotila, M., & Waltimo, O. (1988). Quality of life 4 years after stroke. *Stroke, 19,* 1101–1107.

Ochs, J., Mulhern, R., & Kun, L. (1988). Quality-of-life assessment in cancer patients. *American Journal of Clinical Oncology, 11,* 415–421.

Okun, M. A., Stock, W. A., Haring, M. J., & Witter, R. (1984). Health and subjective well-being: A meta-analysis. *International Journal of Aging and Human Development, 19,* 111–132.

Palmore, E. (1981). *Social patterns in normal aging: Findings from the Duke longitudinal study.* Durham, N.C.: Duke University Press.

Patrick, D. L., Bush, J. W., & Chen, M. M. (1973). Toward an operational definition of health. *Journal of Health and Social Behavior, 14,* 6–23.

Patrick, D. L., Danis, M., Southerland, L. I., & Hong, G. (1988). Quality of life following intensive care. *Journal of General Internal Medicine, 3,* 218–223.

Pearlman, R. A., & Uhlmann, R. F. (1988). Quality of life in chronic diseases: Perceptions of elderly patients. *Journal of Gerontology: Medical Sciences, 43,* M25–M30.

Radloff, L. S. (1977). The CES-D scale: A self-report depression scale for research in the general population. *Applied Psychological Measurement, 1,* 385–401.

Rowe, J. W., & Kahn, R. L. (1987). Human aging: Usual and successful. *Science, 237,* 143–149.

Sackett, D. L., & Torrance, G. W. (1978). The utility of different health states as perceived by the general public. *Journal of Chronic Diseases, 31,* 697–704.

Schipper, H., Clinck, S., McMurray, A., & Levitt, M. (1984). Measuring the quality of life of cancer patients: The functional living index. *Journal of Clinical Oncology, 2,* 472–483.

Seeman, J. (1989). Toward a model of positive health. *American Psychologist, 44,* 1099–1109.

Selby, P. J. (1985). Measurement of the quality of life after cancer treatment. *British Journal of Hospital Medicine, 33,* 267–271.

Selby, P., & Robertson, B. (1987). Measurement of quality of life in patients with cancer. *Cancer Surveys, 6,* 521–543.

Spitzer, W. O., Dobson, A. J., Hall, J., Chesterman, E., Levi, J., Shepherd, R., Battista, R. N., & Catchlove, B. R. (1981). Measuring the quality of life of cancer patients: A concise QL index. *Journal of Chronic Diseases, 34,* 585–597.

Sternberg, R. J. (1987). Liking versus loving: A comparative evaluation of theories. *Psychological Bulletin, 102,* 331–345.

Torrance, G. W. (1982). Multiattribute utility theory as a method of measuring social preferences for health states in long-term care. In R. L. Kane & R. A. Kane, eds., *Values and long-term care,* pp. 127–156. Lexington, Mass.: Lexington Books.

Torrance, G. W. (1987). Utility approach to measuring health-related quality of life. *Journal of Chronic Diseases, 40,* 593–600.

Torrance, G. W., Thomas, W. H., & Sackett, D. L. (1972). A utility maximization model for evaluation of health care programs. *Health Services Research, 7,* 118–133.

Tucker, D. M., & Williamson, P. A. (1984). Asymmetric neural control systems in human self-regulation. *Psychological Review, 91,* 185–215.

Turner, B. F., Tobin, S. S., & Lieberman, M. A. (1972). Personality traits as predictors of institutional adaptation among the aged. *Journal of Gerontology, 27,* 61–68.

Ware, J. E. (1987). Standards for validating health measures: Definitions and content. *Journal of Chronic Diseases, 40,* 473–480.

Watson, D., & Tellegen, A. (1985). Toward a consensual structure of mood. *Psychological Bulletin, 98,* 219–235.

Watson, D., Clark, L. A., & Tellegen, A. (1988). Development and validation of brief measures of positive and negative affect: The PANAS scales. *Journal of Personality and Social Psychology, 54,* 1063–1079.

Wenger, N. K. (1988). Quality of life issues in hypertension: Consequences of diagnosis and considerations in management. *American Heart Journal, 116,* 628–632.

World Health Organization (1948). *Constitution of the World Health Organization.* Geneva, Switzerland: WHO Basic Documents.

Zautra, A., & Reich, J. (1980). Positive life events and reports of well-being: Some useful distinctions. *Journal of Community Psychology, 8,* 657–670.

2

Determinants of Quality of Life in Institutions: Perceptions of Frail Older Residents, Staff, and Families

JODI COHN
JUDITH A. SUGAR

Introduction

Older people are living longer and more of them are residing in long-term care facilities. In 1990, those over 65 years of age represented 12.7% of the U.S. population; by 2020 those over 65 will represent 17.3%. Individuals over 85 years of age, who are the most likely to suffer physical and mental impairments requiring nursing home care, represent the fastest growing segment, one that is projected to quadruple by the year 2030 (U.S. Senate Special Committee on Aging, 1987–1988). Studies by the National Center for Health Statistics estimate that the number of older people residing in nursing homes will increase by 58% from 1978 to 2003 if mortality rates remain constant. Along with this increased utilization of nursing homes, the characteristics of the population are expected to change, resulting in facilities with older and more disabled residents (U.S. Senate Special Committee on Aging, 1990).

Society has tended to define aging as a biomedical problem, focusing on pathologies and physical decrements (Estes & Binney, 1989; Kane, 1989). In assessing life in nursing homes, this approach has been mirrored by a focus on quality of care. While necessary and appropriate, this focus may be overly restrictive. Experts in the field of aging are urging a reintroduction of social concerns to the care of older people (Estes & Binney, 1989; Lyman, 1989), including their care in nursing homes. Ideally, the approach should be multidimensional, including social, psychological, cultural, and environmental factors. A satisfactory quality of life in long-term care facilities depends on much more than quality of care (Institute of Medicine, 1986; Lawton, Chapter 1). Beyond

28

Copyright © 1991 by Academic Press, Inc.
All rights of reproduction in any form reserved.

meeting the basic needs of shelter, care, and food (Maslow, 1968), institutions can do many things to improve the quality of life for their residents.

The present study sought to better understand how quality of life for frail older people in institutions is defined and perceived. This understanding can be enhanced by examining multiple perspectives—those of frail older residents themselves, staff of long-term care facilities, and family of the residents. The perceptions of these interested groups affect the choices made by older persons and their families about facilities, affect policies and procedures that govern the facilities, and, ultimately, affect the development of relevant public policy.

There is a recognition in the literature that these perspectives may diverge (Brennan, Moos, & Lemke, 1988) and that if the perceptions of residents and staff disagree too much, conditions for residents may suffer, and relocation of residents may result. As Lieberman (Chapter 6) demonstrated, this relocation can be particularly hazardous for older people. Families often make the decisions about long-term care placement and have an ongoing role once a relative is institutionalized. Just as a large part of the care of older persons (80%) is provided by families in the community, families demonstrate a continued caring role after institutionalization, as evidenced by their willingness to share or take responsibility for a large number of tasks that include personal care and activities (Schwartz & Vogel, 1990).

However, many of the differences in perceptions may be appropriate. For example, because residents, family, and staff have varying responsibilities, divergent perceptions would be expected. Identifying these differences and the tensions created by them can offer benefits such as better communications between groups, enhanced understanding of different perspectives, or, at least, a sense that someone is listening.

This chapter will describe the background, methods, and findings of this investigation into quality of life. Perceptions of residents, staff, aides, and family members will be compared in order to better understand how they define quality of life and to ascertain the values they give to various factors. This information can aid both practitioners and researchers in identifying areas of disagreement, in recognizing problem areas, and in devising possible solutions.

Literature Review

The existing literature defining or examining determinants of quality of life in the institution is quite limited (Kane & Kane, 1987). Much of the literature on institutionalization has been devoted to the deleterious effects of this phenomenon, including increased dependence, isolation, learned helplessness, and the inability to make decisions (Goffman, 1958; Sommer & Osmond, 1961; Teitelman & Priddy, 1988).

In response to this negative evidence, most research on quality of life for institutionalized frail elderly emphasizes how to improve it, either by institutional interventions or by helping residents adapt to the environment. These published studies generally focus on only one domain: either therapeutic care (Bagshaw & Adams, 1985–1986; Bayer, Bresloff, & Curley, 1986), the social interaction of the residents (Friedman, 1975), or enhanced decision making and autonomy (Langer & Rodin, 1976; Schulz, 1976). The importance of focusing on autonomy was highlighted by the Institute of Medicine study (1986), which recommended increased decision-making opportunities for residents. In the domain of physical environment, Lawton and Nahemow's (1973) competence-environmental press model has offered a widely used framework for evaluating design. Pynoos and Regnier (Chapter 5) indicate that most of the design literature uses a case study approach, resulting in design guidelines and recommendations to improve settings for older people (e.g., Koncelik, 1976), rather than empirical studies.

Another characteristic of the literature is that little attention has been given to residents' perceptions of quality of life. One exception is Kane's study (Chapter 15) on how important autonomy is to nursing home residents and how nurses' aides view autonomy for residents. The study found differences between residents and aides, with aides more likely than residents to rate autonomy items as very important. The order of importance of these items also differed; for example, residents rated control over phone and mail substantially more important than did aides.

Only one other study has attempted to directly elicit residents' perceptions of what affects quality of life. Over 400 nursing home residents from 70 different facilities nationwide were surveyed through a group discussion process by the National Citizens' Coalition for Nursing Home Reform (Spalding & Frank, 1985). Residents were asked to identify quality markers of life and care in a nursing home. Most frequently mentioned was the need for staff with good attitudes and feelings toward the residents. Second in importance were factors contributing to a home like atmosphere, including safety and security. Food—the need for variety, choices, proper preparation, and good service—was mentioned third most often. Other areas of interest included a desire for a broad range of activities, access to high-quality medical care, physicians who communicate well, and cleanliness of food, staff, and facility.

Few studies, other than the one by Kane (Chapter 15), have examined the perspectives of other people, including staff and families, involved in nursing home life. Aides, despite their potential effect on the residents' quality of life, are often overlooked altogether in research on nursing homes (Bagshaw & Adams, 1985–1986; Tellis-Nayak & Tellis-Nayak, 1989; Vladeck, 1980). The studies that have examined multiple perspectives are reviewed here.

Brennan, Moos, and Lemke (1988) compared the viewpoints of older people and "experts" (who were defined as gerontologists and architects involved in designing environments for older adults) on their preferences for physical design characteristics of group living facilities. They found that, indeed, the preferences of the two groups did differ. Experts were more likely to rate specific design features as very important or essential, perhaps because they were attempting to design facilities that would meet the needs of a broad range of older people, while older people's ratings might reflect only their own preferences.

Regarding the views of families as well as professionals, Kane, Bell, and Riegler (1986) surveyed value preferences for alternative patterns of long-term care. Although there were large areas of agreement, students and public officials differed from family members and professionals. The latter two groups were more sensitive to differences among types of care that might be appropriate for different residents. The findings from both of the above studies further validate soliciting the preferences of those groups that are closely involved with long-term care facilities—the residents, staff, and families.

The Present Study

The present study focused specifically on quality of life in the institution as seen through the perspectives of residents, staff, nurses' aides, and families. Multiple domains were examined—including the therapeutic environment, the physical environment, the social environment, and those domains internal to the self (i.e., abilities, autonomy, and morale). The study intended to (1) gather information to make recommendations for designing, planning, and improving procedures in long-term care facilities and (2) stimulate ideas and discussions for future research on this topic.

The following questions were addressed:

1. How do residents, staff, and families define quality of life?
2. What factors do residents, staff, and families believe affect quality of life in the institution?
3. How do perceptions of quality of life differ among the groups?
4. Based on this study, what are some future directions for research and application?

Method

Subjects

A total of 193 people from five different long-term care sites were interviewed for the study: 75 residents, 40 family members, 46 staff, and 32 nursing aides. Residents were sampled from both board and care (N = 42) and skilled nursing (N = 33) levels. Table 1 shows the characteristics of the residents and family members. Table 2 shows the characteristics of the staff and aides. Staff included M.D.'s ($N = 3$), nursing personnel ($N = 12$), social workers ($N = 8$), activities

Table 1 Characteristics of Residents and Family Members

A. Residents (N = 75)			
Sex	Females 73%		Males 27%
	Mean	SD	Range
Age	85.8 yr	6.3 yr	70–99 yr
Length of stay	3.6 yr	3.5 yr	0.5–15 yr

Physical abilities (percentage who do these activities by themselves)

Eating	97%	Transfer to bed	81%
Toileting	86%	Bathing	43%
Dressing	83%		

B. Family members (N = 40)			
Sex	Females 63%		Males 37%
Age	< 50 yr 20%	50–64 yr 50%	> 64 yr 30%

	Mean	SD	Range
Residents' length of stay	3.7 yr	4.0 yr	0.5–15 yr

Frequency of visits	≥ Once a month 95%	< Once a month 5%

personnel (N = 12), administrators (N = 3), rabbis and chaplains (N = 3), and volunteers (N = 5).

Selection of Subjects

To participate in the study, residents had to meet several criteria. They had to be mentally and physically able, and willing, to participate in a 45-minute to 1-hour interview. In addition, 50% of the residents had to have a family member who would also participate in the study.

Various sampling strategies were used because of the diverse characteristics of the sites. In one site, to help give the residents a sense of control over a study that was taking place in their facility, presentations about the project were made. Residents were then given an opportunity to volunteer to participate. In another site, every fifth name was selected from a roster of all residents, and social workers screened out any individuals whom they felt would not be able to complete the interview. In the remaining three sites, the small number of eligible residents and the restrictiveness of the criteria described above severely reduced the potential numbers of subjects. Almost all qualified candidates who met the criteria were tested. Overall, approximately 15% of those approached refused to participate.

We attempted to obtain a selection of different staff positions, because each

Table 2 Characteristics of Staff and Aides

A. Staff (*N* = 46)		
Sex	Females	80%
	Males	20%
Ethnicity	Caucasian	81%
	Black	7%
	Hispanic	2%
	Other	10%

	Mean	SD	Range
Length of service	4.5 yr	3.8 yr	0.5–15 yr
Length of career	9.4 yr	8.5 yr	0.5–44 yr

B. Aides (*N* = 32)		
Sex	Females	94%
	Males	6%
First language	English	41%
	Spanish	47%
	Other	13%
Ethnicity	Caucasian	19%
	Black	9%
	Hispanic	53%
	Other	13%

	Mean	SD	Range
Length of service	5.5 yr	4.6 yr	0.5–18 yr
Length of career	8.9 yr	5.3 yr	0.5–21 yr

Training	Yes	84%
	No	16%

type serves an important function in the nursing home. Some types of staff—social workers, nurses, and activities personnel—were sampled more heavily because they represented a larger portion of the staff. Availability to be interviewed determined the participation of many staff, but it was not the only criterion. While the majority of nurses and nurses' aides interviewed were from the day shift and a smaller number from the swing shift, these shifts represented the periods of greatest interaction between the cognitively alert resident subjects and staff members.

Nurses' aides deliver 90% of patient care in nursing homes (U.S. Senate Special Committee on Aging, 1975) and are responsible for some of the most intimate personal care tasks, giving them the vantage point to observe critical changes in the older persons' conditions or behavior. Because of their distinct perspective, their responses were analyzed separately.

Site Selection

It was not our intention to contrast the quality of life offered by different sites; the groups, rather than the facilities, formed our unit of analysis. Consequently, the data from all sites were pooled for the analyses.

The sites, all within the Los Angeles area, varied in size, levels of care, style of organization, and cultural characteristics. Two sites were under the umbrella of a large, not-for-profit, sectarian facility housing both board and care and nursing home residents. Two other sites were small, for-profit ones—one board and care facility and one skilled nursing facility. The fifth site was the nursing care unit of a large, multilevel facility.

Instrument

The survey instrument was developed to reflect four primary areas of quality of life, namely, therapeutic care, the physical environment, the social-emotional environment, and autonomy. Questions were adapted from several standardized instruments [Lubben, 1988; Neugarten & Havighurst, 1961; Pastalan & Bourestrom, 1975; Thompson, Streib, & Kosa, 1960 (as cited in Mangen & Peterson, 1982–1984)]. Open-ended questions were designed to elicit unconstrained responses about definitions of quality of life, factors influencing quality of life, and recommendations for improvements or changes. Closed-ended questions were used to elicit opinions about the importance of decision making on a variety of matters and the salience of various social contacts. Demographic information was obtained to identify and characterize each group of subjects.

Procedure

Four interviewers, including the senior author, administered the survey to residents, staff, and aides in individual, face-to-face interviews at the participants' facilities. For their convenience, most family members were interviewed by phone.

All interviews were conducted in English. Although 60% of the aides cited another language as their first language, those interviewed were all conversant in English.

Data Analysis

Both quantitative and qualitative methods were used for analyzing the data. Two specially trained raters, other than the authors, categorized participants' verbatim statements by the domains described below. Numbers of comments within categories were then tallied in preparation for statistical analyses.

Categories for Responses

Both style and content of responses were analyzed. Two dimensions defined style: verbosity of responses (how many different comments or thoughts were expressed in each answer) and the tone of the responses (positive or negative). In response to questions about the definition of quality of life, examples of positive statements were: "It's important to feel needed," and "Quality of life is those things that make life joyous and meaningful." Negative tones were seen in statements such as "Everything seems taken away from them," and "This is supposed to be the Golden Age—but it's not, they are caught up in problems."

Domains for the Content of Responses

Six domains were chosen to define the content of the responses. The first domain, care, primarily subsumed the services one might expect a nursing home to provide. Categories of care were: professional care, activities and entertainment, basic needs, and philosophy or ethos. *Professional care* included all comments referring to the type, quality, or characteristics of the professional care at the facility (i.e., medical, nursing, and social work services). *Activities and entertainment* included all comments referring to services intended to stimulate, entertain, or occupy the residents. *Basic needs* included all comments referring to food, laundry, beauty care, warmth, security, or safety. *Philosophy or ethos* included all comments referring to the "atmosphere" the facility tried to create among its employees or residents.

The second content domain was physical environment, which included all comments referring to the physical set-up and characteristics of the facility and its grounds. The third content domain was social-emotional environment, which included all comments referring to the social atmosphere of the facility or emotional aspects of the resident's life (e.g., having visitors, having a staff member who listened to them, etc.).

The final three content domains—ability, autonomy, and morale—focused on comments about personal or psychological aspects of the residents' lives. The ability domain included all comments referring to residents' physical or mental abilities that enabled them to participate in various tasks and activities. The autonomy domain included all comments referring to issues or staff efforts relating to the residents' sense of independence, participation in decision making, or control over their environment. Finally, the morale domain included all comments referring to the residents' enthusiasm, identification with the institution, and positive and negative views that may affect their lives and *how* they address issues and problems.

Results

Do residents feel they have a good quality of life? Residents were asked whether their life in the facility was "contented, comfortable, and meaningful." The great majority (73%) responded "yes" to the question, 21% responded "no," and the remaining 5% responded "yes and no."

Positive comments were significantly more numerous than negative comments [$t(415) = 13.02, p = .001$]. The percentage of positive comments was not significantly different across residents (86%), staff (94%), aides (87%), and family members (94%).

Do perceptions of quality of life differ among residents, staff, and families? The first questions addressed were how residents, staff, aides, and family members would define quality of life and how the groups might differ in their perceptions of its meaning.

Content of the Responses: Differences among Groups

The four groups differed significantly in the content of their responses [$\chi^2 (15, N = 416) = 66.06, p = .001$]. Figure 1 shows the distribution of responses in each of six content domains for the residents, staff, aides, and family members. The greatest differences among the four groups were in morale and care issues.

Morale

When defining quality of life, residents made significantly more comments about morale than did any other group; 38% of residents' comments were about morale, whereas only 17% of the staff's, 13% of the aides', and 14% of the family

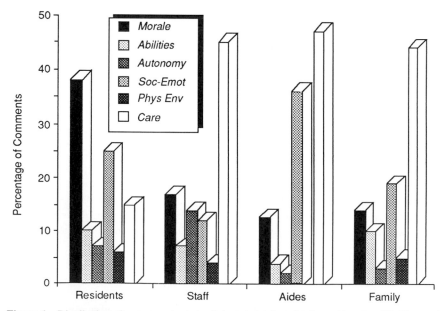

Figure 1 Distribution of responses in each of six content domains for residents, staff, aides, and family members when they were asked to define quality of life.

members' comments were in this domain. Examples of residents' responses were: "Life is what you make it," "Nothing makes me happy as long as I'm not home," and "I couldn't ask for better."

Care Issues

On the other hand, staff, aides, and family members all mentioned care issues significantly more often than did residents. Care issues made up 45% of the staff's comments, 47% of the aides' comments, and 44% of the family members' comments, compared to 15% of the residents' comments. Staff members defined quality of life as ensuring that social and medical wants were met, that life was made more comfortable, and that residents were not talked down to or spoken to in a paternal manner. Aides defined quality of life as ensuring that residents got a shower twice a week, had proper meals, had activities to keep their mind occupied, and received good care, including having a variety of things done for them. Family members envisioned quality of life as having good food, a sense of security, access to medical care and help when needed, and activities and outside stimulation.

Within the domain of care, respondents were asked, "What specifically about [this facility] makes life here contented, comfortable, and meaningful?" Figure 2 shows the distribution of responses for each group for the categories of activities,

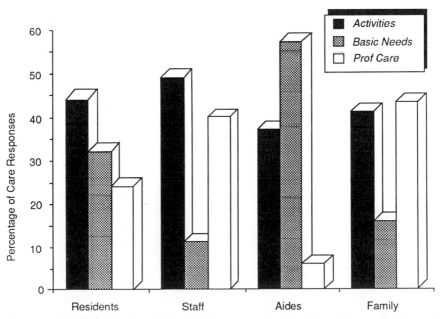

Figure 2 Distribution of responses in each of three categories of care for residents, staff, aides, and family members when they were asked to identify what specifically about the facility affected quality of life.

basic needs, and professional care. A chi-square analysis showed that the groups were significantly different in the distribution of their comments across the three categories [χ^2 (6, $N = 308$) = 52.93, $p = .0001$]. In commenting about care, residents most frequently mentioned activities as contributing to their quality of life, with comments about basic needs mentioned next most frequently, followed by professional care. Family members' and staff responses were most similar, mentioning activities and professional care about equally often; aides mentioned basic needs much more often than any other category of care.

Abilities

Respondents were asked specifically about the extent to which they felt residents' physical problems or health affected their quality of life. Figure 3 shows how each group of subjects rated the importance of physical health to quality of life. The groups were significantly different from one another [χ^2 (6, $N = 186$) = 59.50, $p = .0001$]. Somewhat surprisingly, the majority of residents felt that physical problems were "not at all" important to their quality of life. Staff, aides, and family members, in contrast to the residents, all rated the physical health of residents as important in their quality of life. Aides' responses were most similar to residents', but aides still rated physical health as more important

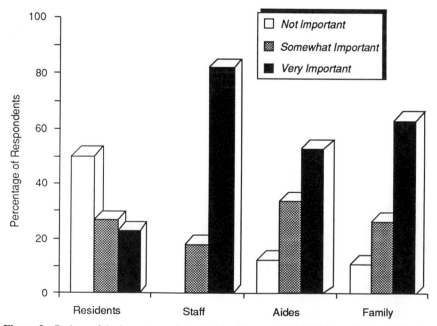

Figure 3 Ratings of the importance of physical health to quality of life by residents, staff, aides, and family members.

than did residents; half of the aides rated it as very important. Most staff members and two-thirds of family members said physical health was "very important." Because this result was surprising, the residents' data were stratified by level of care. Nursing-care level residents indicated that physical health had a greater influence on their quality of life than did the board-and-care residents [χ^2 (2, $N = 70$) = 7.17, $p = .03$].

Social-emotional Environment

A separate set of questions investigated the importance that residents, staff, aides, and family members attach to residents' contacts with family and friends. Respondents were asked to rate the importance of these relationships on a 3-point scale, 1 being "not at all important," 2 being "somewhat important," and 3 being "very important." Figure 4 shows the percentage of residents, staff, aides, and family members who selected "very important" as their response to questions about the importance of contacts with family and friends. Analyses of variance showed a significant difference between respondent groups [F (3, 82) = 6.97, $p = .0003$]. Post-hoc comparisons found significant differences between family and aides and family and staff. Family members felt that relationships were less important than did aides or staff. An additional analysis of variance found a significant difference between the mean percentage of "very important" responses for different types of relationships [F (3, 83) = 17.27, $p = .0001$]. Post-hoc comparisons found that relationships with relatives were rated as significantly more important when compared to each of the other three types of relationships.

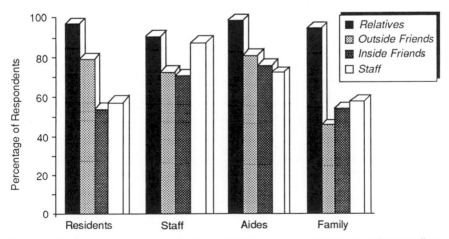

Figure 4 Percentage of residents, staff, aides, and family members answering "very important" on questions about contacts with family and friends.

Autonomy

One structured question specifically addressed perceptions of the importance of residents' decision making. Eleven items were chosen in this domain, representing opportunities for decision making: access to the telephone, a place to be alone, availability of transportation to the community, choice of roommates, having keepsakes nearby, ability to set schedules, frequency of baths, choice of foods, choice of company at meals, choice of where to eat meals, and ability to decorate one's own room. Respondents rated importance on the same 3-point scale used for the questions on social-emotional environment. An analysis of variance on the "very important" responses showed a significant difference among groups [F (3, 188) = 6.01, p = .0006]. The mean percentage of people responding "very important" was 54% for residents, 65% for staff, 71% for aides, and 61% for family members. Post-hoc comparisons showed significant differences between residents and staff and residents and aides. In general, residents felt these aspects of their life and environment were less important than did staff or aides.

To examine the order of importance for the 11 items, the percentages of "very important" responses were rank ordered (see Table 3). Although all respondents agreed that access to a telephone was very important to quality of life and that decorating one's own room was not so important, there was less agreement about some of the other items. The items with the largest discrepancies seem to be choice of foods, place to be alone, availability of transportation, and choices with respect to time scheduling. Correlations on the rank order of preferences across items showed that residents were significantly different from family members in their pattern of preferences (r = .66, p < .05), staff were significantly different from aides (r = .74, p < .02), and staff were significantly different from family (r = .84, p < .05). No other comparisons were significant.

Table 3 Autonomy Issues Rank-Ordered by Importance to Residents, Staff, Aides, and Family Members

	Residents $N = 75$	Staff $N = 46$	Aides $N = 32$	Family $N = 40$
Access to telephone	1	3	4	2
Place to be alone	2	7	10	4
Availability of transportation	3	6	5	7
Choice of roommates	4	2	2	1
Having keepsakes nearby	5	5	9	3
Setting schedules	6	10	8	10
Frequency of baths	7	9	4	9
Choice of foods	8	1	1	5
Choice of company at meals	9	4	4	6
Choice of where to eat	10	8	7	8
Decorating own room	11	11	11	11

Content of the Responses: Similarities among Groups

Although residents, staff, aides, and families differed in many ways in their perceptions of quality of life, there were several points of agreement.

Physical Environment
As Figure 1 shows, physical environment was rarely mentioned as an important determinant of quality of life by anyone.

Care Issues
Within the domain of care issues, relatively few responses from any group were about the philosophy or attitude of the facility (2% for residents, 11% for staff, 4% each for aides and families).

Social-Emotional Environment
Although the groups differed in the importance they attached to specific types of relationships, they were generally similar in their overall perceptions of the importance of the social-emotional environment in quality of life, as indicated in Figure 1. Social-emotional environment was the second most common domain for comments about quality of life by residents, aides, and families. Aides mentioned this aspect of life somewhat more frequently than any other group, and staff mentioned it somewhat less frequently than residents and families.

How can the quality of life in institutions be improved? A set of three questions tapped perceptions of what is currently lacking or could be improved in the institutional setting, allowing respondents to voice their recommendations for change. The questions were:

1. What do you miss most from where you were living before? (For family members: What do you think your family member misses most from where he/she was living before?)
2. Do you feel there are ways in which the care could be improved?
3. If you could change three things here to improve the quality of life for yourself and other residents [or you family member], what would those things be?

The first of these questions was asked only of residents and family members, the latter two questions were asked of all groups.

What Is Missed Most from Previous Home?: Differences among Groups

Residents most frequently mentioned missing aspects of their former life that were categorized as social-emotional or as activities (each category represented 24% of their total comments). Examples included: "being able to bake cakes and entertain friends," "going food shipping with a friend," "belonging to an organization and going to meetings," and "having my car and going on Vegas trips."

Conversely, family members perceived that residents missed aspects of their physical environment (23% of their total comments) and aspects of their lives related to basic needs (19% of their total comments). Frequently cited examples centered on two main topics—rooms and food (e.g., "She has a really small room," "She misses her privacy," and "She misses home cooking").

What Is Missed Most from Previous Home?: Similarities among Groups

Both residents and family members talked generally of concerns that crossed the domains of the social-emotional environment, the physical environment, and autonomy (e.g., missing their home life and the comforts of home, being the boss at home and being able to do as one pleased).

Autonomy was mentioned by both groups, but based on the frequency of comments in this domain it was ranked as third in importance. Here, residents' comments focused on both the abstract and the concrete, as reflected in the statements, "I miss my independence, feeling things were my own," and "I miss my checkbook terribly because now I can't give gifts to my children." Family members' concerns were similar; they felt residents missed the freedom to set schedules, being able to come and go, and just generally "being independent."

Some residents (16%) and family members (11%) indicated that they or their relative missed "nothing."

Respondents' Recommendations: Differences among Groups

In response to the second and third questions, "Do you feel there are ways in which the care could be improved?" and "If you could change three things here to improve the quality of life for yourself and other residents, what would those things be?" the average numbers of recommendations made were 1.6 (residents), 2.6 (staff), 2.0 (aides), and 2.8 (family members).

Residents made recommendations about professional care much less frequently (representing only 13% of their comments) than did aides (37%), staff (33%), or family (24%). This pattern was similar to that for the question, "Do you feel there are ways in which care could be improved?" to which 40% of the residents responded "no" or "I don't know." Of those who suggested improvements, many mentioned increasing the number of staff, and some asked that staff improve their demeanor (e.g., "talk more nicely to me"). Others commented on the roommate-matching process—the importance of placing compatible individuals together (e.g., "Don't put a 'schlumper' with a clean person"). Although the topic of professional care ranked third in number of suggestions mentioned, an indication of the topic's relative importance was reflected in the comment that the "care matters more than the physical environment."

Staff members, aides, and family members recommended that additional staff be hired, especially English-speaking staff. Their aim was to assure continuity, particularly on the weekends, and to avoid the use of personnel from the temporary nursing registry. Other recommendations were that staff have more time to spend with residents, staff meetings include *all* staff working with a resident, doctors be trained in geriatrics, and nurses be experienced in long-term care. Families voiced these same recommendations with the addition of having doctors be more available, putting mentally alert residents together, and evaluating the adjustment of new people to the facility after six months.

Respondents' Recommendations: Similarities among Groups

For residents, the domain in which recommendations were most often made was basic needs, representing 31% of their total comments. Aides, with 29% of their responses in this domain, also seemed to feel this was an area ripe for recommendations. Residents and aides, however, differed from staff and families, for whom only 13% and 14%, respectively, of recommendations were in the domain of basic needs. Comments by both residents and aides about basic needs were overwhelmingly about food. Examples included: "We want better food and choice of foods," "Vary the soup," "There is too much chicken," and "Let the residents choose the recipes." Other recommendations by aides focused on the need for more basic supplies, namely linens and diapers.

Residents, staff, and families who made more recommendations for improving the physical environment than did aides discussed the need for private and bigger rooms, but each had other specific recommendations: larger bathtubs and stall showers (residents), "a honeymoon cottage for married couples" and "enough space to have visitors at all hours" (staff), and "larger closets" and "more privacy" (families).

Discussion

The perceptions of residents, staff, aides, and families differ when it comes to defining quality of life. In the present investigation, residents' perceptions of quality of life primarily focused on their morale or attitude. On the other hand, staff members, aides, and family members defined quality of life primarily in terms of care. Furthermore, major differences were found among the groups in their ratings of the importance of physical health, of the importance of social contacts other than relatives, and of specific items over which they might have control.

Overall, each group tended to define quality of life in terms of domains over which they held responsibility, and which therefore validated their roles. For example, residents defined quality of life in terms of their morale or attitudes, and aides defined quality of life in terms of caring and felt that the frequency of baths (one of their responsibilities) was significantly more important than people in other groups did. Staff, aides, and family members all rated physical health as more important to residents' quality of life than did residents themselves. With respect to social networks, although all groups rated relatives as most important, staff rated themselves almost equal in importance to relatives, and family members rated the importance of friends outside the facility lower than did residents.

In general, residents and staff tended to differ in their perceptions more than did residents and aides or residents and families. Staff, rather than residents, family members, or aides, are likely to carry the most power in the organization. Therefore, the finding that staff and resident perceptions about autonomy issues and social contacts differ may mean that staff policies and efforts may not always be in concert with actions that enhance residents' quality of life.

Alternatively, this might be viewed as a necessary distinction. Staff are responsible for the overall quality of life experienced generally by all residents, whereas residents focus primarily on their own individual needs. It is therefore possible that the staff opinions reflect what is best for residents as a group rather than for the specific individual (e.g., encouraging residents to eat in the main dining room versus eating alone in their own rooms).

Aides, perhaps because of the amount of contact they have with residents, often voiced reactions that were more similar to residents than to other staff members. In the present study, the perceptions of nurses' aides often differed from other staff members' perceptions, suggesting that aides need to be considered as a group distinct from other staff.

Another possible explanation for the differences is that the definitions and perceptions of quality of life change with age. Residents in our study averaged 85 years of age, while most family members were less than 65. For example, significantly more family members than residents rated physical health as very important in determining quality of life. This pattern of responses approximates that of a sample of 1536 community-dwelling Canadians aged 65 and older, 74% of whom rated their health as good to excellent, despite the fact that at least 80% of the group indicated they had at least one health problem (Health Promotion Directorate, 1988). Perhaps older people are more likely to accept functional limitations as part of the aging process and more able to cope with them than other groups perceive. Some of our residents' comments exemplified this—"You have to adjust," "Physically, it's as comfortable as they can make me," and "Doctors here make it as nice as they can for you."

The authors of this study have noted, as have other researchers (e.g., Kane, Bell, & Riegler, 1986), that residents tended to recommend changes in areas that they may perceive as most mutable. Residents may reflect a possible sense of control by defining quality of life predominantly in terms of their own morale or attitude, concentrating on their own responsibility for creating a good quality of life because they do not feel the institution can be changed enough to do so.

Other examples of their perceived sense of control may be reflected in the concerns they voiced about food, roommates, and professional care, for example, rather than the more fixed aspects of the physical environment (e.g., room decor).

In interpreting the results, it is important to note that the institutions we surveyed were in many ways exemplary; thus, they are unlikely to be representative of all long-term care facilities. The average length of service was unusually long for staff (4.5 years) and particularly for nurses' aides (5.5 years), given that many nursing homes experience at least 75% turnover of nonprofessional staff per year (Vladeck, 1980). Another piece of evidence indicating that these were high-quality facilities is the small average number of recommendations for change in the facility. Staff averaged 2.6 recommendations, while residents and aides averaged only 1.6 and 2.0, respectively, although all respondents were asked for 3 recommendations.

The positive characteristics of these facilities may have affected the responses obtained, particularly the lack of importance residents attributed to professional care in affecting their quality of life (see Figure 2) and the finding that 40% of the residents did not feel care could be improved. Residents, having these basic needs met, might have been better able to define quality of life in a more philosophical or self-determined way or in terms of positive attributes—for example, activities and contact with the outside world—that gave them satisfaction (Maslow, 1968; Turnbull, 1972).

Also, in interpreting the results, it may be important to acknowledge the differences between the effects of age-related changes and the effects of living in an institution. Complaints about quality of life, such as the inability to get out as frequently, could be a function of stage of life, independent of the institution.

Other factors that may have affected our findings relate to the difficulties of interviewing institutionalized individuals. Questions of the competency of impaired individuals and the validity of the results arise, as does the potential of a "halo effect" (i.e., that the fear of retribution for negative comments could have resulted in a tendency toward only positive responses to our questions). Other research supports the notion that older people might be unwilling to criticize or offer alternatives to their current housing conditions (Carp, 1975). However, our data contained a number of authentic criticisms and thus did not seem to reflect this tendency.

Practical Implications

A critical step in improving quality of life involves examining how various groups define and perceive the concept and then, wherever possible, working toward reconciling or accommodating their differences by encouraging discussion between the groups. Our findings underscore the importance of involving all groups in discussion and policy making. For example, because residents feel that basic needs are more important determinants of quality of life than do staff, different pressures might be felt on the nursing home. Alternatively, if both residents and family acknowledge the importance of activities, a more successful outcome may be achieved.

Perceptions of quality of life can be viewed as adaptive or maladaptive. One way to use the present results is to work to formalize and encourage the positive perceptions and behaviors and rule out the negative ones. For example, if aides tend to befriend residents who lack families, perhaps specific efforts could be made to identify and work with residents who do not have relatives. Conversely, many residents appear to feel they must relinquish long-established roles that they enjoyed. A number of residents indicated a lack of opportunity for (1) baking and entertaining visitors and (2) participating in meetings and clubs as they had in the community. Some residents seem to benefit from having a quasi-formal role in the daily workings of the facility, for instance, a healthy resident assisting staff with the care of more impaired residents. Opportunities to continue these roles would help "normalize" residents' lives.

Recommendations for Future Research

Defining quality of life is a difficult task. No simple, single definition of quality of life was forthcoming from the respondents in this study; quality of life means different things to different people. Definitions of quality of life include aspects of care, the social-emotional environment, the physical environment, abilities, autonomy, and morale and appeared to reflect the exemplary nature of the residents' current housing situation. Individuals differed from one another in their perceptions of quality of life, and many included several domains in their definition. All of these facts indicate that the concept of quality of life is multidimensional.

The present study examined a greater range of factors that might affect quality of life than has any other study to date. In considering the concept of quality of life, exploring the range of possible factors should lead to a better understanding on which to base subsequent studies of individual factors. Research should now be directed toward constructing a model of quality of life that takes into account the data presented here on differences among groups, as well as individual differences in perception. The preliminary analyses of this study comparing board and care and skilled nursing residents support further study of within-group differences.

Secondly, we need to know what underlying mechanisms account for the different patterns of perceptions observed in the present study, such as the function of age in altering perceptions of quality of life as described above.

A third area of research suggested by the present study is the effect of individual coping styles and attitudes on definitions and perceptions of quality of life. We found residents' morale and attitude toward their institutionalization to be quite important to their own definition of quality of life. These areas of research have yet to be explored.

Conclusion

Throughout this study, a continual theme surfaces: the tensions inherent in even the best of institutions—the tension between needs and preferences for independence, individualization, and control expressed by residents and families and the limits set by an institution that must serve many individuals, invariably within financial and resource constraints. These implicit trade-offs were expressed by residents in their comments about missing their freedom and privacy but also in their comments about feeling reassured in knowing they would be cared for and relieved of household responsibilities. Family members indicated a similar awareness of the trade-offs of roommate problems and loss of privacy, for example, with the social benefits derived from living in a group situation.

Hands-on staff—nurses, social workers, and activity personnel—often act as mediators of these tensions between the administration, residents, and family. Many expressed mixed feelings of being caught between the residents' needs and the institutions' legitimate limitations. These conditions imply a need for ongoing dialogue; for example, residents' tolerance for the limitations could be enhanced by understanding the reasons for the restrictions (e.g., that rising costs might necessitate fewer bus trips for resident activities, or that it would be too costly and unwieldy to have an individual birthday party for each resident).

Many aspects of long-term care facilities can be improved. Some of the desired changes admittedly entail costs—more staff, better-educated staff, private rooms, and so on—but others represent only nominal expenditures—control over meal choices and personal spending choices. The costs of these changes, in terms of both finances and increased demands on the organization, must be balanced with the benefits of enhanced quality of life.

Acknowledgments

We are grateful to the Borun Center for Gerontological Research for financial support and to Timothy LeFedre, M.D., of the Motion Picture Home; Bill Mathias of Beverly Enterprises; Sheldom Blumenthal of the Jewish Homes for the Aging; and Wanda Ewing and Miriam Goldsmith of Hayworth Terrace, who made this study possible. Many thanks to Marcia Cogan, Jo Raksin, and Jeff Shafiroff for interviewing respondents; to Mary Jackson for data analyses; and to Jim Birren, Donna Deutchman, Kate Wilber, Jim Lubben, and Pauline Robinson for critical comments on earlier drafts. Last, but not least, we greatly appreciate the cooperation of residents, staff, aides, and family members who gave their time and energy to participate in our study.

References

Bagshaw, M., & Adams, M. (1985–1986). Nursing home nurses' attitudes, empathy, and ideologic orientation. *International Journal of Aging and Human Development, 22,* 235–246.

Bayer, M., Bresloff, L., & Curley, D. (1986). The enhancement project: A program to improve the quality of residents' lives. *Geriatric Nursing, July/August,* 192–195.

Brennan, P. L., Moos, R. H., & Lemke, S. (1988). Preferences of older adults and experts for physical and architectural features of group living facilities. *The Gerontologist, 28,* 84–90.

Carp, F. (1975). Ego defense or cognitive consistency effects on environmental evaluations. *The Gerontologist, 30,* 707–711.

Estes, C. L., & Binney, E. A. (1989). The biomedicalization of aging: Dangers and dilemmas. *The Gerontologist, 29,* 587–596.

Friedman, S. (1975). The resident welcoming committee: Institutionalized elderly in volunteer services to their peers. *The Gerontologist, 15,* 362–367.

Goffman, E. (1958). Characteristics of total institutions. *Symposium on preventive and social psychiatry.* Washington, D.C.: U.S. Government Printing Office.

Health Promotion Directorate (1988). *The active health report on seniors.* Ottawa: Health and Welfare Canada.

Institute of Medicine Committee on Nursing Home Regulation (1986). *Improving the quality of life in nursing homes.* Washington, D.C.: National Academy Press.

Kane, R. A. (1989). The biomedical blues. *The Gerontologist, 29,* 583.

Kane, R. A., & Kane, R. L. (1987). *Long-term care: Principles, programs, and policies.* New York: Springer.

Kane, R. L., Bell, R. M., & Riegler, S. Z. (1986). Value preferences for nursing home outcomes. *The Gerontologist, 26,* 303–308.

Koncelik, J. A. (1976). *Designing the open nursing home.* Stroudsburg, Penn.: Dowden, Hutchinson and Ross.

Langer, E., & Rodin, J. (1976). The effects of choice and enhanced personal responsibility for the aged. A field experiment in an institutional setting. *Journal of Personality and Social Psychology, 34,* 191–198.

Lawton, M. P., & Nahemow, L. (1973). Ecology and the aging process. In C. Eisdorfer & M. P. Lawton, eds., *The psychology of adult development,* pp. 619–674. Washington, D.C.: American Psychological Association.

Lubben, J. E. (1988). Assessing social networks among elderly populations. *Family and Community Health, 11,* 42–52.

Lyman, K. A. (1989). Bringing the social back in: A critique of the biomedicalization of dementia. *The Gerontologist, 29,* 597–605.

Mangen, D. J., & Peterson, W. A., eds. (1982–1984). *Research instruments in social gerontology,* vols. 1–3. Minneapolis, Minn.: University of Minnesota Press.

Maslow, A. (1968). *Toward a psychology of being.* New York: Van Nostrand Reinhold.

Schultz, R. (1976). Effects of control and predictability on physical and psychological well-being of the institutionalized aged. *Journal of Personality and Social Psychology, 33,* 563–573.

Schwartz, A. N., & Vogel, M. E. (1990). Nursing home staff and residents' families role expectations. *The Gerontologist, 30,* 49–53.

Sommer, R., & Osmond, H. (1961). Symptoms of institutional care. *Social Problems, 8,* 254–263.

Spalding, J., & Frank, B. W. (1985). Quality care from the residents' point of view. *American Health Care Association Journal, July,* 3–7.

Teitelman, J. L., & Priddy, J. M. (1988). From psychological theory to practice: Improving frail elders' quality of life through control-enhancing interventions. *Journal of Applied Gerontology, 7,* 298–315.

Tellis-Nayak, V., & Tellis-Nayak, M. (1989). Quality of care and the burden of two cultures: When the world of the nurses' aide enters the world of the nursing home. *The Gerontologist, 29,* 307–313.

Turnbull, C. M. (1972). *The mountain people.* New York: Simon and Schuster.

U.S. Senate Special Committee on Aging (1987–1988). *Aging America: Trends and projections.* Washington, D.C.: U.S. Dept. of Health and Human Services.

U.S. Senate Special Committee on Aging (1990). *Developments in Aging, 1989,* vols. 1, 2, pp. 237–238. Washington, D.C.: U.S. Government Printing Office.

U.S. Senate Special Committee on Aging, Subcommittee on Long Term Care (1975). *Nursing home care in the United States: Failure in public policy.* Supporting paper no. 4: *Nurses in nursing homes, the heavy burden,* pp. 372–381, 94th Congress, 1st Session.

Vladeck, B. C. (1980). *Unloving care—The nursing home tragedy.* New York: Basic Books.

3

Measurement of Quality of Life in the Frail Elderly

SHARON B. ARNOLD

Introduction

The age distribution of our population is changing rapidly. The elderly, defined as persons over 65 years of age, are becoming an increasingly larger subgroup. And within the elderly population, the proportion of persons aged 75 and older is growing even more rapidly. Since those persons 75 and older, often called the "old-old," are at greater risk of chronic disease and functional disability (Cornoni-Huntley *et al.*, 1985), policymakers view these changing demographics with alarm. The frail elderly use higher rates of health and social services (Soldo & Manton, 1985), which may have serious implications for public expenditures in an era of decreased fiscal resources. Policymakers are increasingly asking clinicians and social scientists to justify the benefit of additional health and social services on this target population.

An increasingly important aspect of gerontological research is the development and evaluation of interventions designed to improve the health and social status of elderly people and their primary informal caregivers. Thus, in general, an important mechanism by which the goals of clinicians and social scientists can be targeted, and their efforts evaluated, is through an assessment of the quality of life of the population they are seeking to help. Since clinicians and social scientists are increasingly being asked to justify the benefit of additional services, the measurement of health status and quality of life is becoming increasingly important. Extrapolating from the reasons to measure health status as described by Ware, Brook, Davies, and Lohr (1981), several reasons exist for attempting to measure the quality of life of the frail elderly. These include:

- *Evaluating the efficiency or effectiveness of interventions.* Any attempt to improve the health or social status of elderly individuals should result in an

Copyright © 1991 by Academic Press, Inc.
All rights of reproduction in any form reserved.

improvement in their quality of life. For example, a medical intervention that simply prolongs life without improving the quality of that life may not be an advantage.

- *Assessing the quality of health care.* Quality of life measures are one of the outcome measures that can be used to assess quality of care.
- *Estimating the needs of a population.* Measuring the quality of life of the frail elderly can provide information about service needs requiring some type of program intervention. For example, finding deficits in social activities in a group of frail elderly may point to the need to develop programs and activities to increase social interaction.
- *Assessing the impact of the environment on quality of life.* Research on the aspects of physical and social environment that are most conducive to high quality of life would enable the creation of better-designed housing and service environments in the future.
- *Improving clinical decisions.* Information on an individual's quality of life can provide important additional information to a clinician in determining a course of therapy.
- *Understanding the causes and consequences of differences in quality of life.* Because differences in the components of quality of life are likely to vary among individuals, interventions are not likely to benefit everyone equally. It is important to study and understand not only the differences in quality of life but differences in preferences as well.

Historically, quality of life has been viewed as a very abstract concept, and more concrete measures (such as mortality or restricted-activity days) have been used both for program planning and for assessing the effectiveness of health and social services. However, as understanding of the importance of more sensitive and relevant outcome measures has grown, and with increasing ability to measure accurately such concepts as quality of life, many researchers and practitioners are turning to quality of life measures to assess health and social program interventions. This is particularly appropriate for the frail elderly, who generally suffer from multiple chronic conditions that are unlikely to be cured by clinical interventions but for whom quality of life improvements are entirely possible.

In the present chapter, the literature on quality of life measures is reviewed with a focus on those measures that are appropriate for use in the frail elderly. First, the literature is reviewed to determine whether there is consensus on a definition of quality of life and to define quality of life. Then, an outline of the characteristics of measures is presented, highlighting aspects of those characteristics that make a measure more or less desirable for assessing quality of life in the frail elderly. Finally, several currently available measures of quality of life are discussed and critically reviewed to determine the extent to which they are practical for use in the frail elderly.

Defining Quality of Life

Defining such an abstract and personal concept as the *quality of life* is inherently complex and involves both objective and subjective elements. Objective elements include financial resources, health status, functioning, and social contacts, among others. These attributes are relatively easy to measure and consistently defined. In contrast, elements such as happiness, life satisfaction, and self-esteem are highly subjective and difficult to define or measure. Thus, we find a variety of definitions of quality of life occurring in the research literature that often reflect the perspectives (and professional orientations) of the authors. Clinically oriented researchers tend to define quality of life in terms of health status or functional ability. Kaplan (n.d.), for example, defines quality of life as the impact of disease and disability on daily functioning. Other researchers take a broader perspective to include: (1) both physical and material well-being; relations with others; social, community, and civic activities; personal development; and recreation (Ferrell, Wisdom, & Wenzl, 1989); (2) material comforts; work; health; active recreation; learning, and education (Flanagan, 1982); (3) social, physical, emotional, and intellectual functioning; life satisfactions; and health perceptions (Pearlman & Uhlmann, 1988); (4) life satisfaction; self-esteem; and general health and functioning (George & Bearon, 1980); or (5) freedom; happiness; financial security; achievement of ambition; activity; and well-being (Bulpitt & Fletcher, 1985).

As can be seen by the sampling of definitions provided here, quality of life is often defined broadly to include many different concepts, although there is considerable overlap in the elements included in different definitions. The majority of researchers appear to agree that any definition of quality of life should consider the following attributes:

- physical functioning and symptoms
- emotional functioning and behavioral dysfunctioning
- intellectual and cognitive functioning
- social functioning and the existence of a supportive network
- life satisfaction
- health perceptions
- economic status
- ability to pursue interests (e.g., job, hobbies) and recreations
- sexual functioning
- energy and vitality

It is noteworthy that health status is always a key component of quality of life as defined in the literature. This is hardly surprising. For example, Flanagan (1982) reports that health was considered important to quality of life by 95 to

98% of adults in each of six age and sex groups in a study of the major factors affecting the quality of life of adult Americans. However, health status is rarely the only aspect of quality of life included in definitions. Other frequently listed components include happiness and well-being, social activities, and financial security.

Measurement Characteristics

The difficulties experienced in defining the quality of life are compounded when attempts are made to develop quality of life measures. In fact, measures of quality of life are often more narrowly focused around more objective criteria, and many are predominantly measures of health status. Clearly, given the range of definitions of the quality of life and the diverse reasons for attempting to measure it, no one measure will be useful for all purposes. The characteristics of a desirable measure depend on the reason for measurement, the population of interest, and the resources available to collect data.

Some of the reasons for measuring quality of life have been discussed in the previous section; they include (1) evaluating the effectiveness of interventions; (2) assessing quality of care; (3) estimating the needs of a population; (4) improving clinical decisions; and (5) understanding differences in quality of life. Each of these purposes has implications for the type and important characteristics of the measure to be selected.

In particular, measures that will form the basis for making decisions about individuals must necessarily be more precise than those that describe population attributes. Evaluating the effectiveness of interventions, especially when comparing the effects of different interventions on overall quality of life, may necessitate an aggregated measure of quality of life. Conversely, when the goal of measurement is needs assessment, a measure with several subscales of the concepts of interest may provide more relevant information.

The population of interest is also an important consideration in selecting measures of quality of life. An understanding of the extent of variation within the population is important in determining the sensitivity necessary. Thus, for example, a measure that does not allow fine distinctions between quality of life at the lower end of the continuum may not provide the specificity needed to capture small but meaningful differences in quality of life in the severely chronically ill.

Finally, the resources available to measure quality of life will influence the selection of the measure. In general, longer and more comprehensive assessment instruments are also more costly to field. Self-administered questionnaires are generally less costly than interviewer-administered questionnaires because of the training requirements and additional manpower required to perform the interviews. Observation of an individual's behavior also may be used to determine presumptive quality of life when it is not possible to question the subject or a proxy. In principle, when resources are limited, it is advisable to use a well-tested measure that is more narrowly defined to ensure that the information obtained is of high quality.

Some of the criteria by which to evaluate measures include practicality, content and scaling, aggregation, reliability, and validity (Ware, 1984). Each of these issues are discussed in turn.

Practicality

In order for a quality of life measure to be used, it must be practical for administration in the population of interest. Aspects of practicality to consider include the burden placed on respondents, the choice of respondent, the method of administration, and likely refusal rates or rates of missing data.

Respondent burden is a significant issue, especially in research involving the frail elderly, who may be more vulnerable than other segments of the population either due to physical or cognitive deficits or through the isolation brought about by disease or living situation. Respondent burden takes into account both physical and emotional burdens. The physical aspect of burden includes the time and effort required by frail individuals to respond. Any attempt at measurement will involve some burden on the part of the respondent, but the length and complexity of the instrument should be minimized to the extent possible, in order to limit the burden. Emotional burden includes any negative feelings or emotions that surface as a result of the content of the instrument; for example, an instrument that includes questions of social functioning may include questions about the extent of time spent with friends and relatives, which may exacerbate the individual's feelings of loneliness.

It is also important to consider appropriate respondents to the questionnaire when selecting measures for use with the frail elderly. The measure can be designed to elicit information from the subject (the elderly person), a family member or significant other, or a health care provider who knows the subject. While obtaining information directly from the subject is often most desirable, this may not always be possible due to the high rate of cognitive dysfunction among the frail elderly. It is important to remember, however, that information provided by any person other than the subject is likely to be biased because it is filtered through the respondent's beliefs and prejudices. For example, previous research has shown that physicians are likely to rate their patients as being in poorer health than the patient perceives (Maddox & Douglass, 1973). In addition to asking a proxy respondent about the elderly person, observation can be used to assess quality of life. However, using an independent observer to assess quality of life is problematic, since there is not necessarily a close relationship between the observer's and the subject's assessment of the components of quality of life.

The method by which the assessment instrument is administered is another important consideration when selecting measures for use with the frail elderly. Quality of life instruments can be self-administered or administered through a personal or telephone interview. Aside from the not insignificant differences in cost between the different methods of administration, there are implications for both data quality and response rate in the selection of administration method. While self-administered questionnaires are usually less expensive, they tend to result in higher rates of missing data, possibly due to the respondent not understanding the questions. Nonetheless, self-administered questionnaires tend to be the best way to handle issues that are extremely personal (such as sexual functioning) because the respondent is not required to discuss the response with another individual. Interviews are the most expensive means to collect health status information; however, the researcher can ensure that the respondent understands the questions and that all responses will be usable. For frail and isolated seniors, personal interviews may provide the additional benefit of interaction with another individual. Telephone interviews combine many of the advantages of self-administered interviews (including anonymity) with some of the human interaction of a personal interview.

Rates of refusal and missing data are problems that plague all data collection attempts. The content, length, and method of administration of the instrument can influence the rates of refusal and missing data and should be considered in the selection of instruments.

Content and Scaling
The content of a measure and the way in which scores are assigned so that they reflect differences in quality of life are important aspects to consider in the selection of a measure. The combination of individual item responses into a score to transmit important information is the scaling technique. Since one of the goals of measurement is to illustrate variation among individuals, a scaling technique that assigns every individual the same score is obviously not very useful. In addition to simply illustrating variation, the score obtained also should be able to capture clinically meaningful differences between individuals. Obviously, the way a measure is scaled will have a significant impact on its usefulness for a given population. For example, when considering the quality of life of the frail elderly, where poor health is likely to negatively affect the quality of life score, one would generally desire a different content than when assessing the quality of life of teenage athletes. Because the two populations are widely different along the dimension of physical health, their scores are likely to be "clumped" at either end of the distribution, and any differences within a population would be masked.

Aggregation
Another issue to consider when evaluating measures of quality of life is the extent to which the score reflects the aggregation of many concepts, or whether each concept is measured and scored separately. Aggregate scores provide a common denominator by which to judge the outcomes and effectiveness of different interventions by translating all aspects of quality of life into one measure.

The disadvantage of aggregate scores is that there is rarely consensus about how to combine information from different concepts of quality of life (e.g., physical functioning and intellectual/cognitive functioning) and about the appropriate weight to assign to each of the concepts. There may well be age-related differences in preferences regarding the relative importance of different aspects of quality of life. The incorporation of information obtained from a series of separate scales may provide more information but is often more complex to understand.

Reliability

When assessing an individual's quality of life, the instrument used should provide consistent information over time, provided the individual's true status has not changed. The reliability of a measure refers to the proportion of true score (as opposed to random noise) that is reflected in the measured score. While all measures contain some noise, the higher the reliability coefficient, the more confident one can be that the score reflects information that will be consistent from one administration to another. However, the reliability actually required in a measure depends on its use; for example, an instrument used for clinical decision making needs to have higher reliability than one used for population comparisons.

There are two aspects of reliability that are often reported for measures of health status and quality of life. These include test–retest reliability and internal consistency reliability. Test–retest reliability measures the agreement between responses obtained at two points in time, usually in the form of a correlation coefficient. One disadvantage of test–retest reliability is the necessity of requiring repeated administrations of the instrument, leaving open the possibility of bias due to recall or to changes in the trait being measured. However, it is the only measure of reliability that is possible for single-item measures, and it is often reported in the literature. Internal consistency reliability measures the correlation across items in a scale, determining the extent to which the items in a scale measure the same concept.

The internal consistency reliability of a measure varies with the length of the measure, and longer questionnaires generally have better reliability. Additionally, questionnaires that are administered to a larger sample will appear to have higher reliability than those administered to a smaller sample because of the smaller standard error of measurement. A common statistic used to report internal consistency reliability is Chronbach's alpha (Chronbach, 1951). Chronbach's alpha is a function of the homogeneity of items and the number of items in a scale and can range from 0 to 1.0, with 1.0 indicating perfect reliability. In general, reliability scores of at least 0.50 to 0.70 are considered adequate for group comparisons, while 0.90 is considered essential for individual comparisons (Ware, 1984).

Validity

While reliability measures the consistency of information obtained from the instrument, validity measures the ability of the instrument to measure the attributes of concern. In other words, the ability to walk a block may not be a valid quality of life measure for a frail elderly person. A number of different measures of validity exist, which focus on different aspects of validity. These include content validity, convergent and discriminant validity, construct validity, and concurrent or predictive validity.

Content validity measures the extent to which the instrument incorporates a comprehensive definition of quality of life into the scope and content of the measure. For a measure to have high content validity, it must contain items relating to the range of quality of life concepts. To the extent that a measure focuses on only one aspect of quality of life, it cannot be said to have high content validity.

Convergent and discriminant validity measure the relationship between individual items and the scale and are often evaluated using measures of item–scale correlation. Discriminant validity measures the extent to which the items correlate more highly with the hypothesized scale than with another scale; convergent validity measures the extent to which each of the items correlate roughly equally with the scale.

Construct validity examines the relationship between the score obtained on the quality of life measure and alternative measures for which a relationship is hypothesized. For example, a measure of quality of life should be correlated with a measure of physical health or social functioning, since those have been defined as aspects of quality of life. Similarly, since there is no theoretical basis to assume that blonds have more fun, and thus better quality of life, we would not expect for there to be a relationship between quality of life and hair color. The measurement of construct validity requires a clear delineation of hypotheses about the relationship between the measure of interest and other measures.

Finally, concurrent and predictive validity are two other aspects that are important to measure. Concurrent validity measures the functional relationship between quality of life and other variables, such as use of health care services. A related concept, predictive validity, is concerned with the extent to which the measure of quality of life can predict future action or behavior. For example, an individual with low quality of life at present may use greater health and social services in the future.

A Review of Selected Quality of Life Measures

Quality of life is a broad term that incorporates a number of objective and subjective aspects of an individual's life, taking into account not only the physiological and medical changes produced by the intervention, but also the impact on patient functioning and well-being. In order to evaluate the effectiveness of interventions aimed at improving the quality of life of frail elderly persons and their primary caregivers, comprehensive measures of quality of life must be utilized. Because there is no absolute theoretical model of what constitutes quality of life, measures must approximate our understanding of the elements of

Table 1 Selected Quality of Life Measures

Measure	Population	Administration	Reliability	Validity
Sickness Impact Profile	Extensive use in many populations, including chronically ill and frail elderly	Interviewer and self-administered versions	Extensive data available	Extensive data available
Older Americans Resources and Services Instrument	Frail elderly	Most experience obtained from interviewer-administered version	Extensive data available	Extensive data available
RAND Health Status Measures	Community-dwelling population, including elderly and those with chronic disease	Self-administered	Extensive data available	Extensive data available
Quality of Well-Being Scale	Numerous populations, including chronically ill	Interviewer and self-administered versions	Extensive data available	Extensive data available
Reintegration to Normal Living Index	Rehab patients	Interviewer-administered	Limited	Limited
City of Hope Medical Center Quality of Life Survey	Cancer patients	Interviewer-administered	Limited	Limited
Perceived Quality of Life Scale	Former intensive care patients	Interview-administered	Limited	Limited
Subjective Well-Being Instrument for the Chronically Ill	General population and cancer patients	Interviewer-administered	Limited	Limited

this very abstract concept. There is currently little certainty about what should be measured when assessing quality of life, which is a complex attribute requiring a multidimensional approach to measurement. Because of the many potential aspects of quality of life, there is good reason to select a measure based upon the target population and the reason for measurement itself. While there are some aspects of quality of life that may be applicable for all situations, time and resource constraints will often dictate that only a limited number be measured. Thus, selecting the concepts that most directly relate to the situation at hand will improve the efficiency of the endeavor.

In this section, several existing measures of quality of life are described, which vary along a number of dimensions. They were designed for various populations, including those with chronic diseases, those with heart disease or diabetes, cancer patients, and the general population. They vary from short to long, from simple to complex. They also vary regarding the extent to which their reliability and validity has been documented. Table 1 briefly illustrates some of the major characteristics of these measures. Included in the review are measures with extensive subscales that assess a range of concepts, as well as those that measure an aggregate global quality of life concept. Table 2 illustrates the range of attributes of quality of life measured by these instruments.

The Sickness Impact Profile (SIP)

SIP is an extensive instrument designed to evaluate the impact of chronic illness on patient quality of life and functioning (Bergner, Bobbit, Carter, & Gibson, 1981). Its original purpose was to evaluate the effectiveness of health services and provide information that could be used for evaluation, program planning, and policy formation. Its original design and development took place at the University of Washington, Seattle, under the direction of Marilyn Bergner and Betty Gilson.

The instrument, which can be either interviewer- or self-administered, consists of 136 items in 12 categories or domains. These include:

- ambulation
- mobility
- body care and movement
- social interaction
- alertness behavior
- emotional behavior
- communication
- sleep and rest
- eating
- work

Table 2 Attributes Assessed in Quality of Life Measures

	Physical functioning	Emotional functioning	Cognitive functioning	Social functioning	Life satisfaction	Health perceptions	Economic status	Recreation	Sexual functioning	Energy and vitality
Sickness Impact Profile	X	X	X	X		X		X		X
Older Americans Resources and Services Instrument										
RAND Health Status Measures	X	X	X	X		X	X	X		
Quality of Well-Being Scale	X	X	X	X	X	X	X	X	X	X
Reintegration to Normal Living Index	X			X			X			
City of Hope Medical Center Quality of Life Survey				X						
Perceived Quality of Life Scale	X	X	X	X	X	X	X	X		
Subjective Well-Being Instrument for the Chronically Ill		X								X

- home management
- recreation and pastimes.

For each question, the respondents are instructed to respond according to how they feel on a given day due to their health.

The SIP has been used extensively in the past decade, and its reliability and validity is well established. Test–retest reliability was evaluated using data from four subsamples of patients: rehabilitation medicine outpatients and inpatients, speech pathology inpatients, outpatients with chronic health problems, and members of an HMO who reported no illnesses. The test–retest reliability, using different interviewers, forms, and administration procedures among a variety of subjects, was high. The reliability of the overall score ranged from 0.75 to 0.92. The authors report that the test–retest reliability did not differ by interviewer, form, or administrative procedures. Internal consistency, measured by Chronbach's alpha, was high at 0.97 (Bergner et al., 1981).

Validity of the SIP was measured in a number of ways. Initial construct validation included an examination of the relationship of the SIP score with self-assessment of dysfunction and with other measures of functioning, which were fairly high. For example, the relationship between the SIP score and self-assessment of dysfunction was 0.69 and between the SIP score and clinician assessment of dysfunction was 0.50. Convergent and discriminant validity were analyzed using the multitrait–multimethod technique and were reported as good. The validity of the SIP was assessed by comparing the SIP score with objective clinical data for patients with total hip replacement, hyperthyroidism, and rheumatoid arthritis. The correlations between the clinical measures and the SIP measures ranged from moderate ($r = 0.41$) to high ($r = -0.84$). Finally, the validity of the SIP was assessed through the use of pattern and profile analyses of SIP sensitivity. The authors were able to obtain a consistent profile of dysfunction for several diagnoses, including total hip replacement and hyperthyroid patients.

While the considerable experience with the SIP in a number of populations (including the elderly) is an advantage to its use in a frail elderly population, the emphasis of the SIP on health status results in a limited view of quality of life. Additionally, with its considerable length and interviewer training required, the SIP could be quite costly to use in many settings.

The Older Americans Resources and Services (OARS) Instrument

The OARS is a comprehensive instrument designed to assess the multidimensional functional status of elderly persons in order to guide program evaluation and resource allocation. It was developed by a multidisciplinary team of individuals at the Duke University Center for the Study of Aging and Human Development and has since been used extensively in numerous settings and for many purposes, including clinical intake, evaluation, population surveys, and longitudinal studies (Duke University Center for the Study of Aging and Human Development, 1978).

In addition to basic demographic information, the 70 questions of the OARS instrument encompass the following five domains:

- *social resources,* including marital and living status, social activities, existence of a confidant, and the perceived adequacy of social resources
- *economic resources,* including employment status and income from various sources, income ownership, use of social programs, insurance coverage, and perceived adequacy of personal resources
- *mental health,* including psychic distress and organic diseases
- *physical health,* including perceived health, use of health care services, chronic conditions, use of supportive devices and prostheses, physical exercise, and use of medications
- *functional status,* including activities of daily living (ADLs) and instrumental activities of daily living (IADLs)

The responses to the questions in each of the five domains are translated into a 6-point scale (where 6 indicates total impairment and 1 indicates total independence in functioning). The scale for each domain can then be combined in a variety of ways (Kane & Kane, 1981).

The OARS instrument has most often been used as an interview guide, with trained interviewers administering the questionnaire. Reliability has been extensively studied and appears to be good (Kane & Kane, 1981). Test–retest reliability was assessed during the development of the OARS scale using data from 30 community-dwelling individuals who were administered the scale approximately five weeks apart; correlations coefficients for each domain ranged from 0.32 (mental health) to 0.82 (physical health). One reason that test–retest reliability may have been so low is that one-third of the subjects reported experiencing a major event between interviews.

The OARS instrument appears to have high validity. The items were selected by experts in the field of gerontology and measurement to represent fully the five domains. The ratings obtained closely mimic professional assessment of the individual obtained by clinicians. Finally, the instrument is able to discriminate among institutionalized and community-dwelling individuals.

Some of the disadvantages of the OARS instrument for use in a frail elderly population include the length of the survey (it can take up to 45 minutes to complete) and the expense involved in training interviewers and raters. Consequently, an attempt has been made to shorten the OARS instrument, as evidenced by Pfeiffer's Functional Assessment Inventory (Pfeiffer, Johnson, & Chiofolo,

1980, reported in Kane & Kane, 1981), which includes questions on the same domains and many of the key components of the OARS instrument.

The RAND Health Status Measures

The RAND Health Status Measures were developed by John Ware and his colleagues at the RAND Corporation as part of the Health Insurance Experiment (Brook *et al.,* 1979; Stewart, Ware, & Brook, 1981). The Health Insurance Experiment was designed to test the effects of different levels of cost sharing on health care utilization and on health status outcomes. A major focus of the experiment was the development of reliable and valid health status measures that could detect small but important changes in health status in a general community population. Measures were developed for the following aspects of health status:

- *physical health,* including self-care limitations, mobility limitations, physical functioning, role functioning, and leisure activities
- *mental health,* including anxiety, depression, positive well-being, vitality, general health, and self-control
- *social health,* including interpersonal interactions and measures of participation in four areas: family and home, social life, community involvement, and work on major role activity
- *general health perceptions,* including prior health, current health, health outlook, resistance-susceptibility, health worry and concern, and sickness orientation

Extensive reliability and validity information is available for these measures, obtained from various samples of the approximately 8000 persons aged 14 to 65 from six sites enrolled in the Health Insurance Experiment. Both internal consistency and test–retest reliability were measured and found to be quite high. For example, internal consistency for the physical health scales ranged from 0.89 to 0.98. Test–retest reliability (over a four-month period) ranged from 0.92 to 0.99 for those measures tested. Two aspects of validity were tested: content and construct validity. The development of the measures was preceded by an extensive review of the literature on health status measures, and all constructs identified in the literature were included. Construct validity was measured by examination of the associations among other health status measures (both the same dimension, different dimensions, other health status measures, and other variables such as patient satisfaction). Factor analysis was used to test the construct validity of the health status measures, comparing the relationships between the RAND measures and other measures the validity of which had been tested.

Extensive work has recently been done to improve the RAND Health Status

Measures and to make them more practical for use with an older and chronically ill population (Stewart, Hays, & Ware, 1988). New concepts were included to increase the breadth of the measures, the scales were changed to measure a wider range of differences, and some of the longer measures were shortened. The new measures cover a wide range of concepts, including:

- physical functioning
- mobility
- satisfaction with physical functioning
- depression
- anxiety
- loss of behavioral/emotional control
- physiological well-being
- loneliness
- cognitive functioning
- family functioning
- sexual functioning
- social contacts
- role functioning
- general health perceptions
- sleep
- energy/fatigue
- pain.

Tests of the reliability and validity of these new short-form measures are currently being completed, and it appears that the new measures perform as well as the initial measures from which they were derived. Internal consistency reliability was only slightly lower than for the longer scale and ranged from 0.81 to 0.88. The reliability was not substantially different in persons 75 years of age and older, those with serious chronic conditions, and those with depressive symptoms. Construct validity was tested by an examination of the correlations between these new short-form measures and other health measures. The patterns of correlations were similar to that observed with the longer measures.

The RAND Health Status Measures provide a comprehensive view of health status and quality of life, containing many aspects of quality of life that were identified as important in the literature. In addition, they are self-administered and relatively inexpensive to administer. However, there are several issues to consider for use of the RAND Health Status Measures in the frail elderly. Because the instrument is so comprehensive, it is also extremely long. Additionally, it does not provide one global measure of the quality of life; rather, a separate score is calculated for each of the measures. While this may be advantageous in program planning or assessment, it is a more complex measurement strategy than would be desired in some circumstances.

The Quality of Well-Being (QWB) Scale

The QWB scale is designed to measure the quality of life of individuals and translate that into a score that can be used to inform resource allocations across services or programs. It was developed by Kaplan and Bush and their colleagues at the University of California at San Diego as part of a General Health Policy Model (Anderson, Kaplan, Berry, Bush, & Rumbaut, 1986; Balaban, Sagi, Goldfarb, & Nettler, 1986; Kaplan & Bush, 1982). The QWB scale is based on a decision-theory approach to assessment, as opposed to a psychometric approach. The psychometric approach is that most often seen in questionnaires, where items (questions) that measure certain aspects of the concept of interest are identified and the responses directly combined into a score. The decision-theory approach is based upon the definition and quantification of *preferences* for various stages of the concept, which are often rated on a scale of 0 to 1. The score is obtained from the preference assigned to a particular level of functioning, for example. While the decision-theory approach requires that the concept be scaled on a single dimension (e.g., one cannot easily break the measure of quality of life into several components such as physical and social functioning and obtain separate scores for each), it does allow for the incorporation of a preference for mortality into the score.

The QWB score is created by assigning a preference weight to a functional level in three domains—mobility, physical activity, and social activity—and adding that to an adjustment weight that takes into account other symptoms or conditions that might affect quality of life. Possible scores range between 0 and 1.0, with 1.0 indicating the highest possible quality of life.

The functional levels, derived from information obtained from a standardized questionnaire administered by a trained interviewer, indicate a complete range of functional abilities. For example, the functional levels for the social activity domain range from "had help with self-care" to "did work, school, or housework and other activities." The preference weights assigned to these functional levels were derived from the evaluations of the relative desirability of over 400 case descriptions or well-state profiles provided to community-dwelling individuals in several studies. The authors used conjoint analysis and functional measurement based on category ratings of multidimensional stimuli to obtain the weights.

A series of potential symptoms and problems are also used to discriminate between levels of quality of life experienced by persons at similar functional levels. These include coughing; wheezing or shortness of breath; taking medication or staying on a prescribed diet for health reasons; and trouble seeing, or needing to wear glasses or contact lenses. Each of these symptoms or problems has been assigned an adjustment weight, which is derived by the same methods used to derive the preference weights for functional status levels.

Although generic preference weights are used, the authors have demonstrated that no systematic differences exist in the preference weights derived from different demographic groups or groups with differing health status (e.g., rheumatoid arthritis patients compared with the general population) (Kaplan & Anderson, 1988). The QWB scale has been used in elderly populations, and reliability and validity information are available. Using data from a general household survey and a study of patients from a regional burn treatment center, the authors found the score on the QWB scale to be highly correlated to a clinical assessment of health status when the interviewer-administered version of the instrument was used. The self-administered version did not perform as well (Anderson, Bush, & Berry, 1988). Test–retest reliability, calculated using data from a number of populations, was quite high and ranged from 0.78 to 0.99 (Anderson *et al.*, 1989).

The QWB scale is an excellent example of the potential of the decision-theory approach to assessment. Although it focuses on a very narrow definition of quality of life—health-related quality of life—it simplifies the information obtained into a simple score from 0 to 1.0. In this way, the scale allows the direct comparison of changes in quality of life resulting from different interventions that impact different aspects of quality of life. However, the simplicity of the score is also a drawback. The QWB scale is not as effective as other measures in a setting in which program planning and assessment is the focus because it does not provide domain-specific quality of life scores.

The Reintegration to Normal Living (RNL) Index

The RNL index is an 11-item instrument designed to assess the ability of persons who underwent extensive rehabilitation as a result of trauma or incapacitating illness to reintegrate into the community and continue living a normal life. It was created by Wood-Dauphinee and her colleagues at McGill University in Montreal (Wood-Dauphinee, Optzoomer, Williams, Marchand, & Spitzer, 1988).

In the development of the RNL index, the authors identified a number of concepts that related to reintegration: indoor, community, and distant mobility; self-care; daily activity; recreational and social activities; general coping skills; family roles; personal relationships; and presentation of self to others. The resulting index consists of two domains: daily functioning and perceptions of self, with items closely reflecting the concepts related to reintegration. An alternate form of the index allows for the use of wheelchairs or other equipment in completing activities. The index uses a 100-mm visual analogue scale, in which the respondent is asked to indicate what point, along a line anchored by opposing phrases, best describes his or her situation; each item is scored from 1 to 10 points, and the scores from all the items are summed and converted to a 100-point scale.

Initial efforts at testing reliability and validity are promising. Three patient samples were used to test the psychometric properties of the index: (1) patients from two acute care hospitals and one rehabilitation center ($n = 109$), (2) patients newly diagnosed with cancer or myocardial infarction ($N = 70$), and (3) 250 cancer (predominantly lung and breast) patients who were participating in a study examining whether patient profiles could be created that would predict who would do well or poorly in reintegration to normal living and in disease outcomes. The authors report high internal consistency, with an alpha score of .904. They report that the RNL index is responsive to changes in condition and that there is high agreement between scores obtained from individuals and close family members. While agreement between individuals and physicians is not as high, it is more likely due to the physicians' unfamiliarity with the individuals' true situation than to any deficiency in the instrument.

The authors report that the score is marginally related to work status and not related to family status, living arrangements, or presence of problems in living. Therefore, they feel that the index is a good measure of changes in patients' conditions rather than a measure of external factors.

While the RNL index was developed with a different population in mind, it appears promising for use with the frail elderly. It incorporates a comprehensive definition of functioning and quality of life, which include both objective functional ability and patient perceptions, although some changes in items may be required for use in a frail elderly population. It is short and simple to administer, although it requires the use of trained interviewers. More work is required to establish the reliability and validity of the RNL index before its widespread use can be recommended.

The City of Hope Medical Center Quality of Life Survey

The City of Hope Quality of Life Survey was developed by Betty Ferrel at the City of Hope Medical Center in Duarte, California, as an instrument for assessing the outcomes of care for cancer patients in terms of pain management and functioning (Ferrel et al., 1989). It measures quality of life related to the areas of psychological well-being, physical functioning, general symptom control, specific symptom control, and social support. It contains 28 items that are scored using a 100-mm visual analogue scale anchored at both ends.

The authors report limited reliability and validity statistics. One hundred fifty patients were selected; these included cancer patients (with and without pain) and a control group of persons without cancer. Internal consistency reliability was adequate for group comparisons with a Chronbach's alpha score of 0.88 overall and subscale scores ranging from 0.65 to 0.75. A panel of experts in oncology and pain management verified the content validity of the measure. The authors reported a "moderate to strong relationship" between the scores obtained from the survey and other measures of pain and functional status. The survey was sensitive enough to distinguish between patients at different levels of illness and those with and without pain.

Although it was developed for a population of cancer patients undergoing treatment, the City of Hope survey might be adapted for use with the frail elderly. It was designed as an interviewer-administered instrument; and it has the advantage of being relatively short. While many of the questions are not applicable to patients who are not undergoing treatment for cancer, the majority of the remaining questions reflect a well-balanced definition of quality of life. For example, questions ask about enjoyment of life, happiness, feeling useful, and giving and receiving sufficient affection, as well as about health worries and worries about the patient's outcome of disease and the cost of medical care. Some questions refer to energy and strength, the ability to perform instrumental activities of daily living, and whether the amount of sleep received is sufficient. The reliability and validity of the survey will need to be tested in the frail elderly in order to establish its appropriateness for use in that population.

The Perceived Quality of Life (PQOL) Scale

The PQOL scale was designed by Donald Patrick and his colleagues at the University of North Carolina at Chapel Hill to measure the quality of life of post–intensive care users (Patrick, Danis, Southerland, & Hung, 1988). Although there have been numerous studies of the cost-effectiveness of intensive care, which generally focus on outcomes such as decreased mortality and morbidity, and increases in functional status, and employment, Patrick *et al.* sought to identify other, less easily measured benefits of intensive care, such as quality of life.

The PQOL is an interviewer-administered instrument containing 11 items that ask how satisfied the respondent is with health, thinking, happiness, family, help, community, leisure, income, respect, meaning, and work. Respondents are asked to rate, on a 0–100 scale, their satisfaction with each aspect of quality of life queried. The scores for each item are averaged to provide the overall PQOL score. The scale was developed on a sample of 160 persons 55 years and older who had used intensive care in the past. The authors report limited reliability and validity information. Internal consistency reliability was adequate for group comparisons with a Chronbach's alpha coefficient of 0.88. The authors tested the construct validity of the PQOL scale and report that the scores are correlated with behavioral dysfunction as measured by the SIP and with affective status as measured by another scale, the Psychological General Well-being Schedule (Dupuy, 1984).

The PQOL is an innovative instrument for measuring quality of life. It is short, minimizing subject burden. It is comprehensive, incorporating a number of aspects of quality of life. However, much more work needs to be done to establish its validity and reliability before its use can be recommended.

The Subjective Well-Being Instrument for the Chronically Ill

The Subjective Well-Being Instrument, designed by W. Malcolm Gill at the University of Auckland in New Zealand, was intended to be used as a tool for physicians to measure the subjective well-being of their patients (Gill, 1984). The instrument attempts to measure subjective well-being, or quality of life, along the two dimensions of happiness and energy. It is unique in that it consists simply of a list of 50 adjectives (20 that refer to happiness, 20 that refer to energy, and 10 distracter adjectives). Individuals are asked whether the adjectives describe how they feel "right now." The instrument can be scored to give either a total state of well-being net (SOWBNET) score or separate scores for happiness and energy.

Reliability was tested during the development of the instrument with a sample of 100 urban Aucklanders. Immediate test–retest reliability was high, at 0.99. Construct validity was tested by comparing the score with that obtained from another measure of life satisfaction, and a high correlation was reported. The instrument was able to distinguish differences in quality of life that were identified through independent assessments by the researcher. Finally, it was able to detect clinically important differences in the course of treatment for acute leukemia of 35 patients observed over a period of 11 weeks; the instrument was sensitive to changes in quality of life resulting from courses of chemotherapy and changes in patients' clinical conditions.

Although this instrument was not designed for use with the frail elderly and has not been subjected to adequate tests of reliability or validity, it was included in this review because it is an interesting and creative method of assessing quality of life in individuals that may not otherwise be able to complete an extensive questionnaire.

Conclusion

Quality of life is becoming an increasingly important aspect of the evaluation of health and social services, especially in the frail elderly who suffer from multiple chronic conditions and who are unlikely to be cured by interventions but for whom quality of life improvements are entirely possible. The literature contains many references to quality of life. It has been defined quite broadly, often including both objective and subjective elements. Health status is universally considered to be a key element of quality of life, although many other concepts are often included, such as social contacts and resources and psychic well-being.

While various elements of quality of life have been defined, the relative importance of these elements in defining quality of life itself has not yet been determined. While health status is considered a key element and is included in many instruments, it is not clear whether the inclusion of measures of health status reflects it as the most important element or simply reflects our ability to measure health status as opposed to other components. Research is needed to determine those elements that are most important in determining quality of life. It is highly likely that the relative importance of these elements will be different for various age, sex, and cultural groups. Research should focus not only on the similarities in the determinants of quality of life but the differences as well. This will enable the development of more valid measures for various subpopulations.

The field of measurement is changing rapidly, and new measures are being developed constantly. Gerontological researchers can choose, among many available instruments, one that best suits their needs. Some important criteria in the selection of a quality of life instrument include practicality, content and scaling, aggregation, reliability, and validity. No one measure will be useful for all purposes. The researcher must consider the reason for measurement, the population of interest, and the resources available when selecting a measure.

Although the definitions of quality of life are generally broad, measures of quality of life are more narrowly defined and often focus on more objective criteria. In part, this reflects our ability to more easily measure objective concepts such as functioning and social contacts. Several measures of quality of life were reviewed in the present chapter, including the Sickness Impact Profile, the Older Americans Resources and Services Instrument, the RAND Health Status Measures, the Quality of Well-Being Scale, the Reintegration to Normal Living Index, the City of Hope Medical Center Quality of Life Survey, the Perceived Quality of Life Scale, and the Subjective Well-being Instrument. This review was not intended to be comprehensive; it included instruments that range from the complex to the simple. These measures reflect the importance of health and functioning in any measure of quality of life. All of the instruments except two incorporate measures of health; all except one include a measure of functioning. Other concepts frequently included in the instruments include social functioning, happiness, and perceived well-being.

Many measures of health status and functioning have been in use for a number of years and generally have well-demonstrated reliability and validity. Some focus on more global definitions of health and functioning, such as the SIP and the RAND Health Status Measures, included in this review. In general, quality of life measures tend to be less sophisticated and less well-developed than measures of health status and functioning. While these quality of life measures have not undergone the same rigorous development, there are several available that represent innovative methods of assessing quality of life.

Suggestions for Future Research

Currently, few measures exist that comprehensively address quality of life. Of those that do exist, few have demonstrated reliability and validity in the frail elderly. In keeping with the advances in measurement and health status assessment, future research should focus on the development of comprehensive quality of life measures that are reliable and valid as well as appropriate for use in a frail elderly population.

Although it may appear attractive to develop extensive measures that tap all important attributes of quality of life, the practical issues of use should always be kept in mind. Assessment strategies and administration methods should take into account the potential difficulties associated with the assessment of the frail elderly, such as high rates of cognitive deficit and physical impairments that may limit the number and type of items to be included. Additionally, the length of a comprehensive instrument and the high cost of collecting data are sure to pose obstacles to use.

Hundreds of health status assessment instruments have been developed in the last 20 years (Lohr & Mock, 1989), which vary in design and primary target population. However, most of these instruments were designed for and used in research and policy settings. Only recently has interest been generated in the clinical community for methods to assess the health status and health outcomes of patients. Interestingly, geriatrics has been a major user of health status assessment instruments. Researchers focusing on the health status of the elderly have been at the forefront of advances in the development of health status assessment instruments for use in clinical settings. It will be the challenge of those working with the frail elderly to expand the focus of assessment to include quality of life and to lead the field in the development of reliable and valid measures of quality of life.

References

Anderson, J. P., Bush, J. W. & Berry, C. C. (1986). Classifying function for health outcome and quality-of-life evaluation: Self-versus-interviewer modes. *Medical Care, 24,* 454–469.

Anderson, J. P., Bush, J. W., & Berry, C. C. (1988). Internal consistency analysis: A method for studying the accuracy of function assessment for health outcome and quality of life evaluation. *Journal of Clinical Epidemiology, 41,* 127–137.

Anderson, J. P., Kaplan, R. M., Berry, C. C., Bush, J. W., & Rumbaut, R. G. (1989).

Interday reliability of function assessment for a health status measure: The quality of well-being scale. *Medical Care, 27,* 1076–1084.

Balaban, D. J., Sagi, P. C., Goldfarb, N. I., & Nettler S. (1986). Weights for scoring the quality of well-being instrument among rheumatoid arthritics: A comparison to general population weights. *Medical Care, 24,* 973–980.

Bergner, M., Bobbit, R. A., Carter, W. E., & Gilson, B. S. (1981). The sickness impact profile: Development and final revision of a health status measure. *Medical Care, 19,* 787–805.

Brook, R. H., Ware, J. E., Davies-Avery, A., Stewart, A. L., Donald, C. A., Rogers, W. H., Williams, K. N., & Johnston, S. A. (1979). Overview of adult health status measures fielded in Rand's health insurance study. *Supplement to Medical Care, 17,* 21–131.

Bulpitt, C. J., & Fletcher, A. E. (1985). Quality of life in hypertensive patients on different antihypertensive treatments: Rationale for methods employed in a multicenter randomized controlled trial. *Journal of Cardiovascular Pharmacology, 7,* S137–S145.

Chronbach, L. J. (1951). Coefficient alpha and the internal structure of tests. *Psychometrica, 16,* 297–334.

Cornoni-Huntley, J. C., Evans, D. A., Foley, D. J., Suzman, R., Wallace, R. B., & White, L. R. (1985). Epidemiology of disability in the oldest old: Methodologic issues and preliminary findings. Milbank Memorial Fund Quarterly, *Health and Society, 63,* 350–376.

Duke University Center for the Study of Aging and Human Development (1978). *Multidimensional functional assessment: The oars methodology.* Durham, N.C.

Ferrell, B. R., Wisdom, C., & Wenzl, C. (1989). Quality of life as an outcome variable in the management of cancer pain. *Cancer, 63,* 2321–2327.

Flanagan, J. C. (1982). Measurement of Quality of Life: Current State of the Art. *Archives of Physical Medicine and Rehabilitation, 63,* 56–59.

George, L. K., & Bearon, L. B. (1980). *Quality of life in older persons: Meaning and measurement.* Durham, N.C.: Duke University Medical Center, Human Sciences Press.

Gill, W. M. (1984). Subjective well-being: Properties of an instrument for measuring this (in the chronically ill). *Social Science Medicare, 18,* 683–691.

Kane, R. A., & Kane, R. L. (1981). *Assessing the elderly: A practical guide to measurement.* Lexington, Mass.: DC Heath and Co.

Kaplan, R. M. (n.d.). *Quality-of-life measurement.* Washington, D.C.: National Heart, Lung and Blood Institute of the National Institutes of Health.

Kaplan, R. M., & Anderson, J. P. (1988). A general health policy model: Update and applications. *Health Services Research, 23,* 203–205.

Kaplan, R. M., & Bush, J. W. (1982). Health-related quality of life measurement for evaluation research and policy analysis. *Health Psychology, 1,* 61–80.

Lohr, K. N., & Mock, G. A. (1989). *Advances in the assessment of health status.* Washington, D.C.: Council on Health Care Technology, Institute of Medicine, National Academy of Sciences.

Maddox, G., & Douglass, E. B. (1973). Self-assessments of health. *Journal of Health and Social Behavior, 14,* 87–93.

Patrick, D. L., Danis, M., Southerland, L. I., & Hong, G. (1988). Quality of life following intensive care. *Journal of General Internal Medicine, 3,* 218–223.

Pearlman, R. A., & Uhlmann, R. F. (1988). Quality of life in chronic diseases: Perceptions of elderly patients. *Journal of Gerontology: Medical Sciences, 43,* M25–M30.

Pfeiffer, E., Johnson, T. M., & Chiofolo, R. C. (1980). *Functional assessment of elderly subjects in four service settings.* Paper presented at the annual scientific meeting, Gerontological Society of America, November, San Diego, Calif.

Soldo, B. J., & Manton, K. G. (1985). Health status and service needs of the oldest old: Current patterns and future trends. Milbank Memorial Fund Quarterly, *Health and Society, 63,* 286–319.

Stewart, A. L., Hays, R. D., & Ware, J. E. (1988). The MDS short-form general health survey. *Medical Care.* 724–735.

Stewart, A. L., Ware, J. E., & Brook, R. H. (1981). Advances in the measurement of functional status: Construction of aggregate indexes. *Medical Care, 19,* 473–487.

Ware, J. E. (1984). Methodological Considerations in the Selection of Health Status Assessment Procedures. In N. K. Wenger, M. E. Mattson, C. D. Furberg, & J. Elinson (eds.). pp. 87–111. Assessment of Quality of Life in Clinical Trials of Cardiovascular Therapies. Le Jacq Publishing Inc., New York.

Ware, J. E., Brook, R. H., Davies, A. R., & Lohr, K. N. (1981). Choosing measures of health status for individuals in general populations. *American Journal of Public Health, 71,* 620–625.

Wood-Dauphinee, S. L., Optzoomer, M. A., Williams, J. J., Marchand, B., & Spitzer, W. O. (1988). Assessment of global function: The reintegration to normal living index. *Archives of Medicine and Rehabilitation, 69,* 583–590.

4

A Review of the Literature on Interventions and Quality of Life in the Frail Elderly

KATHLEEN M. GENTILE

Recent developments have compelled the medical community to acknowledge the existence of social dimensions in the domain of the practice of medicine (Levine, 1987). Quality of life has emerged as a basic criterion in evaluating the effectiveness of health and medical interventions in the treatment of illness and disability of the elderly population. Why has quality of life emerged as a major concern at this time?

Some chronic diseases—such as heart disease, hypertension, stroke, diabetes, and arthritis—cannot be cured as yet, but the pain associated with them can be relieved and social functioning improved. Maintenance of quality of life has forever been the desired outcome of medical interventions. Technological advances in transplant surgery, heart bypass, artificial organs, and various other ways of prolonging the life of a dying patient have raised questions of application and limitation. Expenditure of personal assets for life-prolonging technology on patients who have lost interactive capacities raises questions of cost-containment and quality of life. There has also been a social movement critical of the health care system, and demands have been made to humanize health care. This convergence of medicine and social dimensions redirects our attention to a new concept of quality of life (Levine, 1987).

The frail elderly are exposed to life situations and circumstances that are likely to reduce independence and increase the need for assistance. With the 65 and older population expected to reach over 35 million people, or 13% of the total population, by the year 2000 (up from 29 million, or 12%, in 1985), the demand for health care and social services will increase proportionally. It is projected that by the year 2020 the 65 and older population will constitute 17% of the total population, or 51 million persons. Within that cohort group, the 85 and older population is expected to increase at a rate double that of the elderly population

Copyright © 1991 by Academic Press, Inc.
All rights of reproduction in any form reserved.

as a whole. Consequently, it is projected that in 2020 there will be at least 7 million persons at least 85 years old, compared with 3 million in 1985. The health care and social service needs of this potentially frail elderly population will stretch the limits of the health care and social service delivery systems.

The resulting negative effects of increased demand for services by the burgeoning population due to the increasing incidence of chronic disability and acute illness can be considered a threat to the quality of life of such individuals (Teitelman & Priddy, 1988). These situations can range from medical to psychological to environmental, in any direction or combination. To reduce the negative consequences of a diminished quality of life, gerontologists have developed appropriate and specific therapeutic interventions that have been successful in reducing these effects, thus improving quality of life for the frail elderly (Teitelman & Priddy, 1988).

The purpose of the present chapter is to review relevant literature on the quality of life of the frail elderly, with particular attention to the types of nonmedical interventions or modifications that may affect the interest or well-being of the individual and, ultimately, his or her quality of life. An effort is made to develop a definition of quality of life integrating psychological, social, spiritual, and environmental dimensions. There will be some discussion of interventions that attempt to bring about improvement in or maintenance of an individual's quality of life. Recommendations for future study of relevant topics and issues related to quality of life in the frail elderly conclude this chapter.

Definitions

For the purposes of this paper, *intervention* refers to a planned manipulation designed to improve the status of the individual or a planned modification to improve the physical environment that, ultimately, will improve the quality of life for the frail elderly. Examples of the diversity of approaches that may be classified as interventions but which are characteristically labeled as activities of specific professional groups or agencies include, for example, adult day care, mental health counseling, housekeeping assistance, assistance in the performance of activities of daily living (ADLs), pain control, physical therapy, conservatorship or guardianship, and assistance in the performance of instrumental activities of daily living (IADLs). Health or social service interventions prevent, minimize, or manage chronic functional disabilities, affording the impaired person the capability of living as full a life as possible.

Reference to the "frail" elderly population includes that portion of the elderly population who suffer from diminished abilities or limitations brought on by injury, chronic physical or mental illness, or acute illness. In addition to those individuals who have limitations of function due to physiological causes, there are those who have limitations arising from social or cultural background and "emotional" trauma due to culturally derived differences and special status, such as widowhood, which might hinder their capacity for unassisted functioning. It is noted in the review of the literature that there are many attempts at modifying the environment with desired outcomes to improve the quality of life of the elderly, but references to these attempts are not found in routine searches of "quality of life" or "intervention" literature, making the identification of relevant studies a difficult task and results somewhat incomplete. It is expected that the terminology will become more specific in the future as quality of life becomes defined as a larger focal point of research and systematic attempts are made to modify it.

Defining Quality of Life

Defining "quality of life" has long been an issue of the humanities, religion, philosophy, sociology, and medical science. Historically, definitions of quality of life have been derived from outcomes of measurements of the structure or process of a medical intervention as opposed to a social functioning model. Consequently, there have been as many definitions and interpretations of quality of life as there have been humanitarians, theologians, philosophers, sociologists, and physicians. The values, ethics, and essence of human life are not easily stated in definable terms or measured by validated instruments; this complicates the measurement, research, and definition-formation processes.

Acknowledging that for some readers there might be some question concerning a relationship or distinction between quality of life and quality of care, this might be the appropriate place to discuss quality of care and clarify its relationship to quality of life. "Quality of care" represents the performance of specific activities in a manner that either increases or at least prevents the deterioration in health status that would have occurred as a function of a disease or condition (Brook & Kosecoff, 1988).

Wyszewianski (1988a) refers to quality of care as the actual determination of whether care is good or bad, appropriate or inappropriate, and well executed or poorly executed (Lohr, Yordy, & Thier, 1988; Siu, 1987). Wyszewianski (1988b) also emphasizes that the structure, process, and outcome of health care resources are elements in a chain bound by causal connections.

Kane and Kane (1988) point out that quality assurance activities in long-term care, due to its very nature, should focus on outcomes, using process measures only when they are related to desirable outcomes. In attempting to unify the literature on quality of care, Donabedian (1988) proposes that quality is proportionate to the attainment of achievable improvements in health. Quality of care assessments essentially provide knowledge of the efficacy of medical interventions, which is only one aspect of quality of life.

Zinam (1989) and Sirgy (1986) studied quality of life in technological and economic development perspectives based on Abraham Maslow's (1954) hierarchy of human needs. Zinam (1989) presented six basic areas of development with corresponding parts of quality of life: (1) ecological—dealing with the safety of our natural environment; (2) military—concerned with peace and security; (3) economic—stressing human material well-being; (4) social—based on social harmony and justice; (5) political—dealing with freedom, human rights, and dignity; and (6) cultural—based on the preservation and fostering of the development of cultural values. If the relationship between any two of these areas is one of substitution or competitiveness, a scheme of trade-offs can be developed. If the components are complementary, no trade-offs are possible.

One element of a societal model of aging proposed by philosopher and gerontologist Harry R. Moody advances the notion that the elderly population has the possibility to live with dignity, determine their own existence, and remain socially integrated, thus enabling them to live their lives in the mainstream of society. The potential and opportunity for growth, development, and continuing engagement are pursued through involvement in community events. Thus, the elderly population is viewed as being capable of making meaningful contributions to society (Hofland, 1989).

Levine (1987) suggests that a contemporary sociological perspective views health care issues as social decisions made by people playing social roles, guided by social values, and located in particular social settings. Until recently, the medical school curriculum, the culture of medicine, and the social organization of health have not allowed this sociological message to be effectively advanced within the medical community (Levine, 1987). Medicine is learning to deal with criticism of the biomedical model and to accept the emergence of quality of life as a major criterion to evaluate health interventions. The concept of quality of life then goes beyond the dimension of health functioning to performance of social roles, mental acuity, emotional states, subjective well-being, and interrelationships (Bergner, 1984; Dupuy, 1984; Haug & Folmar, 1986; Levine, 1987).

McDowell and Newell (1987) define quality of life in terms of both the adequacy of material circumstances and people's feelings about these circumstances. This definition of quality of life distinguishes it from related themes such as life satisfaction, morale, happiness, or anomie, which differ somewhat in their degree of subjectivity. Life satisfaction generally refers to a personal assessment of one's condition, compared to an external reference standard, or to one's aspirations. Morale refers to a person's mental orientation, such as enthusiasm, confidence, sadness, or depression. Happiness generally refers to shorter-term transient feelings of well-being in response to day-to-day events (McDowell & Newell, 1987). Teitelman and Priddy (1988) assert that life satisfaction, self-esteem, and physical health are all key dimensions of quality of life (George & Bearon, 1980).

Changing social circumstances tend to bring changes in the definition of these concepts. For example, there has been an evolution in definitions of quality of life, from viewing it in material terms of income, possessions, and outward symbols of career success toward emphasizing psychological rewards such as satisfaction, personal development, and participation in the community. A person's feelings about his or her circumstances usually take precedence over wealth or environment. The idea that a person's perceived needs rise in proportion to improved material conditions is shown in empirical studies where there is a strong association between objective and subjective indicators of quality of life (McDowell & Newell, 1987). Application of this idea to social programming raises an interesting dilemma. Should social programs be planned on the basis of external indicators, or on the basis of people's subjective responses?

Haug and Folmer (1986) defines quality of life as indicative of general well-being. Among the indicators of a good quality of life are health, sufficient funds, absence of psychological distress, and availability of supportive family and friends. For the elderly, the level of functional ability, both physical and cognitive, should also be taken into account.

Similar concepts are considered in the Institute of Medicine (IOM) (1986) report on the quality of care in nursing homes. This report, which considers quality of care as one aspect of quality of life, posits that an institutionalized person's sense of well-being, level of satisfaction with life, and feeling of self-worth and self-esteem determine quality of life. This includes a sense of satisfaction with oneself, the environment, the care received, the accomplishment of desired goals, and degree of control over one's life.

For example, a resident's quality of life is enhanced by close relationships and interchange and communication with others, including staff, physicians, other residents, family, and friends; by an environment supporting independence and incorporating personal belongings, such as easily accessible public areas, well-designed directional insignia, and personal possessions and furnishings in bedrooms; and by the opportunity to exercise reasonable control over life decisions, such as selection of dining hours, when to see visitors, and inclusion in formulating social activities and times to rise and retire (for contrary indications, see Cohn and Sugar, Chapter 2).

Opportunities for choice are limited somewhat in an institutionalized environment, but not to the extent historically assumed (IOM, 1986; Rodin, 1989). Participation in care planning is one aspect of personal autonomy. An enhanced sense of personal control leads to an increased sense of well-being, as found by Smith et al. (1988). Opportunities to engage in religious, political, recreational (Russell, 1990), or other social activities fosters a sense of worth for the frail elderly person.

Lack of privacy for visits with family or friends, for whatever reason, contributes to lack of self-esteem. Also, the quality and variety of food are often said to be among the most important attributes of quality from the resident's perspective (IOM, 1986).

Essentially then, quality of life in an institutional setting, whether referred to as a nursing home or a long-term care facility, is different from quality of care (Doherty, 1989). Whereas quality of care is measured by the cleanliness of the environment, compliance with regulations, and the type of nursing and medical care provided, quality of life focuses on the attitudinal and affective atmosphere of the facility in addition to quality of care as one component. Behaviors, attitudes, and the atmosphere of a long-term care facility can be enhanced to create a homelike environment for residents.

One approach to the concept of quality of life for residents of an institution has been taken by the Western Gerontological Society (WGS) (Doherty, 1989). The long-term care section of the WGS recognized the need for a nontraditional approach to promotion of a quality of life philosophy by institutional management. In an effort to change the focus of the quality of life outcome of care, an emerging social model to enhance a quality of life philosophy was developed, including guidelines that identify ways in which a long-term care facility can enhance quality of life for the residents through staffing and programming.

The social model focus in predicting the quality of life outcome is on the whole person: assessing relationships between physical, social, cultural, psychological, and environmental aspects. The traditional medical model focuses on disease/illness/diagnosis, thereby treating the disease rather than the person; health and illness are viewed as discrete and separate entities, where control lies with the health care providers since decisions regarding care are made by health care professionals. In the new social model, control lies with the competent individual or responsible party; the health care professional is seen as a therapeutic partner. There is a low level of standardization, and resident rights are strongly emphasized. This model essentially supports the convictions of personal control, opportunities for choice, and independence. The traditional primary intervention of medication and surgery is replaced by alternative appropriate interventions, including psychological, spiritual, social, behavioral, or environmental methods.

Derived from this perspective, quality of life outcomes are determined by the sensitivity to the individuality of each resident, which includes promoting respect and dignity, nurturing resident empowerment, enhancing emotional and mental well-being, maximizing independence and comfort to the resident, and providing a homelike atmosphere as well as a caring and well-trained staff who like working with residents and who want to help them live as comfortably as possible (Doherty, 1989).

As was mentioned earlier, quality of life is an important consideration in medical decisions involving elderly patients using the traditional medical model. Quality of life in elderly outpatients suffering from chronic disease was determined to be a multidimensional construct involving not only health but, more importantly, such nonmedical factors as relationships and finance, environmental factors, and psychological and socioeconomic factors. In a study by Pearlman and Uhlmann (1988a), elderly patients with chronic disease considered their quality of life to be good enough that they had no major complaints. In contrast, the physicians rated their patients' quality of life as being significantly worse. This lack of understanding by physicians of their patients' perceptions has previously been seen (Pearlman & Uhlmann, 1988a). Patients in this study emphasized medical care, health-related problems, and interpersonal relationships as factors affecting quality of life.

These results are consistent with a previous survey in which 70-year-old Americans identified critical incidents that influence quality of life (Flanagan, 1982). Financial concerns, psychological distress (depression and anxiety), and relationships also were significantly correlated with patient quality of life. Pearlman and Uhlmann (1988a) characterized patient quality of life as a multidimensional construct that is more complex than a model based simply on health and functional disability.

We must remember, however, that the differences found by Pearlman and Uhlmann (1988a) might be due to different responsibilities of medical staff and patients. When physicians attend to improvement of physical health and functioning it allows a patient the ability and opportunity to fulfill personal needs. Further research is needed that addresses the discrepancy between physician and patient opinions of health status and quality of life.

Quality of life definitions differ according to perspectives, but within each definition lies a thread of commonality. Themes of privacy, control and independence emerge as detractors from the traditional medical model of quality of life. It is apparent from the literature reviewed here that contemporary thoughts on quality of life for the frail elderly lean toward a more holistic, socially integrated definition, acknowledging the role of psychological, spiritual, social-behavioral, and environmental interventions in the maintenance or enhancement of quality of life for the frail elderly but not eliminating the role of health functioning or status as an essential dimension in measuring quality of life.

Measurement

Measurement of quality of life outcomes is problematic, as presented by Arnold (Chapter 3); however, it is necessary in evaluating the effectiveness of any selected interventions or in determining population needs. The specificity of desired outcomes dictates the type of measure selected. As Arnold suggests, when comparing the effects of different interventions on the quality of life, an aggregated measure of quality of life may be necessary. Considerations of instrument length, methods of administration, content and scaling, and reliability of the measure influence selection of the appropriate measurement instrument.

Currently, measures of quality of life frequently utilize objective criteria with respondents such as staff, physicians, or family caregivers, rather than subjective criteria sampling populations of frail patients. These differing criteria offer predictably different outcomes and, consequently, different standards of quality of life.

Interventions

Interventions may be implemented at the institutional level in long-term care facilities or acute care centers, and also in community- or home-based settings. The essential health care and social service interventions can be similar, but the settings where the service is performed can differ. This section describes the multiplicity of interventions that, when implemented, can positively affect the quality of life for the frail elderly. The dimensions of interventions range from sociological to psychological to spiritual and environmental.

Emerging from the concepts of life satisfaction and well-being are the interventions that support or rehabilitate psychological dysfunction or forms of mental health, for example, cognitive impairment, dependence, powerlessness, or helplessness (Teitelman & Priddy, 1988). Dependence, for example, is the need for personal intervention by another in order to sustain life and maintain living arrangements. Dependence may arise for reasons of physical ill health or frailty but can also apply to the frail elderly with mental health dysfunctions. Of the mental disorders, senile dementia of the Alzheimer's type is the most common cause of dependence in old age.

It is important to assess a person's capacity to live independently, to determine the level of care needed and thus the degree of intervention that is necessary to sustain independence. The degree of dependence will influence services required by the patient and, thus, the cost of home or institutional care. The degree of dependence is also an indicator of the severity of the mental disorder and appropriate treatment regimens implemented (Gurland, 1977).

The prime assessment instruments to determine dependence (or in the more positive language, the determination of independence) are the Index of Independence in Activities of Daily Living and the Instrumental Activities of Daily Living Scale (Gurland, 1977, 685). The ADL index assesses performance in bathing, dressing, toileting, transfer, continence, and feeding. The IADL scale assesses ability to telephone, shop, prepare food, keep house, do laundry, use transportation, manage medication, and handle finances. There are some modified versions of these instruments that have been used to measure dependence, but no advantage has been shown over the original versions (Gurland, 1977).

For the purposes of planning and monitoring the delivery of supportive services (interventions) to the dependent elderly, it is useful to assess dependence not only using the ADL–IADL measures but also in terms of the amount and types of services required (Gurland, 1977). Traditional social service interventions, including meal delivery, housekeeping chores, transportation, adult day care, senior centers, companion visits, and more, have served the frail elderly extensively over the past two decades. Interventions of this type have allowed the frail elderly to retain some form of independence and to remain in familiar environments while adjusting to the changes dictated by chronic disabilities or rehabilitation from acute illness or surgery.

Family support systems play an important role in designing and implementing a care program for the frail elderly. Supportive family members or friends performing services for the frail individual have the potential of postponing or eliminating the need for institutionalization.

Other research findings reach similar conclusions, effectively arguing that interventions, the objectives of which include enhancement of quality of life, control enhancement, and increased autonomy, generally are successful (Collopy, 1988; Hofland, 1988). Using research findings to improve the quality of life for residents in a long-term care institution, Wells and Singer (1988) established committees of residents, staff, and families to develop and implement procedures to improve the quality of life. The staff and residents completed a questionnaire to evaluate the social climate of their institution as it was at the time and as they would have liked it to be. Social climate was measured along three dimensions: interpersonal relationships, personal growth and development, and organizational factors. Results indicated that residents wanted more responsibility and self-direction and improved physical comfort, including privacy and sensory satisfaction. They valued opportunities to express feelings and concerns, to have influence within the institution, and to be not unduly restricted by regulations. Staff also gave priority to independence and physical comfort for the residents.

These results were used as a catalyst for organizational discussions; as purposeful connections with residents, staff, and families; and as a focus point for forming committees. Committees focused on the areas that the social climate scale had indicated were most important. Committees included separate staff, resident, and family committees and a joint resident and staff committee. Issues of control, the environment, right to privacy, liaison between family and home, and communication were handled by the committees. The nonadversarial approach to this model, its recognition of the needs and rights of residents, line staff, management, and families, and its systematic attention to problem solving and conflict resolution provided a means for a progressive institution to translate its values and mission into action (Wells & Singer, 1988). This was a unique approach to the problem of quality of life within the institutional setting.

An intervention that has been shown to improve the overall well-being of elderly persons is the process of life review. The concept of life review as a universal adaptive process naturally occurring in old age was identified almost 25 years ago by Robert N. Butler. Butler (1974) saw the life review process as a means to successful reintegration, which provided new significance and meaning to an individual's life. Clinical case studies, reminiscing groups, auto-biographical experiences, life histories, and multiple other forms of reminiscing have all been included in the rubric of life review.

Some researchers, who have studied life review empiricially, have found it lacking as an adaptive procedure; failure to distinguish life review from its many other forms has diminished the value of life review as a beneficial process for the frail elderly population (Haight, 1988). Others have stated that the nature of the integrative process of life review needed to be defined in order to articulate more fully its intrapersonal and interpersonal dimensions, while others believe that the concept of reminiscence and its relationship to other affective processes must be clearly delineated (Haight, 1988).

Haight (1988) set out to prove that elderly people who participate in a struc-tured process of life review will improve in overall well-being as compared with those elderly people who participate in a friendly visit or the testing process only. Well-being was defined and operationalized through life satisfaction, psychologi-cal well-being, depression, and activities of daily living variables. Life satisfac-tion and psychological well-being were the only two dependent variables affected significantly by the life review process in this sample population. A look at the life review process as a therapeutic intervention potentially holds value for the frail elderly population. Although the results of Haight's (1988) study can only be generalized to similar populations of homebound elderly subjects, the use of structured life review as a therapeutic intervention holds promise for improving the quality of life for the frail elderly (Birren & Deutchman, in press).

Another area for beneficial intervention was studied by Linn and Linn (1981), who found that of 120 terminally ill cancer patients who received counseling for up to 12 months after diagnosis, counseled patients changed significantly in comparison to controls in a favorable direction by 3 months. The patients were studied on quality of life variables (alienation, depression, locus of control, life satisfaction, and self-esteem) as well as functional status and survival. Compared by age, those 60 and over were more disabled and were less satisfied with life. With counseling intervention, over time there was some improvement in patients over 60, but not to the extent seen in patients under 60 years of age. Although the authors were somewhat disheartened by this study, expansion of these kinds of counseling services for the recovering or terminally ill patient does hold some promise for positive intervention.

The subject of religion and its impact on the older person has not been examined extensively in the literature. In studies in which the correlates of life satisfaction and well-being have been examined, attention has been placed on factors such as social support, socioeconomic status, and health. In over 30 years of research on subjective well-being of older Americans, Larson (1978) found no mention of the possible impact of religion on well-being.

Religious factors were found to be significantly related to morale, independent of the effects of health, social support, and financial status (Koenig, Kvale, & Ferrel, 1988). Despite a slight decline with age in performance of religious activities and in attitudes for the sample as a whole, respondents age 75 and over who were actively involved in religious behaviors or intrinsically committed to a spiritual belief system were significantly more likely than the less religious to achieve high morale scores. Studies in which the relationship between religion and well-being in late life has been examined, especially those comparing the young and the old-old, are scarce. Several have shown positive correlations between adjustment and religious attitudes or beliefs, and similar associations have been found with religious behaviors, such as church attendance (Koenig *et al.*, 1988).

Blazer and Palmore (1976), studying a cohort of older persons over an 18-year span in the Duke Longitudinal Study of Aging, reported that as persons aged, correlations between religious attitudes and behaviors and personal adjustment increased in strength, which suggests that religion may have a particularly important impact on adjustment of persons who survive in their 70s and 80s. Why are these associations so strong? Religion may have been more fully integrated into the lives of the cohort age 75 and over at a time when its impact on culture and society was greater than it is today. One explanation for this is that the cohort group is described as a "generation of immigrants whose lives were rooted in the ethnic community and ethnic institutions" (Koenig *et al.*, 1988). Another explanation for the association between religion and the older cohorts is that, as people grow older, their personal resources become less abundant. Self-perceived control over situations and life in general may decline. If it is assumed that religious resources are relatively less influenced by aging factors or personal control, then the older religious person may have a more durable source of support and comfort, which may facilitate adaptation to life changes (Koenig *et al.*, 1988).

While data are often collected as to affiliation with a religious denomination (Koenig *et al.*, 1988), detailed information on levels of involvement in the religious community is not widely gathered. It is also important to remember that collecting data on religious involvements and affiliations does not reflect the intrinsic religiosity or spirituality of an individual. Attending religious services or affiliation with a denomination does not directly translate to a spirituality that acts as a psychological support mechanism for an elderly person.

In addition to the psychological, sociological, and spiritual interventions that assist the frail elderly person in maintaining a normal life-style, interventions within the physical environment have the intended effect of allowing the individual to maintain a functional independence. No matter where an elderly lives—at home, in an extended-care facility, or temporarily in an acute care hospital—the physical environment should maximize the person's independence, choices, opportunities for social interaction, privacy, safety, and security (Tilson, 1989).

There are several factors that must be considered in the interaction between the individual and the environment, including: (1) reduced physical activity and autonomic nervous system dysfunction; (2) the "senile gait" and other mobility problems and barriers to accessibility; (3) visual impairment and legibility factors within buildings; (4) cognitive disorders and orientation to spaces regarding their color and predictability; and (5) increased physical vulnerability and the need for a building secure enough to keep out intruders or uninvited visitors (Pastalan & Paulson, 1986). Design of an environment appropriate for the frail elderly goes beyond the physical dimensions of walls, ceilings, and rooms (see Pynoos and Regnier, Chapter 5). It relates to the qualities of privacy, autonomy, sense of place, and environmental mastery. In the institutional setting, provision of opportunities for expression of these aspects is the responsibility of the administration and staff; in the home setting, it is the responsibility of the family members, case manager, and/or social worker responsible for the management of care.

Interventions that contribute to an improvement or enhancement of quality of life for the frail elderly can be classified into four types (Okun, 1990): (1) control-enhancing interventions, which focus on increasing the older person's sense of personal control over his or her environment; (2) social activity interventions, which focus on providing opportunities for social interaction; (3) psychoeducational interventions, which provide structured opportunities for specific subpopulations of older adults to increase their knowledge and skills; and (4) a "potpourri" of miscellaneous treatments providing a variety of social interactive and environment-enhancing opportunities.

Recommendations

Consensus on a definition of quality of life precedes any coordinated effort to systematically define and classify interventions that will affect quality of life. If we can reliably conclude from research that a particular intervention results in an improvement in quality of life for the frail elderly, replication of that intervention would indicate an improvement in quality of life.

Practical issues that need to be addressed at a future time include the importance of communication skills in the matrix of quality of life determinants. The manner of communication with the frail elderly becomes an important factor in their perception of control and autonomy, and thus quality of life. The mode of communication is important for the staff member, who must remember that affective toning, condescension, level of information, and recognition of language dissimilarities and cultural barriers affect the behavior, emotion, and comfort of the elderly person.

Communication with the nonverbal or dementing patient offers special challenges for those who need to obtain information. Agitation, aggressive behavior, and shouting typify the symbolic or nonverbal communicative skills that are open for interpretation.

Problems of determining appropriate treatment programs or appropriate intervention regimens sometimes occur because of cultural or ethnic differences. Culturally symbolic meanings of appearance, language, dress, food, order, or overt behavior affect assessment, intervention, and evaluation.

Further research and exploration is needed in psychological, sociological, spiritual, and environmental interventions as factors in quality of life measures. Many of the relevant research topics are studied by the other authors in this volume and should be referred to for specific background and current findings. Suggested topics for consideration should include, among others, aspects of supportive social networks; design of physical environments in institutions; utilization of the elderly in designing appropriate physical environments; effects of federal health benefit policy on the health care and socialization of the institutionalized elderly; and adequacy of quality of life measurements within diverse ethnic and cultural groups.

If the goal of interventions is to enable the frail elderly to live as independently as possible, whether institutionalized or cared for in the home, realizing their full potential and growth and maintaining a personally acceptable quality of life, researchers need to construct measures the outcomes of which accurately predict quality of life for the frail elderly.

References

Bergner, M. (1984). The sickness impact profile. In N. K. Wenger, M. E. Mattson, C. D. Furberg, & J. Elinson, eds., *Assessment of quality of life in cardiovascular therapies.* New York: LeJacq.

Birren, J. E., & Deutchman, D. E. (in press). *Guiding autobiography groups for older adults: Exploring the fabric of life.* Baltimore, Md.: Johns Hopkins University Press.

Blazer, D., & Palmore, E. (1976). Religion and aging in a longitudinal panel. *The Gerontologist, 16,* 82–85.

Brook, R., & Kosecoff, J. B. (1988). Competition and quality. *Health Affairs, 7,* 150–151.

Butler, R. N. (1974). Successful aging and the role of the life review. *Journal of the American Geriatrics Society, 22,* 529–535.

Collopy, B. J. (1988). Autonomy in long term care: Some crucial distinctions. *The Gerontologist, 28* (Suppl.), 10–17.

Doherty, E., ed. (1989). *New images: Quality of life in a long term care facility.* Denver: Colorado Gerontological Society.

Donabedian, A. (1988). Quality assessment and assurance: Unity of purpose, diversity of means. *Inquiry, 25,* 173–192.

Dupuy, H. J. (1984). The Psychological Well-being (PGWB) Index. In N. K. Wenger, M. E. Mattson, C. D. Furberg, & J. Elinson, eds., *Assessment of quality of life in cardiovascular therapies,* pp. 170–88. New York: LeJacq.

Flanagan, J. C. (1982). Measurement of quality of life: Current state of the art. *Archives of Physical and Medical Rehabilitation, 63,* 56–59.

George, L. K. & Bearon, L. B. (1980). *Quality of life in older persons: Meaning and measurement.* New York: Human Sciences Press.

Gurland, B. J. (1977). The assessment of the mental health status of older adults. In J. E. Birren & K. W. Schaie, eds., *Handbook of the psychology of aging*. New York: Van Nostrand Reinhold.

Haight, B. K. (1988). The therapeutic role of a structured life review process in home-bound elderly subjects. *Journal of Gerontology, 43,* P40–P44.

Haug, M. R., & Folmar, S. J. (1986). Longevity, gender, and life quality. *Journal of Health and Social Behavior, 27,* 332–345.

Hofland, B. F. (1988). Autonomy in long term care: Background issues and a programmatic response. *The Gerontologist, 28* (Suppl.), 3–9.

Hofland, B. F. (1989). Value and ethical issues in residential environments for the elderly. In D. Tilson, ed., *Aging in place: Supporting the frail elderly in residential environments*. Glenview, Ill.: Scott, Foresman Professional Books on Aging.

Institute of Medicine (1986). *Improving the quality of care in nursing homes*. Washington, D.C.: National Academy Press.

Kane, R. A., & Kane. R. L. (1988). Long-term care: Variations on a quality assurance theme. *Inquiry, 25,* 132–146.

Koenig, H. G., Kvale, J. N., & Ferrel, C. (1988). Religion and well-being in later life. *The Gerontologist, 28,* 18–28.

Larson, R. (1978). Thirty years of research on the subjective well-being of older Americans. *Journal of Gerontology, 33,* 109–125.

Levine, S. (1987) The changing terrains in medical sociology: Emergent concern with quality of life. *Journal of Health and Social Behavior, 28,* 1–6.

Linn, B. S., & Linn, M. W. (1981). Late stage cancer patients: Age differences in their psychophysical status and response to counseling. *Journal of Gerontology, 36,* 689–692.

Lohr, K. N., Yordy, K. D., & Thier, S. O. (1988). Current issues in quality of care. *Health Affairs, 7,* 6–18.

Maslow, A. (1954). *Motivation and personality*. New York: Harper and Row.

McDowell, I., & Newell, C. (1987). *Measuring health: Guide to rating scales and questionnaires*. New York: Oxford University Press.

Okun, M. A., Olding, R. W., & Cohn, C. M. G. (1990). A meta-analysis of subjective well-being interventions among elders. *Psychological Bulletin, 108,* 257–266.

Pastalan, L. A., & Paulson, L. G. (1986). Importance of the physical environment for older people. *Journal of the American Geriatrics Society, 33,* 874.

Pearlman, R. A., & Uhlmann, R. F. (1988a). Quality of life in chronic disease: Perceptions of elderly patients. *Journal of Gerontology, 43,* M25–M30.

Pearlman, R. A., & Uhlmann, R. F. (1988b). Quality of life in the elderly: Comparisons between nursing home and community residents. *Journal of Applied Gerontology, 7,* 316–330.

Rodin, J. (1989). Sense of control: Potentials for intervention. *Annals of the American Academy of Political and Social Science, 503,* 29–42.

Rowe, J. W., & Kahn, R. L. (1987). Human aging: Usual and successful. *Science, 237,* 143–149.

Russell, R. V. (1990). Recreation and quality of life in old age: A causal analysis. *Journal of Applied Gerontology, 9,* 77–89.

Sirgy, J. J. (1986). A quality-of-life theory derived from Maslow's Developmental Perspective: 'Quality' is related to progressive satisfaction of a hierarchy of needs, lower order and higher. *American Journal of Economics and Sociology, 45,* 329–341.

Siu, A. L. (1987). The quality of medical care received by older persons. *Journal of the American Geriatrics Society, 35,* 1084–1091.

Smith, R. A., Woodward, N. J., Wallston, B. S., Wallston, K. A., Rye, P., & Zylstra, M. (1988). Health care implications of desire and expectancy for control in elderly adults. *Journal of Gerontology, 431,* P1–P7.

Teitelman, J., & Priddy, J. M. (1988). From psychological theory to practice: Improving frail elders' quality of life through control-enhancing interventions. *Journal of Applied Gerontology, 7,* 298–315.

Tilson, D., ed. (1989). *Aging in place: Supporting the frail elderly in residential environments.* Glenview, Ill.: Scott, Foresman Professional Books on Aging.

Wells, L. M., & Singer, C. (1988). Quality of life in institutions for the elderly: Maximizing well-being. *The Gerontologist, 28,* 266–269.

Wyszewianski, L. (1988a). Quality of care: Past achievements and future challenges. *Inquiry, 25,* 13–22.

Wyszewianski, L. (1988b). The emphasis on measurement in quality assurance: Reasons and implications. *Inquiry, 25,* 424–436.

Zinam, O. (1989). Quality of life, quality of the individual, technology and economic development. *American Journal of Economics and Sociology, 48,* 55–68.

II

The Physical World and Quality of Life in the Frail Elderly

5

Improving Residential Environments for Frail Elderly: Bridging the Gap between Theory and Application

JON PYNOOS
VICTOR REGNIER

We shape our dwellings and afterwards our dwellings shape us.
—WINSTON CHURCHILL

Introduction

Housing for the elderly is one of the most important yet unappreciated issues confronting our society. Housing for all age groups bears significantly on the quality of life. It affects physical health, status, friendship formations, and access to neighborhood services. Older persons place special importance on housing because they are likely to spend more time in it, have more difficulty taking care of it, and have stronger psychological attachments to it (having lived in the same place for many years) than their younger counterparts. If there is a poor fit between the capabilities of older persons who have become frail and their environments, they may give up activities unnecessarily or carry them out in a dangerous manner, both of which can contribute to accidents, isolation, and premature or unnecessary institutionalization.

Environment–behavior researchers typically approach the problem of understanding the relationship between the physical environment and the behavior of older persons by developing theories and accompanying methodologies to test their validity. Designers and planners, however, are often faced with the need to make decisions and judgments with scanty data that rarely resemble testable research hypotheses. Intuition and the ability to problem solve often take precedence over rigorous application of empirically based research findings or an elaborate theoretical framework. Consequently, there is a wide gap between

The Concept and Measurement of
Quality of Life in the Frail Elderly

Copyright © 1991 by Academic Press, Inc.
All rights of reproduction in any form reserved.

environment–behavior theory and everyday necessary decisions that must be made to manage or design the physical environment.

This chapter attempts to bridge the gap between the theoretical framework researchers use to understand the environment and the practice or application of decisions by designers and planners. After discussing why this gap exists, 12 principles for environments for frail older persons will be presented. Each principle is accompanied by a series of interventions or strategies intended to provide researchers, designers, and planners with ways to implement them. A final section discusses the impact of policies and regulations on achieving the principals and suggests a strategy to conduct better applied research on environmental interventions.

Lawton suggests that research in environment–behavior has four principal orientations: (1) an orientation to place—which involves a focus on specific places or settings; (2) an orientation to design—which focuses on the creation and shaping of the setting and the objects used by people; (3) an orientation to social–psychological processes—which recognizes the primary interest of behavioral and social science researchers (i.e., in psychological processes as they relate to the environment); and (4) an orientation to policy—which recognizes the relationship between the environment and the national/regional/local plans and strategies that have been established to respond to social and environmental problems.

The two domains this chapter attempts to address are those orientations to design and management/programs/policy. In organizing the responses to various principles, we have chosen to discuss implications for purpose-built new housing and the existing home environment where appropriate. The latter category, often overlooked in the literature, is important because of the strong preference of the great majority of older persons to age in place and the increasing emphasis on home care services for the frail elderly.

Social and Behavioral Science Models

Theory building in environment–behavior research has been based on classic approaches to psychology (Lewin, 1951; Murray, 1938). The most useful and widely recognized framework cited by design researchers is the competence-press model of Lawton and Nahemow (1973). In this model, "adaptive behavior and positive affect are treated as outcomes of environmental demands that are commensurate with the bio-behavioral competence of the person" (Lawton, Altman, & Wohlwill, 1984). The corollary to this model, the "environmental docility hypothesis," as described by Lawton, "holds that as competence decreases, behavior becomes increasingly determined by factors outside the person (i.e., the environment)." The simplicity of this model and its application to the range of housing types older people inhabit makes it a particularly powerful conceptual tool.

Perhaps the most successful attempt to apply Lawton's framework to actual environmental situations is the Kahana congruence model of person–environment interactions (Kahana, 1974). Kahana's model seeks to transform Lawton's competence-press model into a process of matching the environment and its qualities with the personal needs of the individual. The congruence between these two domains is assumed to lead to positive well-being.

Others who have attempted to expand the Lawton model have done so by establishing very elaborate frameworks that dimensionalize the environment in more exacting ways (Carp & Carp, 1984; Golant, 1984). These attempts have led to more comprehensive approaches but have raised as many measurement questions as they have resolved. Their utility for designers and policymakers has been limited to date because they are not easily translated into practical guidelines that can be used to shape the environment. One exception is the work of Moos and his colleagues (Moos & Lemke, 1980; Moos, Lemke, & David, 1987). They have developed an instrument that measures the qualities of the physical environment and program characteristics. Called the Multiphasic Environmental Assessment Procedure (MEAP), it is a comprehensive method for assessing supportive residential environments. Although this approach to bridging the gap between theory and application is promising, the model's complexity has made it difficult for designers and policymakers to use.

Designers and Policymakers Are Case Study Oriented

Designers and policymakers typically resolve problems through the application of handbook guidelines and code requirements that establish prescriptive solutions based on accepted norms. This information is often gathered from isolated examples that are applied without the benefit of any adjustment or interpretation. Furthermore, the level of competence and specific needs of the individual often vary, and solutions that are appropriate for one level of impairment are often either over- or undersupportive for individuals at another level. In the typical handbooks, suggestions for planning and design are rarely organized or conceptualized as principles. In some cases, guidelines are presented as checklists that address only specific elements and do not address underlying common characteristics of design elements affecting older people. For example, the issue of grasp and manipulation is usually accompanied in such checklists by a recommendation to use lever door handles; however, windows, water faucets, heat controls, cabinet locks, and jar openers, which all share the same principle, are rarely mentioned.

Guideline Organization Schemes

Guidelines embrace a range of organizational schemes. The approach of some publications is to organize information by "scale level," ranging from features within the unit (private) to community-level considerations (public) (Green, Fedewa, Johnston, Jackson, & Deardorff, 1975; Zeisel, Epp, & Demos, 1977; Zeisel, Welch, Epp, & Demos, 1983).

A second approach organizes guidelines so as to correspond with the requirements for specific rooms (AIA Foundation, 1985; Aranyi & Goldman, 1980; Calkins, 1988). This is appealing to architects because design often begins with the process of "programming" the building through assigning and specifying special requirements for specific rooms. A third approach organizes information around the process of implementation (Chambliss, 1989; Welch, Parker, & Zeisel, 1984). In this approach, guidelines are organized to match the sequence that normally accompanies the development of a project. The information is general in nature at the beginning of the process, when decisions are conceptual; later, more specific choices are made with detailed data about application.

A common denominator of all these organizational approaches is their link with the process of design and policy making. The most useful and effective applied research usually deals with an important design or policy variable. For example, reimbursement or cost controls can determine what features are to be included in a building (Pynoos, 1990), while an important architectural consideration such as building circulation can be powerful in organizing design theory and practice. In the latter regard, Howell's (1980) work on the relationship between circulation and sociability directly communicates the positive social outcomes associated with common spaces tethered to main circulation spaces. Typically, it is driven by one important variable, rather than a comprehensive examination of how the environment supports use. It therefore does not address the multiplicity of factors that should be considered if the environment is to truly serve the broader needs of residents.

Twelve Encompassing Principles

It is the contention of the authors that the design, planning, and management of residential settings for older persons could be improved by bridging broad theory and application. Toward this end, 12 specific principles are identified that have surfaced in the design and policy application literature. These principles will be used to create a research framework that attempts to be sensitive to management/program and environmental design concerns, rather than being led by theory building at the expense of application. Because this framework is informed by the range and types of decisions and considerations made by designers and policymakers, it represents a conduit through which social science-based research can more tangibly influence the management, program, policy, and design arenas.

The 12 principles are based on common themes in the literature (Cohen *et al.*, 1988; Lawton, 1975, 1986; Regnier & Pynoos, 1987). They were selected because they have a universal or timeless quality about them. While they have particular relevance for older persons, these principles are also applicable to other segments of the population. Although some are present and identified in the work of Cohen *et al.* (1988), as they relate to nursing homes, and others are recognizable from the theory sections of textbooks that deal with environmental effects, we are not familiar with a comprehensive list of those that address both the design and program/policy areas.

Each of the 12 principles is accompanied by a rationale explaining in broad terms why it is important. This discussion is followed by design and management/program interventions that provide examples of how the principles can be applied. These interventions are intended to be illustrative and do not represent an exhaustive list. Many of the principles are interdependent, and some are conflicting. Others represent ends of a continuum. For example, "privacy" and "social interaction" address two opposite aspects of the environment. "Safety" and "challenge" have a similar conflicting quality. These interrelationships are referred to in cautionary notes that follow the presentation of the principles involved and their related interventions. The final section of the chapter discusses the importance of broader macropolicy for both implementation of the principles and the design and management/program interventions.

Applying these 12 principles will vary depending on the flexibility available in making major adjustments in planned environments or modest improvements to existing dwelling units. Table 1 rates each of the 12 variables with regard to the

Table 1 Relevance of 12 Principles within Planned and Existing Environments

	Environmental context	
Environment behavior principles	Planned environment	Retrofitted existing
1. Privacy	X	O
2. Social interaction	X	X
3. Control/choice/autonomy	X	X
4. Aesthetics/appearance	X	O
5. Personalization	X	O
6. Orientation/way finding	X	O
7. Safety/security	X	X
8. Accessibility and functioning	X	X
9. Stimulation/challenge	X	X
10. Sensory aspects	X	X
11. Adaptability	X	X
12. Familiarity	X	O

X = High relevance
O = Low relevance

two environmental contexts that are the foci of this chapter. For example, privacy, which is an important and critical concern in planned group living arrangements, may be less relevant within an existing home environment where it is a major attribute. Although all principles are deemed important, the table reveals a number of issues that are implicit within an existing home environment and therefore may be less important to address within that context.

Privacy:

Provide opportunities for a place of seclusion from company or observation where one can be free from unauthorized intrusion. This is important because: It provides a sense of self and separateness from others. Privacy is usually provided by having one's own dwelling unit within which there is a bedroom or study. Sometimes privacy is achieved by methods such as: (1) informing others not to interrupt when one is working on a project; (2) putting a "do not disturb" notice on a door; (3) taking the phone off the hook; and (4) using an answering machine to screen calls even when the person being called is present. Altman (1977) defines privacy as "the selective control of access to the self." When asked what privacy means, individuals often respond: "being alone," "no one bothering, distracting, or disrupting me," "controlling access to information," and "controlling access to space." It becomes difficult to maintain or enforce these boundaries as an older person becomes more frail and dependent on other persons for help in such tasks as bathing or toileting. The ultimate loss of privacy occurs, however, when an older person has to move in with children, share a house with someone else, or share a room with one or more unrelated individuals whom he or she has not known previously.

According to Archea (1977), "no matter how we conceptualize privacy, we cannot escape the fact that the behavior required to attain or maintain it occurs in an environment for which the physical properties can be specified." The physical environment can be used to channel and obstruct the visual and auditory information upon which the regulation of privacy depends. For example, features such as walls, doors, mirrors, and windows can either facilitate or inhibit the flow of information an older person can acquire. These physical properties can also affect what others can learn about an older person by controlling the probability that his or her behavior can be monitored.

Design and Management/Program Interventions in Planned Environments

1. Provide private spaces where one can be alone, such as carrels in libraries or places in which private conversations can occur without interruption.
2. Provide individual sleeping and toilet/bathing areas whenever possible.
3. Install hospital locks on bedroom and bathroom doors.
4. If bedrooms are shared, divide rooms in such a way that individuals have

as much visual and auditory privacy as possible through the use of biaxial plans, room dividers, and furniture arrangement.

5. Install gradients, such as shades or blinds, on windows that allow older persons' privacy.
6. Reinforce the principles of privacy through rules such as requiring staff to knock on doors before entering and covering residents before and after assisting them with a bath.
7. Provide outdoor retreat or meditation spaces where residents can be alone and commune with nature.

Caution: Concern over the safety of some frail persons may require some surveillance on a regular basis. Environments that allow privacy should also provide opportunities for social interaction.

Social Interaction:

Provide opportunities for social exchange and interaction. This is important because: One of the fundamental reasons for creating communal environments is to establish the opportunity for creative social relationships between individuals (Rosow, 1967). These relationships can facilitate problem solving and emotional development, as well as motivate individuals to engage in more stimulating and lively experiences. Older people without peer associations can experience isolation, which may lead to depression. Social interaction can reduce isolation and increase life satisfaction by allowing the older person to share problems, life experiences, ideas, and everyday events with someone who also benefits from the exchange. Governmental policies that established purpose-built, age-segregated elderly housing did so primarily to create normative environments where peer associations encourage older people to help one another. The attractiveness of this aspect of the environment is clearly demonstrated in retirement communities that have appealed to a broad social and economic slice of the elderly, representing a life-style that involves sharing life experiences through organized and informal means in communities that range in size from several hundred to over 20,000 persons.

Design and Management/Program Interventions in Planned Environments

1. Design communal spaces so they allow opportunities for chance encounters that can lead to friendships.
2. Develop residential unit corridors with places to sit, rest, and talk with fellow residents.
3. Design spaces for several levels of participation such as direct contact between friends, chance encounters between potential friends, and vicarious watching of activities.

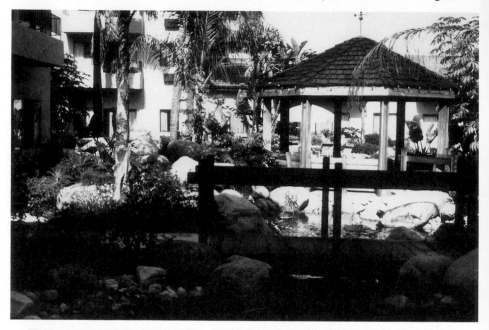

Figure 1   This shaded outdoor sitting area is adjacent to the living areas of this complex. The stream and landscaping provide an interesting and varied setting in which to relax and interact with fellow residents.

4. Specify spaces that support intermittent and informal contact such as hospitality lounges, bulletin kiosks, and waiting areas that overlook or are connected to activity areas.
5. Design lounge areas to resemble intimate residential places in scale and character. Features such as bookcases, fireplaces, and unique furnishing items should be used to establish a specific character.
6. Management should take responsibility to program spaces that require joint activities. Crafts, outdoor games, and planned events require creative management to effectively engage residents.
7. Capitalize on opportunities for residents to watch interesting activities such as gardening, daily deliveries, and maintenance activities on the site and within the building.
8. Arrange several types of related activities near places where residents are likely to visit on a daily basis, like the mail alcove or the dining room. A comfortable chair where residents can wait for mail to arrive and a desk for posting a letter can support the mail area. A pre-dining lounge with activities can increase opportunities for social exchange.

9. Encourage families and friends to visit by providing comfortable visitors' spaces, play areas for grandchildren, and sleeping accommodations.

Caution: Designing environments for social interaction requires adequate opportunities for maintaining one's privacy or separation from others.

Design and Management/Program Interventions in the Home Environment

1. Create a neighborhood connection by adding features such as a porch or bay windows to look in and out.
2. Add features such as flower boxes, mail boxes, personalized front doors, and play equipment for grandchildren or neighborhood children that function as symbols of life, individuality, and openness.
3. Provide transportation to and from community activities.
4. Encourage community institutions such as churches and synagogues, which have traditionally provided opportunities for social exchange, to reach out to older frail members.
5. Support friendly visiting from old friends and acquaintances within the dwelling unit or at local community places, such as senior centers.
6. Promote involvement in passive activities, such as music, as well as service activities (e.g., health counseling/peer group associations).
7. The family is often the most important and immediate source of contact. Training family members about the problems that result from conditions such as memory loss or creating peer groups for caregivers to cope with an aging family member can provide bridges for social exchange.

Control/Choice/Autonomy:

Promote opportunities for residents to make choices and control events that influence their lives. This is important because: Older persons are more alienated, less satisfied, and more task dependent in settings that are highly restrictive, regimented, or promote dependency. On the other hand, actually having control, feeling that one is in control, or having a sense of mastery are enhancing characteristics (Langer & Rodin, 1976). Controlling aspects of one's social and physical environment has been embraced by social psychologists as a fundamental basis for positive social adjustment. Independence, which is frequently the single most cherished aspect of life for the frail, has its basis in choice, control, and autonomy.

Design and Management/Program Interventions in Planned Environments

1. Specify easily manipulatable individual controls for heating, air conditioning, lighting, and window shades in residential units.

2. Allow residents to furnish and decorate their own rooms.
3. If residents must share a bedroom, allow them to choose their room-mate(s).
4. Provide locks on doors and clear rules about intrusion.
5. Provide architectural features that allow residents to "preview" rooms and activities before they enter a public space.
6. Provide residents with choices concerning mealtimes, seating at meals, and daily schedules.
7. Encourage residents to participate in house meetings and resident commit-tees, as well as to be involved in planning facility activities.

Design and Management/Program Interventions in the Home Environment

1. For frail older persons who are experiencing difficulties in carrying out tasks (e.g., cooking, bathing), assess the usefulness of environmental modifications to restore their ability to function independently prior to arranging services.
2. Changes in the individual's home, such as rearranging furniture, installing grab bars, or acquiring new lighting fixtures, should be made with the participation of the older person. Whenever possible, choices of products or devices, as well as alternative solutions, should be provided so that the older person experiences a sense of participating in the final solution.

    Caution: Choice/control must be congruent with competence.

Aesthetics/Appearance:

Design environments that appear attractive and provoking. This is important because: The overall appearance of the environment sends a message to older persons and their family and friends about that person's physical, mental, and spiritual state of well-being (Hartman, Horowitz, & Herman, 1987). Housing environments that are institutional or dehumanized in appearance suggest that inhabitants share that same set of characteristics. Housing that is designed around familiar and supportive behavioral settings also provides clues to residents about how that environment can be used to enhance comfort and social interaction.

Design and Management/Program Interventions in Planned Environments

1. Design the appearance of the setting so it is consistent with the idea of a residential environment. Styles that have a historic place in the vernacular architecture of a region are generally comfortable and familiar.
2. Certain housing elements/features reinforce the iconography of the house. Perhaps the most commonly agreed upon form is the pitched roof. Other

features, such the front porch and the fireplace (hearth), also transmit a very direct and clear message about its residential qualities.

3. The scale of the housing form and the way in which it is detailed also provide overt clues about its residential form. Housing linked by enclosed, double-loaded corridors, which relies on the commercial detailing of windows, doors, and balconies, often appears commercial rather than residential in character.

4. Landscaping plays an important role in relating housing to nature while referencing the outside world of color and texture and the natural forces of wind, light, and rain.

5. Interior furnishings are very important. They can reference time, place, and culture in ways that architecture alone may not be able to. Interior design treatments that focus on symbolic objects or settings can create interest and add variety.

6. The life experiences of older people provide another opportunity for enriching the environment with objects, elements, and settings that reference the past.

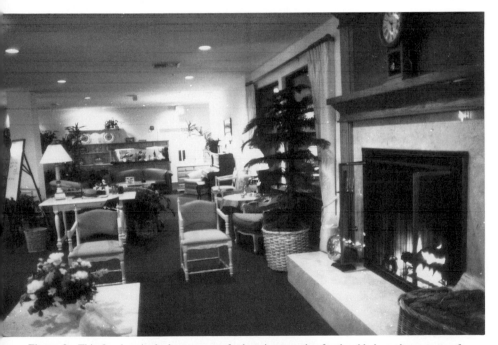

Figure 2 This fireplace in the lounge area of a housing complex for the elderly evokes a sense of home and family, contributing to the residential quality of the building.

7. Appliances and aids such as grab bars, handrails, and fixtures should
    appear attractive and "normal" rather than symbolic of institutional and
    hospital-like settings (see Fernie, Chapter 7).

Caution: Although artistic expression is an important part of any designed
environment, the focus should be on fostering community and feelings of self-
worth and not on the creation of an anonymous architecture that gains its effect at
the expense of these qualities.

Personalization:

*Provide opportunities to make the environment personal or individual and to
mark it as the property of an individual.* This is important because: Self-
expression or personalization reinforces an older person's sense of identity, as
well as expressing this identity to others. It is also a way of demonstrating to
others that the space is occupied by a single, unique individual. Personalization
is a compelling, intrinsic feature of living in one's own home. Claire Cooper has
written, for example: "The furniture we install, the way we arrange it, the
pictures we hang, the plants we buy and tend, are all expressions of our images of
ourselves, all are messages about ourselves that we want to convey back to
ourselves and to the few intimates that we invite into this, our house" (Cooper,
1974). Encouraging someone who is frail to personalize the exterior and interior
of his or her apartment or unit may help alleviate the sense of anonymity or a
negative image associated with a setting (Becker, 1977). It may also provide a
sense of competency and mastery of the environment as well as greater levels of
environmental stimulation. Participation in the process of personalizing the environment itself can also produce positive outcomes.

Design and Management/Program Interventions in Planned Environments

1. Allow residents to decorate the entrance to their units.
2. Permit residents to display personal and meaningful objects in their rooms,
    add storage space, and choose the colors for their walls.
3. Design units that create flexibility through wall placement and that have
    sufficient space to allow furniture to be arranged in more than one way.
4. Allow residents to use their own personal items such as furniture and rugs,
    which have emotional value and represent personal aesthetic choices.
5. Provide areas for the display of an individual's mementos.
6. Assist residents in altering their units when they desire change or variety.
7. Provide outside areas where individuals can plant individual gardens.
8. Provide opportunities, such as wall niches and "memory walls," so that
    individuals can display some of their items in semipublic or public areas.

Caution: Design solutions and administrative policies need to be developed
that facilitate the positive effects of personalization while minimizing the chaos

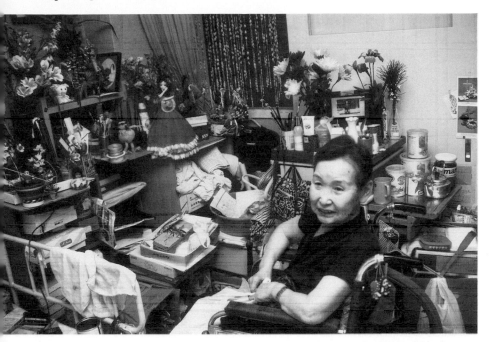

Figure 3 Even in the limited space of her ward in a nursing home in Japan, this resident has personalized her environment.

that might result if everyone plans their own environment without respect to others.

Orientation/Way Finding:

Foster a sense of orientation within the environment that reduces confusion and facilitates way finding. This is important because: Feeling lost or disoriented within an environment is a frustrating and frightening experience that can affect one's sense of perceived competency and well-being (Weisman, 1987). Larger-scale housing environments often rely on winding corridors, elevators, and compact, double-loaded corridors that can exacerbate feelings of disorientation. Older people with cognitive problems can experience great difficulty in orienting themselves within an anonymous, featureless environment.

Design and Management/Program Interventions in Planned Environments

1. Select a footprint or floor plan for the building that is not disorienting. Circular and/or highly symmetric corridor plans can be disorienting because there are too few differentiations.

2. Maps that help to reinforce one's "cognitive map" of a setting can be useful in entry spaces and on floors where reorientation is needed.
3. Signs, graphics, and architectural differentiation in the form of wall treatments and objects can provide landmarks for orientation.
4. Provide features that allow residents to orient themselves with regard to the surrounding context, such as windows that open to a unique feature of the external environment (e.g., a garden or view).
5. Atrium features within buildings provide the option of looking through the setting to the other side and thus make it easier to place two aspects of the building within the same mental construct.
6. Courtyard housing, although sometimes symmetrical in plan, can benefit from views into the courtyard, which can provide order in the same way as an atrium plan.

Safety/Security:

Provide an environment that ensures each user will sustain no harm, injury, or undue risk. This is important because: Elderly not only experience a high rate of home accidents but also more than twice the number of resulting deaths compared with other age groups (Pynoos, Cohen, Davis, & Bernhardt, 1987). The most serious accident-related problems result from falls and burns. Research suggests proper design can help prevent many accidents and lessen the severity of injury.

Design and Management/Program Interventions in Planned Environments

1. Safety features such as grab bars, handrails, nonslip flooring, and ramps should be built into planned environments in an unobtrusive and nonstigmatized manner. For example, grab bars or handrails made of wood or colored materials may be more acceptable than those made of metal, which could appear institutional in character.
2. The environment should be designed so that it is resilient and less dangerous for older persons who may experience a fall. In this regard, round edges on furniture and fixtures and carpeting that absorbs impacts rather than hard floor surfaces should be specified.
3. The environment should compensate for sensory losses. For example, greater susceptibility to glare could contribute to a fall. This might be compensated by features such as overhangs, north-facing skylights, and window shades.

Design and Management/Program Interventions in the Home Environment

1. Modifying unsafe furniture, finishes, and fixtures may allow older persons to keep items of sentimental value and thereby reduce resistance to making

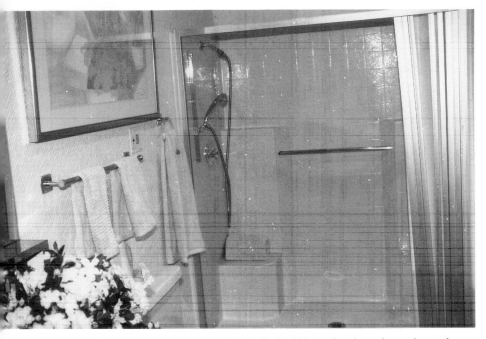

Figure 4 Safety features such as grab bars and handrails should be unobtrusive and attractive, such as these in a congregate housing complex.

the home safer. For example, rather than removing slippery throw rugs, firmly secure them.

2. Safety and security throughout the home can be enhanced through the installation of a number of items, such as smoke detectors, security alarm systems, door peepholes, outdoor lights, and locking devices on doors and windows.

3. Provide bathtub and shower temperature controls that regulate unpredictable water temperature swings. These can protect the older person from accidental burns and scalds.

4. Reduce dangerous clutter by eliminating unnecessary items and improving storage capacity.

5. Particular attention should be paid to supportive railings, nonslip floor surfaces, and lighting on stairs and in bathrooms because accidents are likely to occur in these places.

Caution: Safety and security can conflict with efforts to provide stimulation/challenge or personalization. Efforts to improve safety and security in the home environment should take into consideration the need for control, choice, and autonomy.

Accessibility and Functioning:

Consider manipulation and accessibility as the basic requirements for satisfying concerns about functionality. This is important because: Older people often experience problems manipulating the environment (windows, doors, HVAC equipment, appliances) due in part to chronic disabling diseases such as arthritis. Reach-capacity and muscle-strength impairments can affect stooping, bending, sitting, and standing. These limitations can literally handicap a frail, older person, making it difficult to navigate and fully utilize an environment (Noelker, 1982). Adaptations to the environment that make it easier to manipulate can begin to overcome this major problem, as can the specification of fixtures, equipment, and devices that are designed to be manipulated by individuals with limited grip capacity or twisting ability. Ambulation can become a problem, making it harder to get from one place to another without frequent rest stops. Making the environment convenient and easy to access for both individuals and caregivers will often facilitate a higher level of use.

Design and Management/Program Interventions in Planned Environments

1. Within the dwelling unit, the major rooms that require careful planning are the bathroom and the kitchen, where the ability to manipulate the environment and to carry out activities of daily living are often impaired by conventional equipment and standard designs.
2. Specifying special equipment and appliances that are designed with manipulation control and safety in mind can resolve many potential problems.
3. Reach capacity is a problem that many older, shorter females experience. Closets, storage areas, and shelves should be designed for ease of access.
4. Controls for HVAC systems, water valves, doors, windows, and lighting often require handle adaptations or replacement fixtures that are easy to turn, twist, or pull.
5. Travel distances also can be a problem. A compact, centralized plan can help minimize difficulties, but the setting should also be planned to include convenient seating opportunities for rest.
6. Level changes can be harder for the older person to manipulate safely; therefore, the need to introduce spatial variety and hierarchy is best explored in ceiling-level changes and the manipulation of this aspect of the environment.
7. Avoid changes in level between floor materials, between rooms, and

between indoor and outdoor spaces. This helps ambulatory older adults avoid tripping and falling; it also makes the environment safer for those with ambulation impairments and easier for those who are wheelchair bound.

Caution: Considering manipulation and accessibility as preemptory criteria can lead to building plans and unit designs that are unchallenging and appear suited for "sick" people. The need to balance challenge with support is a subtle but important aspect of design.

Design and Management/Program Interventions in the Home Environment

1. Changes in floor levels are often a major problem to overcome in the home environment. Adequate handrails positioned in strategic places can facilitate movement.
2. Changes in grade often occur between the front door and the street, where surfaces can be wet and slippery. Falling on pavement can be traumatic. Handrails located at the appropriate level and designed for good grasp control are important.
3. Older people will often create a "control center" near a couch or favorite chair that centralizes access to light switches, television remote devices, telephone instruments, and reading materials. Cords from various devices, throw rugs, and other living room furniture items can make this setting unsafe.
4. Reaching the restroom in the middle of the night is also a problem. Strategically placed night lights can help make this trip a safer one.
5. Bathrooms and kitchens are often rooms where the most severe safety problems exist. Changes that make it easier to access food, cutlery, dinnerware, and pots and pans can help avoid unnecessary risks associated with climbing on a step stool or back problems that may result from retrieving a heavy pot from a deep drawer under the counter.
6. Making improvements in the home often requires capital and coordination with semiskilled and skilled workers. Programs for making home modifications should be structured to overcome the problems many older people face in coordinating the delivery of services and paying for environmental improvements.
7. Unlike the leaky roof or the heating system that malfunctions, home modifications oriented toward safety do not always seem "necessary" to the older person. A positive attitude regarding safety is important to pursue so that adjustments can be made before a change in resident competency leads to an avoidable accident.
8. Assessment procedures that involve the family in making changes or

negotiating safety features with the older person can also facilitate implementation.

Stimulation/Challenge:

Provide a stimulating environment that is safe but challenging. This is important because: It keeps the older person active, alert, and aware. Stimulation can be viewed in a number of ways, one of which is sensory. Color, smells, surface textures, and sounds give environments a richness of character that often reinforces their individuality and complexity. Spatial variety and hierarchy can also enhance the experience of an environment. The challenge of fitting other people, plants, and animals into a stimulating physical setting is the essence of making an environment a memorable place. A lack of stimulation is often considered boring and monotonous, leading to inactivity and depression. One difficulty in designing safe environments is that challenge is often reduced. An appropriate degree of challenge is highly desirable. Institutional environments are often faulted for their lack of variety or for their sensory monotony. A stimulating environment is especially important to combat boredom, a common problem of persons with mobility impairments.

Design and Management/Program Interventions in Planned Environments

1. Encourage variety and complexity in hallways by using pictures, photographs, and artwork.
2. Provide an environment rich in texture, color, and pattern.
3. Provide outside views that vary at different times of the day, on different days of the week, and during different seasons. Activities that are observable from the inside, such as children playing, street traffic, and pedestrian flow, are especially interesting.
4. Provide seating in areas where residents can watch others as well as participate in activities.
5. Allow contact with other living things by including aviaries, bird cages, fish tanks, rabbit hutches, and dog houses.
6. Provide spaces for a range of mentally and physically stimulating activities such as dance, music, crafts, and swimming.

Design and Management/Program Interventions in the Home Environment

1. Dramatize time changes such as daylight, seasons, and daily weather by adding such features as window boxes, skylights, corner windows, and french doors.

2. Add features—such as greenhouses, aquariums, aviaries, vegetable gardens, and bird baths—that may promote productivity, alertness, and activity.

Sensory Aspects:

Changes in visual, auditory, and olfactory senses should be accounted for in environments. This is important because: Older people with age-related losses often experience problems with vision and hearing that can place them at a disadvantage in the environment (Hiatt, 1987). When environmental conditions involve high levels of sound and low lighting levels, socialization and manipulation of the environment can be impaired.

The amount and source of light can cause problems that affect basic visual acuity and glare. Color distortions brought about by the aging of the eye muddle color distinctions and mute color differences. The use of natural light in combination with indirect artificial lighting can have pleasing and effective results.

Design and Management/Program Interventions in Planned Environments

1. Lighting levels should not change abruptly, because contrasts in light level could cause glare, which could be exacerbated by accommodation delays.
2. Create small alcoves for personal conversation that eliminate confusing background noise and support effective communication.
3. Control reverberation by specifying sound-absorptive materials that minimize the disruption of background noise.
4. In assembly areas where sound control is harder to achieve, high-technology adaptations could be used to resolve problems.
5. Gardens that provide stimulation through fragrance and pungent smells can complement the repertoire of experiences available to the older person.

Design and Management/Program Interventions in the Home Environment

1. Since the eyes of an older person are sensitive to glare, light from exposed windows should be controlled through the use of exterior overhangs or window treatments (e.g., louver-type shades, shading tints).
2. Difficult-to-read instructions or numbers on appliance controls such as on stoves, thermostats, telephones, and washing machines should be replaced with larger, easy-to-read graphics.
3. It is likely that the level of illumination will need to be increased, with special attention to task-related activities (e.g., cooking, reading, sewing). This may require additional outlets as well as fixtures.
4. Illuminated light switches can be used to help locate them when entering a dark room.

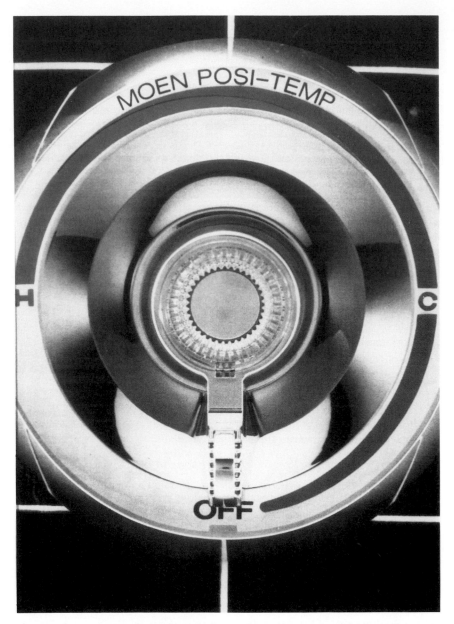

Figure 5 Large letters and numbers with good contrast make it easier for older persons to see controls. This shower/bath mechanism also includes an easy grasp lever.

Adaptability:

An adaptable or flexible environment can be made to fit a specific new use or situation by modification. This is important because: As older persons age and become more frail, they often find that the setting within which they live no longer fits their capabilities (Steinfeld, 1987). Consequently, some older persons carry out activities in unsafe environments, give up some tasks, or move to another setting in spite of their strong preference to stay in the same place. For a setting to meet the diminished capabilities of frail older persons it must either include supportive features (e.g., ramps, grab bars, handrails) or be able to be retrofitted. Unfortunately, many housing units cannot easily be adapted to the changing needs of older persons because of stairs, bathrooms being located on only one floor, and other problems associated with accessibility. Such problems are particularly difficult for older frail persons who use wheelchairs. In addition, the availability of modifications is limited by inadequate reimbursement policies and the lack of an adequate delivery system for home modifications.

Design and Management/Program Interventions in Planned Environments

1. Employ the concept of adaptable housing to accommodate the needs of older persons as they age and become more frail. This will allow moderately disabled older persons to remain in their own units. Areas of particular concern are the entrance, kitchen, and bathroom. For example, bathroom walls could be framed so they will safely receive grab bars and handrails when they are considered necessary.
2. The changing level of disability for an individual may require that grab bars and handrails inside and outside be phased into a project as residents age and the need for these supports increases.
3. Adaptable housing standards require that corridors, doorways, and critical dimensions within bathrooms and kitchens be wide enough to be adaptable for the use of wheelchair-bound residents, if necessary.
4. Provide some units for severely disabled residents so that even if they cannot remain in their own units they can be accommodated within the same facility.
5. Design the kitchen and bathrooms with adequate lateral storage for supplies and utensils.
6. Specify heavier-than-normal towel racks that can be solidly attached if older residents choose to use these to steady themselves.

Design and Management/Program Interventions in the Home Environment

1. Improve the system for financing and carrying out home modifications.
2. Reduce the reluctance of some older persons to make changes by making

available products that are attractive and "normal looking" in appearance rather than products that are constructed out of institutional materials and appear to be made for hospital and nursing home settings (see Fernie, Chapter 7).

3. Provide educational programs to the general public concerning hazards and problems in the home and what can be done to remedy them.
4. Improve environmental assessment procedures for the home, and train professionals in their use.
5. Provide zoning options or conditional-use permits that allow accessory apartments to be placed in single-family residential areas. This can encourage other persons who need housing to live with frail older persons and provide services or assistance.
6. Consider a universal design approach to single-family housing that includes features such as nonslip flooring, grab bars, accessible bathrooms, and adjustable kitchen counters and shelving. Such housing should also allow the flexibility to live on a lower-level floor should that be necessary.

Caution: These adaptations could conflict with efforts to create a homelike, personalized environment.

Familiarity:

Environments that use historical reference and solutions that are steeped in tradition can provide a sense of the familiar. This is important because: For some older people, moving from one setting to another can be disorienting, especially when there is little continuity between these places (Hunt & Pastalan, 1987). Bringing personal objects and possessions that constitute a familiar frame of reference is a way to create continuity (Becker, 1977). The environment should also constitute a familiar frame of reference in which rooms have a vernacular reference point.

Design and Management/Program Interventions in Planned Environments

1. Design social lounge spaces that appear to be like conventional, residentially scaled living rooms in terms of furniture selection and decor.
2. Policies that allow furniture and other important objects to be a part of the residential living unit help foster a sense of continuity with the past.
3. Landscape treatments that include mature trees and plant materials make a connection with nature that evokes familiarity through a natural context.
4. Rooms that constitute places with differing roles or expectations provide both variety and a sense of continuity within the environment. For example, a game room, parlor, and billiards area all sanction different

forms of behavior and dress. Informal and formal settings provide variety and choice.

5. Foster a sense of continuity through management and personnel policies.

Regulatory/Policy Implications

Our ability to implement these environment–behavior principles and their accompanying design and management/program interventions is significantly affected by government policy. Reimbursement policies, regulations, land-use zoning, and building codes all influence what is built and how it is managed, as well as the availability of programs. In many instances, these policies have been moving in directions that make it more difficult rather than easier to create environments that will improve the quality of life for frail older persons (Pynoos, 1990).

Reimbursement

Government reimbursement policies influence costs; therefore, they directly impact the size and variety of spaces, the quality of construction, and the overall scale of many buildings. The underlying philosophy of the privacy principle suggests, for example, that assisted-living or nursing home complexes should include a large proportion of one-bedroom units. A facility based on this principle is likely to be more costly to construct than a conventional complex, in which persons share rooms. There could be long-term cost savings in managing a more appropriately designed facility; however, the major benefits are likely to be improved staff morale and resident satisfaction. The latter are outcomes that are difficult to quantify. Consequently, if current government policies continue, better-quality environments are likely to be achieved in settings that cater to middle- to upper-income residents, rather than to those who have lower incomes and must rely on SSI or Medicaid. Such economic constraints force us to accept less-than-optimal solutions that create a two-tiered system: one for those able to pay and another for the poor. For example, in lieu of creating private rooms in low-cost housing, we attempt to devise ways to divide space.

As noted earlier, there is also inadequate reimbursement for home modifications that can assist older persons to stay in their current residences. Home modification programs are particularly important given the preference of older persons to age in place and the environmental barriers inherent in their homes.

Codes

The construction costs of buildings are often inflated by highly restrictive building codes that can serve as constraints to innovative design solutions. The explicit

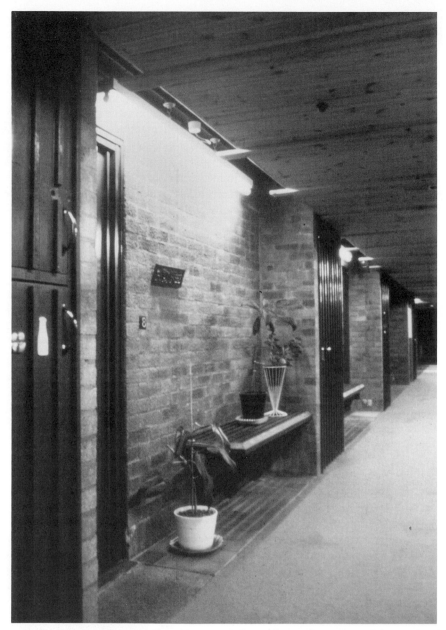

Figure 6 European treatments of corridors, which frequently use plants, natural light, wood and brick surfaces, and indirect lighting are difficult to use in this country because of problems with codes.

purpose of building codes has been to ensure safety and durability as well as to protect against fires, accidents, and structural failures. Institutional settings, like nursing homes, experience the tightest controls related to such features as exits, hallways, corridors, and fire doors. Many of these codes are derived from outmoded assumptions that are not congruent with the residential types of environments which better meet the needs of most frail older persons. Unfortunately, most code provisions employ specification standards (i.e., identifying specific permissible materials) as opposed to performance standards (identifying a minimum level of performance).

New materials cannot be introduced under specification standards without modifying the building code or convincing local, state, or regional authorities of their acceptability. It is especially difficult to obtain code approval for the use of natural materials such as wood—because of concerns regarding combustibility—or brick or stone—because of concerns regarding their abrasive surface texture. It is also difficult to introduce attractive features, such as fireplaces, that in any way increase the perception of problems with fire safety. Efforts to gain exceptions to codes can result in long and costly delays with no assurance that approvals will be forthcoming. Consequently, many of the code requirements established to protect the public welfare also have limited our ability to experiment with ideas.

On the other hand, codes can be important in improving safety and accessibility. For example, the Fair Housing Amendment Act of 1988 will increase accessibility in multiunit housing, especially for those in wheelchairs, allowing more disabled and elderly persons to age in place. However, codes have often ignored features that could improve safety for older and younger persons alike. For example, while local codes pertaining to single-family homes often require handrails on stairs, there is a great deal of variation in their placement. Moreover, there are virtually no local codes that require single-family housing to have such features as grab bars in showers or bathtubs, even though they would improve safety for all age groups.

Regulations

While codes may unnecessarily add to the cost of buildings or ignore features that might improve the quality of life of frail older persons, many recently imposed cost-saving regulations appear very shortsighted. For example, during the early 1980s, HUD imposed cost-containment regulations on Section 202 housing for the elderly that reduced the size of units, mandated that at least 20% of the units be efficiencies, reduced allowable common spaces, disallowed elevators in buildings that were two stories high, eliminated balconies, and reduced the possibility of using materials, such as brick facing, that architects often specify for durability and because of the residential character it references. These cost-saving restrictions make it more difficult for older persons to age in place and result in buildings that are much less residential in appearance than publicly subsidized buildings constructed in earlier times.

Directions for Future Research

Our attempts to loosen government purse strings or create more flexibility in codes would be greatly enhanced if we were able to demonstrate that following the 12 environment–behavior principles and their accompanying design and program interventions would significantly improve the quality of life for frail older persons. It must be pointed out, however, that there is not yet a strong research base on which to predict the effect of the interventions on the lives of older persons, the extent to which one intervention will be more important than another one, nor the degree to which a particular intervention will interact with another. Nevertheless, following the method proposed by Zeisel (1981), the authors think that the proposed principles and interventions could be useful in carrying out applied research that would have a double impact on the world of theory building and design innovation. In Zeisel's approach, the building and its subcomponents become the hypotheses and establish the research agenda. The best example in this regard is the Captain Eldridge Congregate House, which contains 20 design behavior hypotheses that are created as a result of the way in which the environment is structured to support, protect, and connect residents. Facilities need to be developed that include the provision for testing hypotheses regarding the effect of the social and physical environment on the behavior and well-being of residents, staff, and visitors. For example, a series of research questions could be formulated around a principle such as personalization (Becker, 1977). Who chooses to personalize their environment and under what conditions? To what extent does personalization extend to spaces outside the individual unit? What effects does individual personalization have on the elderly residents, staff, friends, and relatives? What effects does group personalization have on group cohesiveness and a sense of community? How does personalization affect interaction patterns and the development of friendships?

Because of the complexity of buildings and their overall costs, it is difficult to conduct controlled studies of how different spaces are used, although this can be done on a small scale. In lieu of such experiments, the authors suggest a three-step research approach. First, potential users or residents should be involved in early design stages to gauge their attitudes toward particular features such as the building facade; orientation toward the street; size and location of common space; color; and personalization of unit entrances (Hartman, Horowitz, & Herman, 1987; Regnier, 1986). Second, planners and designers should hypothesize how they believe different aspects of a building will be used or viewed by the residents in the form of a behaviorally based architectural program. Third, postoccupancy evaluations should be conducted to better understand how residents actually respond to what has been designed. A similar method could be employed to research how older persons respond to increasing frailty in terms of adapting to or making changes in their existing home environments. In this way, increased knowledge should be gained concerning the relative importance and interrelationships of the proposed principles and the impact of design and management/program interventions.

Summary

The environment is an important component of the quality of life, especially for frail older persons who are more dependent on it than their more healthy counterparts. Unfortunately, many environments are planned, built, and managed with little attention to the needs of older persons. The above discussion has stressed the importance of establishing clear principles, such as providing privacy, promoting social interaction, and fostering way finding. Such principles can be linked to interventions that designers, planners, managers, older persons, and policymakers can use. Many of these principles will interact and some may conflict with each other. The interventions and strategies to implement the principles will therefore require that architects, planners, managers, and older persons themselves be not simply technicians but problem solvers.

Attempts to improve the quality of life for frail older persons must be viewed in the context in which government policy places constraints on what is built and how it is managed. Policy often affects the amount of money available, the materials that can be used, layouts, and staffing. Policy affecting environments for frail older persons could be improved if the principles and their accompanying interventions could be proven to save costs and improve the quality of life. In order for this to occur, much more systematic research needs to be conducted on the impact of environmental interventions on the quality of older persons' lives.

References

AIA Foundation (1985). *Design for aging: An architect's guide.* Washington: AIA Press.

Altman, I. (1977). Privacy regulation: culturally universal or culturally specific? *Journal of Social Issues, 33,* 66–87.

Aranyi, L., & Goldman, L. (1980). *Design of long term care facilities.* New York: Van Nostrand Reinhold.

Archea, J. (1977). The place of architectural factors in behavioral theories of privacy. *Journal of Social Issues, 33,* 116–137.

Becker, F. D. (1977). *Housing Messages.* Vol. 30 of Community Development Series. Stroudsberg, Penn.: Dowden, Hutchinson and Ross, Inc.

Calkins, M. (1988). *Design for dementia: Planning environments for the elderly and confused.* Owings Mill: National Health Publishing.

Carp, F., & Carp, A. (1984). A complimentary/congruence model of well-being or mental health for the community elderly. In Altman, Lawton, & Wohlwill, eds., *Elderly people and the environment*. New York: Plenum Press.

Chambliss, B. (1989). *Creating assisted living housing*. Denver, Colo.: Colorado Association of Homes and Services for the Aging.

Cohen, U., Weisman, J., Ray, K., Steiner, V., Rand, J., Toyne, R., & Sasaki, S. (1988). *Environments for people with dementia: Design guide*. Washington, D.C.: Health Facilities Research Program.

Cooper, C. (1974). The house as symbol of self. In J. Lang *et al.*, eds., *Architecture and human behavior*. Stroudsberg, Penn.: Dowden, Hutchinson and Ross, Inc.

Golant, S. (1984). *A place to grow old: The meaning of environment in old age*. New York: Columbia University Press.

Green, I., Fedewa, B., Johnston, C., Jackson, W., & Deardorff, H. (1975). *Housing for the elderly: The development and design process*. New York: Van Nostrand Reinhold.

Hartman, C., Horowitz, J., & Herman, R. (1987). Involving older persons in designing housing for the elderly. In V. Regnier & J. Pynoos, eds., *Housing the aged: Design directives and policy considerations*. New York: Elsevier.

Hiatt, L. G. (1987). Designing for the vision and hearing impairments of the elderly. In V. Regnier and J. Pynoos, eds., *Housing the aged: Design directives and policy considerations*. New York: Elsevier.

Howell, S. C. (1980). *Designing for the aging: Patterns of use*. Cambridge, Mass.: MIT Press.

Hunt, M. E., & Pastalan, L. A. (1987). Easing relocation: An environmental learning process. In V. Regnier and J. Pynoos, eds., *Housing the aged: Design directives and policy considerations*. New York: Elsevier.

Kahana, E. (1980). A congruence model of person–environment interaction. In M. P. Lawton, P. G. Windley, & T. O. Byerts, eds., *Aging and the environment: Directions and perspectives*. New York: Garland STPM Press.

Langer, E., & Rodin, J. (1976). The effects of choice and enhanced personal responsibility for the aged. *Journal of Personality and Social Psychology, 34*.

Lawton, M. P. (1975). *Planning and managing housing for the elderly*. New York: Wiley and Sons.

Lawton, M. P. (1986). *Environment and aging*. Albany, N.Y.: Center for the Study of Aging.

Lawton, M. P., & Nahemow, L. (1973). Ecology and the aging process. In C. Eisdorfer and M. P. Lawton, eds., *Psychology of adult development and aging*. Washington, D.C.: American Psychological Association.

Lawton, M. P., Altman, I., & Wohlwill, J. (1984). Dimensions of environment behavior research. In Altman, Lawton, & Wohlwill, eds., *Elderly people and the environment*. New York: Plenum Press.

Lewin, K. (1951). *Field theory in social science*. New York: Harper and Row.

Moos, R., & Lemke, S. (1980). The multiphasic assessment procedure. In A. Jegar and B. Blotnick, eds., *Community mental health: A behavioral ecological perspective*. New York: Plenum Press.

Moos, R., Lemke, S., & David, T. (1987). Priorities for design and management in residential settings for the elderly. In V. Regnier and J. Pynoos, eds., *Housing the aged: Design directives and policy considerations*. New York: Elsevier.

Murray, H. (1938). *Explorations in personality*. New York: Oxford University Press.

Noelker, L. (1982). Environmental barriers to family caregiving. Paper presented at the Annual Meeting of the Gerontological Society of America, November.

Pynoos, J. (1990). Public policy and aging in place: Identifying the problems and potential solutions. In D. Tilson, ed., *Aging in place: Supporting the frail elderly in residential environments,* pp. 167–208. Glenview, Ill.: Scott, Foresman and Company.

Pynoos, J., Cohen, E., Davis, L. J., & Bernhardt, S. (1987). Home modifications: Improvements that extend independence. In V. Regnier and J. Pynoos, eds., *Housing the aged: Design directives and policy considerations*. New York: Elsevier.

Regnier, V. (1986). Congregate housing for the elderly: An integrative and participatory planning model. In T. Vonier, ed., *Proceedings of the research and design '85 conference*. Washington, D.C.: American Institute of Architects.

Regnier, V., & Pynoos, J., eds. (1987). *Elderly housing: Design directives and policy considerations*. New York: Elsevier.

Rosow, I. (1967). *Social integration of aged*. New York: Free Press.

Steinfeld, E. (1987). Adapting housing for older disabled people. In V. Regnier and J. Pynoos, eds., *Housing the aged: Design directives and policy considerations*. New York: Elsevier.

Weisman, G. (1987). Improving way-finding and architectural legibility in housing for the elderly. In V. Regnier and J. Pynoos, eds., *Housing the aged: Design directives and policy considerations*. New York: Elsevier.

Welch, P., Parker, V., & Zeisel, J. (1984). *Independence through interdependence*. Commonwealth of Massachusetts: Department of Older Affairs.

Zeisel, J. (1981). *Inquiry by design*. Monterey, Calif.: Brooks Cole Publishing.

Zeisel, J., Epp, G., & Demos, S. (1977). *Low-rise housing for older people: Behavioral criteria for design*. Washington, D.C.: U.S. Government Printing Office, HUD-483, September.

Zeisel, J., Welch, P., Epp, G., & Demos, S. (1983). *Mid-rise elevator housing for older people*. Boston: Building Diagnostics.

6

Relocation of the Frail Elderly

MORTON H. LIEBERMAN

Introduction

Thirty years of published reports on relocation of the elderly address two core issues: What are the effects? And what characteristics of individual persons or conditions of the relocation explain the observed effects? The present chapter reviews what we now know about these two central questions and how we have come to understand the issues. To accomplish these goals, all published studies have been reviewed. What kinds of studies exist? And, perhaps most importantly, how cumulative is the knowledge gained across such studies? Addressing these questions requires an examination of both methods and concepts in order to determine the adequacy of the accumulation.

Although the central concern of this chapter is neither to review nor make recommendations about the social policy implications of relocation research but to discuss how and why much of the empirical data has been generated, it is necessary to understand the origins of a public concern with how, when, under what conditions, and with what strategies the infirm elderly should be moved.

The chapter is divided into two sections. The first section is organized around Table 1, which summarizes published empirical studies. The author has chosen to present these studies on the basis of a time line rather than to divide them into familiar and, in this investigator's mind, not useful study types. Categories used in previous reviews include forced versus voluntary relocation; mass versus individualized transfers; and movement from the community to congregate living, from one institutional setting to another, or from a congregate setting to community living. As will become apparent later in the chapter, there are conceptual and methodological problems in assessing and defining voluntary versus involuntary movement in the absence of homogeneity when studies are categorized as similar, despite wide variations in the population characteristics of the relocated samples. For example, studies examining community moves to institutional settings range from investigations of psychiatrically ill populations moving

The Concept and Measurement of
Quality of Life in the Frail Elderly

Copyright © 1991 by Academic Press, Inc.
All rights of reproduction in any form reserved.

Table 1 Relocation Studies

Author	Type of relocation[a]	N	Control[b]	Death rate experiment versus control	Other outcome measures	Comments
Aleksandrowicz (1961)	I-I, fire	40	P	20.0% vs. 7.5%	—	—
Lieberman (1961)	C-I, homes for the aged	640	P	24.7% vs. 10.4%	—	—
Bortner (1962)	VA	65	—	—	Catell 16 PF	Length of residence, differences based primarily on selection
Aldrich (1964); Aldrich & Mendkoff (1963)	I-I	43	P	36.0%	Psychiatric evaluation	Differential mortality based on personality
Pihkanen & Lahdenpera (1963)	I-I	108	X, 116	3.0% vs. 14.0%	—	Questionable equivalence of control group
Carp (1966)	C-C	190	—	5.0%	Self-report	Nonfrail elderly
Anderson (1967)	C-I	101	X	—	Self-esteem	Cross sectional, institutional vs. waiting list; serious differential sample attrition
Jasnau (1967)	I-I, mental hospital	141	P	56.3% vs. 44.0%	—	Noncomparable sample
Stotsky (1967)	I-I, psychiatric patients	141	X	4.0% vs. 12.0%	—	—
Kasteler et al. (1968)	C-C, urban renewal	48	X, 267	—	Interview: poorer adjustment and attitudes	—
Kral et al. (1968)	I-I	54	—	—	Symptoms, plasma cortods	Psychiatrics and men, > death rate

(Table continues)

Table 1 (*Continued*)

Author	Type of relocation[a]	N	Control[b]	Death rate experiment versus control	Other outcome measures	Comments
Killian (1970)	I-I, state hospital	253	X, 253	6.7% vs. 2.4%	—	Aged > death rate
Lawton & Yaffe (1970)	C-C, apartment complex	103	X	6.0%	Health	Health > death rate
Markus et al. (1971)	I-I	393	P, X	18.0%	—	Nonmover, not comparable
Goldfarb et al. (1972)	I-I	70	X, 176	28.0% vs. 38.0%	Psychiatric exam	Mortality linked to CBS
Pino et al. (1978	C-I, I-I	—	X	—	Functional, physical	ADL and life satisfaction improvement; illness > death
Silberstein (1979)	I-I	137	P	13.0% vs. 37.0%	—	—
Csank & Zweig (1980) (see also Zweig & Csank, 1975)	I-I	—	P	49.0% vs. 39.0%	—	Chronic brain syndrome subgroup affected
Haddad (1981)	I-I	398	—	8.2% vs. 8.4%	Behavioral adjustment, psychiatric, health	3 types of transfer, noncomparable samples
Wells & MacDonald (1981)	I-I	56	—	—	Social network, life satisfaction, Pamie	Social network hypothesis not demonstrated
Dube (1982)	I-I	50	P	—	Orientation, cognition, memory	Inadequate statistical analysis

	C-C				ADL, days ill/in bed	Decrements ADL and illness
Ferraro (1982)	C-C	200	X	—	ADL, days ill/in bed	
Lieberman & Tobin (1983)	I-I, home for the aged	45	P	9.0%	Health, cognition, social, emotional	52% deteriorated, 46% unchanged, 2% improved
Lieberman & Tobin (1983)	I-I, mental hospital patients	427	C, 100	18.0%	Health, cognition, social, emotional	56% deteriorated, 24% unchanged, 20% improved
Lieberman & Tobin (1983)	I-I, mental hospital	85	P	0.02%	Cognition, health, social, emotional	49% deteriorated, 30% unchanged, 21% improved
Nirenberg (1983)	I-I, nursing home	40	—	—	ADL, cognition, morale	Low-functioning > negative outcome; high-functioning > improvement
Eckert & Haug (1984)	C-C, SROs	—	X	—	Self-perceived physical, functional well-being	Trends, movers, lower ADL, higher well-being
Shamian et al. (1984)	I-I, nursing home	20	X, 16	—	ADL, health, behaviors	9 weeks, temporary, no differences
Anthony et al. (1987)	I-I	25	X, 14	—	Behavior observation	> depression and dysfunctional behavior
Pruchno & Resch (1988)	I-I, room transfer	207	X, 353	—	Level of competence	Death rate highest among noncompetent
Bonardi et al. (1989)	I-I, intact social system	—	—	—	Functional levels	Highest death, prior move relocated > depression, > withdrawal

[a] I-I, institution to institution; C-I, community to institution; C-C, community to community.
[b] P, prior death rate of population; X, contrast group, not relocated; WL, awaiting move to institution.

moving from community to psychiatric hospitals, to relatively healthy elderly moving into institutional settings because of social needs.

Several conventions were chosen as criteria for entry into Table 1. Each represents a single study rather than a single publication. Outcome rates are recalculated, deleting subjects under 60 years of age. Studies of urban renewal and migration and movement of elderly into retirement communities are generally excluded. Most subjects in these cases do not fit the criteria of frail elderly. However, several studies involving the movement of elderly from community to communal settings (such as the work of the Philadelphia Geriatric Center) contain many frail elderly; these studies have been included. The entries in Table 1 provide information on type of relocation, characteristics of the control group (if available), characteristics of the population moved, measurable impact of the relocation, death rates, and other measures of impact, such as morbidity and measures of psychological and social behaviors.

The second section provides an analytic look at the processes and mechanisms that account for or explain the observed effects of relocation. Included are: (1) individual resources or capacities, including personality types, locus of control, coping strategies, and cognitive capacities; (2) cognitive appraisal, expectations, or meaning of the relocation; and (3) environmental characteristics and changes in the environment as the source of relocation stress.

Most of the empirical studies, and much of the controversy associated with relocation of the frail elderly, is centered on a single effect variable: excess mortality. Mortality rates are obviously associated with levels of physical disability. Difficulty in attempting to accumulate findings across studies (most relying on relatively small samples) arises because mortality rates will differ radically from one study to another depending upon the level of physical disability and illness prior to the relocation. Unless precise and matched control groups are available, comparisons across studies are difficult to make.

It is possible that the wrong questions have been asked. To study the effects of relocation in terms of theoretical and practical significance requires an investigation of the effects of such relocation relative to the prior functioning of the person. If effects are conceptualized on a continuum relative to where the individual was prior to the relocation, it becomes clear that the degree of impact (whether positive or negative) is best represented as movement on some measure, be it physical, psychological, or social. Individuals in relatively good health prior to relocation may develop increased symptoms or increased disability; their social patterns may change, or their psychological and psychiatric conditions may alter. Such "movement" in either direction may represent more change than the simple observation that highly debilitated and frail elderly are dead subsequent to the environmental change.

The difficulty in developing experimental conditions using a true random group in a clinical trial study makes it imperative that anchoring be done for changes based upon individual functioning prior to relocation. This does not preclude the necessity of contrast groups, but, by and large, such groups represent control conditions that are far from ideal.

Forced versus voluntary relocation is another important issue. Although it has become increasingly popular to attribute the effects of relocation on the voluntariness of the move, the vast majority of the studies summarized in Table 1 were classified as involuntary. With the exception of several that examined the movement of individuals from the community to old age homes, the majority of voluntary relocations involve studies of community to apartment complexes or to congregate living settings, representing populations that are not comparable to those moving to nursing homes. Thus, meaningful comparisons across studies on this variable are not possible.

Along with the development of empirical studies has been the periodic appearance in the scientific literature of critical reviews of studies of relocation. Many, starting with the earliest available (Blenkner, 1967), have repeatedly pointed to problems raised in the present chapter. The interested reader should refer to Blenkner, 1967; Borup, Gallego, and Heffernan, 1979; Coffman, 1981; Kasl, 1972; Laughton and Nahemow, 1973; Lieberman, 1969, 1974; and Schulz and Brenner, 1977. All conclude that method and design problems severely restrict firm conclusions that relocation increases the likelihood of excessive mortality. However, when making comparisons, one must take into account that these reviews utilized somewhat different data bases. For example, comparison of the cited references in Borup and Gallego (1981) and Coffman (1981) reveals some lack of correspondence between the cited evidence. Obviously, this is attributable in part to the particular criteria the reviewer uses in selecting evidence. Unfortunately, however, it also appears, at times, that there is an absence of reasonable scholarship in searching out relevant studies.

Most of the above reviews raise common methodological issues. For example, highlighted by all were questions about the adequacy of the contrast, or control, groups. Generally, there are two types of contrast groups used to evaluate the effects of relocation: (1) baseline data on populations prior to the move and (2) contrasting samples drawn from individuals who are not relocated. Since, with one minor exception, no relocation studies manage randomized designs, the distinction made in the literature by some of the reviewers between baseline information and what has been incorrectly termed experimental studies using a contrasting group appear to be questionable. Often in studies involving the movement from one institutional setting to another, the groups chosen for relocation compared with those not chosen may differ in important characteristics that can affect outcome rates. Similarly, of course, other sources of bias arise when one looks at past rates of mortality along with changes that can and have occurred in institutional populations (e.g., increased average age of institutionalization).

Studies do differ in how well measured the contrast groups are; most rely on similar institutions using simple demographic comparisons. A few have directly assessed the control sample using the same set variables measured in the relocated sample. In the absence of true randomization designs, which are unlikely to be logistically feasible, the quality of effect evidence depends on the similarity between the relocated and contrast group. Too often in the studies reviewed, possible bias due to selection differences was an equally plausible hypothesis to account for the sample differences.

Some reviewers point to the problems in comparing "apples and oranges" when relying on a distinction of forced versus voluntary relocation. A quick review of Table 1, however, suggests that almost all of the studies involved forced relocation. The few that are clearly not forced involve other conditions that make it difficult to evaluate this variable across studies. As will be discussed later in this chapter, reliance on subject testimony to index whether a move is voluntary may be problematic.

Another condition used to account for differences among studies' rates of impact is preparation prior to relocation. All studies with the exception of three studies representing disaster-caused relocations (Aleksandrowicz, 1961; Kowalski, 1978; Silverstone & Kirschner, 1974) involve some level of preparation of the elderly prior to relocation. It has been a canon in relocation policy (not necessarily based upon good empirical evidence) that, prior to moving the frail elderly, extensive methods for preparing them to anticipate the move are critical. Despite the lack of sound empirical evidence, all studies of relocation of the frail elderly, with the few exceptions mentioned, involve populations that had undergone some form of preparation making it impossible to meaningfully evaluate the effects of this "experimental manipulation" across diverse studies. Some of the studies summarized in Table 1 report on experimentally generate level or type of preparation, but few, if any, involve the null condition (i.e., no preparation).

Conceptual Explanations and Relocation Effect

How has the field attempted to explain the differences in the impact of relocation? The evidence suggests that there are instances where relocation has the "feared impact" (i.e., increase in excessive mortality compared with a contrast group). In studies that have expanded the evaluation to include the individual level of well-being assessed by measures of physical health, psychological health, and social functioning, the range of evidence for the negative effects of relocation becomes somewhat more apparent. It is useful to remind ourselves that not only are there negative effects but, depending on the study cited, evidence exists that some people improve in their functioning subsequent to relocation. In general, rates of improvement are not as high as are negative impacts, but they still exist and are observable. There are several major factors that need to be taken into account as sources of influence on observed positive and negative changes subsequent to relocation. Since relocation involves the change from one environmental setting to another, the influence of environment qua environment must be assessed. If the relocation involves moving from the community to an institutional setting, one must consider that institutions obviously differ widely in the quality of their services and their potential for enhancing functioning. If the relocation involves moving from one institutional setting to another, it is again reasonable to assume that in some instances the institution to which people move may be a highly beneficial environment capable of enhancing conditions or even "countering" relocation effects.

The conceptual underpinnings of relocation as a stress rests upon fundamental principles well documented in the history of stress research: that the ability to anticipate future events, to experience feelings about such events, and to form attachments—to other people, to places, and to things—are fundamental human characteristics. Because of such attachments, losses as well as potential losses can critically affect psychological and physical functioning. In short, *because of its symbolic meaning, relocation is a potential stressor for many under this view.*

An alternative explanatory construct is that relocation, a major life-space change, constitutes a crisis because it demands new adaptive efforts in a new environment. Relocation constitutes a stress to the degree that it disrupts customary modes of behavior and imposes a need for strenuous psychological work. From this perspective, relocation presents the individual with the need to abandon many assumptions about the everyday world, with the challenge of replacing them with others. This may involve new mechanisms for relating to and filling needs in a social world that are either not in the individual's current repertoire or require considerable efforts to accomplish. *This view of relocation as a stress, then, is one of overload of capacity required to meet the new demands.*

The ideal world for a reviewer would provide studies reflecting measurements of environments and environmental discrepancy (the amount of environmental change actually experienced by a relocatee), as well as assessment addressing directly or indirectly the meaning hypothesis. Such a data base of studies would make the task of generalizing across investigations a reasonable and meaningful one. Then, observations that studies differ markedly in outcome magnitudes, leaving aside error effects due to method and design, would provide the necessary data base for making meaningful statements about the effects of relocations, the conditions under which they occur, and the individuals they involve. Unfortunately, the accumulated studies of relocation do not begin to approach this ideal. What follows is a summary of the efforts of past reviews in organizing the empirical literature.

Coffman (1981), foremost among the previous reviewers, contributed most to distinguishing relocation studies on the basis of imputed stress. He compared relocation studies involving a disrupted population (e.g., involved when an institution had closed down or its members were redistributed) with studies in which an intact social structure was maintained. Although the imputed distinction between what he calls Type 1 and Type 2 studies is open to serious question (since it is based upon indirect evidence rather than direct measurement of environments), the results reported by Coffman suggest that the condition under which the change takes place and the type of change itself are linked to mortality rates (the only outcome measure Coffman considered in his review).

Schulz and Brenner (1977) present a cognitive framework to explain the observed differences in the impact of relocation among various studies. They suggest that (1) the greater the choice the individual has in being relocated, the less negative the effects of relocation; (2) the more predictive the new environment is, the less negative the effects of relocation; and (3) an individual's response to relocation is mediated by the difference in environmental controllability between pre- and postrelocation environments. Unfortunately, as is similar to the dilemmas faced by Coffman, evidence across studies providing either for Coffman's framework of disruptive and integrative environmental changes or information permitting the reviewer to designate differences in studies based upon cognitive variables is severely limited. In short, despite the availability of conceptual models to explicate the source of stress associated with relocation, as well as the existence of models and measurements, the available empirical studies generally do not permit reasonable assessment of either Coffman's or the Schulz–Brenner hypothesis.

Factors Affecting Relocation Outcomes

This section reviews studies that provide information on processes associated with outcome. Three areas are considered: (1) the symbolic meaning of the relocation, (2) the environmental change hypothesis, and (3) the risk factors.

Exploration of the Meaning Hypothesis— Anticipations and Expectations

Three general strategies are used to examine the relationship between expectations, anticipations, and relocation outcomes. Analyses are available both between and within studies where samples are differentiated on the basis of forced versus voluntary relocation (Ferrari, 1963; Wolk & Tellen, 1976; Zweig & Csank, 1975). No study has measured directly the underlying psychological variable, controllability. Unfortunately, the studies that do exist are sufficiently flawed, limiting confidence in the general conclusions that can be drawn about the effects of voluntary/involuntary relocation. When the comparisons are within a study, the comparability of the subsamples can be seriously questioned. For example, in the Wolk and Tellen (1976) study, those moved involuntarily in all likelihood were in much poorer health than those who had a choice; and in the Schrut (1965) study, those who moved from community to institutional settings compared with apartment dwellings constituted populations with different health and functional levels. Attempts to compare across studies falter because the overwhelming majority of involuntary studies contain more debilitated people than do samples of voluntary movement.

Even in these few voluntary move studies of relocation from community to homes for the aged for social reasons, the "voluntariness" of the move is open to question. Tobin and Lieberman (1976) and Lieberman and Tobin (1983) compared the movement from community to homes for the aged with three other relocation settings. They found that in the move from community to homes for the aged the elderly had more positive feelings about leaving the setting they were living in, did not anticipate many losses, and anticipated high levels of satisfaction once they were relocated. Such positive responses and the sense that they were in control of the situation were further supported by analyses of a specially constructed thematic apperception test (TAT) reflecting institutional themes (Lieberman & Lakin, 1963). Stories told by subjects (those who had applied to and had been accepted by the institution) attributed much more control to the elderly person portrayed in various stages of entering and living in an institution. Comparisons, however, between this relocation study and those in which respondents reported much less control and felt they were "forced" to move did not reveal outcome differences. Furthermore, responses to the same TAT cards after living in the institution six months demonstrated considerably less "control themes," including choice in entering the institution, raising questions about the validity of the Time 1 measures. Assessment, based only on self-report used in most voluntary/involuntary studies, may reflect socially desirable responses and/or defensive postures.

What about studies that directly assess anticipations and expectations? Lieberman and Tobin (1983) utilized identical methods in three relocation studies: (1) "unwilling old ladies" (involving the closing of an institution and residents moving to another radically different type of institution), (2) "home for life study" (involving "volunteer" applicants to homes for the aged), and (3) the "Institutionalized Elite" (involving selected samples of elderly living in a state mental hospital's special geriatric ward who were relocated to a variety of institutional settings). There were major differences in conscious appraisals of threat and loss in the studies, although differences in long-term adaptation (based on changes in physical, psychological, and behavioral measures) were not found. Analyses of individual differences within each of the three studies revealed that there were no substantial linkages between measures of threat or loss and outcome. Level of threat intensity was linked to increased depressive reactions (measures taken two months after relocation); however, there was no relationship between reactions and outcome (i.e., one-year adaptation).

Lieberman and Tobin (1983) pursued an alternative strategy for measuring threat and loss, one not dependent on conscious responses open to social desirability bias. To measure threat, difference scores were computed measuring the level of cognitive performance on two sets of TAT cards, the standard Murray TAT and the institutional TAT. Levels of cognitive performance on these TATs were found to be equivalent for a community-living sample of elderly matched to those awaiting entrance into institutions. Threat was defined as poorer cognitive performance on the institutional TAT compared with the Murray TAT.

The indirect method to assess loss relied on an analysis of loss themes in early memories. Findings comparing those awaiting institutionalization with control groups suggest that elderly about to be relocated experience significantly more threat and loss. However, no evidence was developed that variations in threat and loss were substantially associated with outcomes (one-year morbidity, mortality, psychiatric disability, and social-behavioral assessments) or with most measures of reactions (based on two to three months' postrelocation). Threat and loss were significantly associated with affect and self-perception. Such reactions, however, did not predict one-year outcomes.

Evidence has been gathered in a variety of relocation studies on preparation that is assumed to impact on the relocatees' cognitive sets. As indicated earlier, almost all studies involve preparation. Thus, the ability to compare across studies to determine the effects of preparation and the implied cognitive restructuring is severely limited. Studies by Jasnau (1967), Bourestom & Pastalan (1975), and Zweig and Csank (1975) have been cited by some reviewers as providing evidence for the efficacy of preparation in reducing negative outcomes. The problems of comparable samples, particularly since studies did not test the null hypothesis, and of the sample biases that occurred in the cited studies make it impossible to clearly determine whether preparation has a measurable effect on relocated samples.

Our review of the available evidence does not support the hypothesis that cognitive sets (i.e., the meaning of relocation to the respondent) have an impact on outcome. However, given the substantial empirical and conceptual research on cognition and stress, we would probably be foolhardy to discard this as a viable hypothesis for further research.

The Environmental Discrepancy Hypothesis

The simple form of this hypothesis views relocation as a stressor because it requires or demands new adaptive efforts; relocation constitutes a stress to the degree that it disrupts customary modes of behavior and imposes a need for strenuous psychological work. Many problems are encountered in relocation research that attempts to put into operation and test this relatively straightforward hypothesis. Several "artifacts" must be taken into account prior to utilizing data for testing the hypothesis. Most significantly, the effects observed in a relocation study may not result from environmental change or discrepancy but rather may be a product of the quality of the prior and post environments. The relationship between behavior and environment is well known, and thus some of the observed effects noted in our review of the relocation research can be attributed to a hypothesis more parsimonious than that of environmental discrepancy. A second major artifact, particularly in those studies that have followed populations from communities to institutions, has come to be known as the "waiting list" effect. Several studies have demonstrated that some effects previously thought to be attributable to living in an institution or associated with environmental change are in fact characteristic of samples waiting to enter institutions. It is not the environment per se under those conditions, but rather the effects attributable to the symbolic characteristics of what it means to become an institutionalized person (Sherwood and Glassmann, 1974; Tobin & Lieberman, 1976).

Difficulties of Conceptualizing and Measuring Environments

To some, environment implies physical attributes: size, pathway for mobility, and complexity. To the social geographer it may imply accessibility to transportation and community resources. For social psychologists, the environment may consist of the significant personal world that surrounds an individual for the formal and informal rules, regulations, and obligations of social interaction—the normative rules of behavior and contingencies for reward and nonreward. To sociologists, environments may reflect the basic structural aspects of society and, particularly when the focus is on the elderly, the ability of the environment to maintain role behavior. Not only do conceptual frameworks of environments differ, but methods of measurement vary considerably. The work of Moose (1974), for example, utilizes well-developed schedules asking respondents for information about the environment. Lieberman and Tobin (1983) base their social-psychological categorization of environments on observer ratings of the institutional environments.

Relocation studies report a variety of assessment strategies as well as conceptualization of environment. Bourestom and Tars (1974) used a quasi-experimental comparative method to examine the effects of environment and the movement of one group of elderly to a radically new environment (defined as new staff, new programs, and new people), and they contrasted this with a moderate change where elderly were moved to a new building but the staff and patients remained the same. No measures were taken directly, but it was assumed that these two conditions were the active ingredients and could account for the observed differences in outcomes. Other investigators (e.g., Markson & Cumming, 1974), in a large study of movement of mental hospital patients, utilized formal characteristics, staff–patient ratios, and institution size as a proxy for environment.

Lieberman and Tobin (1983) examined environments directly measuring environmental characteristics before and after relocation. They employed a variety of strategies. Their first study was based upon the assumption that individuals differ in the ease with which their preinstitutional life-styles fit into the particular demands of the specific institution. Intensity of relocation stress was defined using an assessment model of institutional demands based on personality characteristics of successful elderly living in the institution (judgments of success based upon elderly who had lived in the institution for at least three years and were currently functioning at social, psychological, and physical levels to meet admission standards). Those about to be relocated were studied to determine how well their personalities matched those of the successful "old-timers." A positive relationship was found between congruence and low rates of negative one-year outcome.

In their study of the institutionalized elite, Lieberman and Tobin (1983) assessed needs at Time 1. At Time 2, ratings based upon observation were used to assess environments in 26 different institutions. Eleven dimensions were developed on the basis of the observational ratings: achievement, individuation, dependency, warmth, affiliation, recognition, stimulation, physical attractiveness, cue richness, tolerance for deviancy, and adequacy of health care. It was found that the quality of the new environment contributed substantially and significantly to the level of adaptation. An overall test of the fit hypothesis could not be calculated because the number of subjects mismatched (Time 1 needs and Time 2 environment) was low. They tested the variant of the Lawton environmental docility hypothesis by dividing their sample into those showing high and low signs of aging. Those showing many signs of aging were least responsive to environmental contingencies, and their adaptation was not based upon the characteristic quality of the environment; conversely, those who showed few signs of aging demonstrated that the level of adaptation measured one year after relocation was highly contingent upon environmental characteristics.

In the "death of an institution" study, Lieberman and Tobin (1983) evaluated 427 patients who were moved from a large state mental hospital geriatric wards to 142 different facilities. The methods used in the previous study (Institutional Elites) were used to assess both Time 1 and Time 2 environments. Analysis based upon one-year outcomes found that environmental discrepancy had a significant impact on future adaptation. Elderly who were moved into environments similar to those whence they came were likely to maintain stability; environmental discrepancies, on the other hand, produced adaptational instability. This instability, however, when coupled with certain environmental characteristics, often led to improvement; similar levels of environmental discrepancy, in the context of nonfacilitating environments, led to deterioration.

Overall, the evidence does suggest that environmental discrepancy as a source of stress is a viable hypothesis. It is, however, not a straightforward hypothesis since discrepancy alone does not appear to have consistently negative effects. The findings from the Lieberman and Tobin group of studies suggest that, akin to many other stressors, moves can be both facilitative as well as debilitating. A comparative analysis by Lieberman and Tobin (1983) of the contribution of various classes of variables (individual resources, expectations, personality, and environment) found that environmental variables account for most of the variation across studies in explaining differences in adaptation. That environment plays a large role in adaptation seems a reasonable conclusion, and, thus, using the level of environmental discrepancy to index stress intensity is a supportable hypothesis. The simple hypothesis, however, that the imputed effects of relocation, assessed by indexing morbidity, mortality, and maladaptation, are linked directly to the amount of environmental change is not borne out by the empirical research.

Risk Factors

Even a casual reading of the various research literatures on stress and adaptation would reveal a rich and complex chain of investigations characterizing person variables mediating the effects on stress and adaptation. Unfortunately, this research history is not echoed in the relocation literature. Relocation studies examining risk factors have overemphasized prior physical health and cognitive functioning. In large part this emphasis has been dictated by preoccupation with mortality as the single outcome of interest. It has been found that elderly who are in poor physical health and/or who have serious cognitive deficits are more likely to be among the group of individuals who are dead within one year after relocation. Such repeated findings do little to add to our conceptual understanding of relocation.

A minority of investigators have addressed more classical issues found in the stress literature. Aldrich (1964) and Aldrich and Mendkoff (1963), as well as Lieberman, Tobin, and their colleagues, examined personality assessed prior to relocation as predictors of negative consequences associated with relocation. Both studies found that certain personality types put individuals more at risk than others. In a few studies, positive associations between prerelocation characteristics—such as affective states—and coping strategies are reported (Lieberman & Tobin, 1983). The sparsity of studies in this area, however, precludes even modest generalizations.

Pruchno and Resch (1988) and Lieberman and Tobin (1983) examined the relationship between person characteristics and environment and reported similar findings about the relationship among environmental discrepancy, the stressor, and person characteristics. Those more vulnerable to the stress generated by environmental discrepancy are the more intact elderly.

Future progress in the study of risk factors requires attention to several currently clouded conceptual areas. Lieberman and Tobin (1983) have suggested that adaptive characteristics among the elderly may be age-specific. Comparing their findings with studies on stress in younger populations, they found that characteristics adaptive in the elderly may be different from, and at times opposed to, the same characteristics shown to mitigate stress responses in younger populations.

The complexity of the problem of investigating characteristics of individuals and their relationship to the environment, specifically as relates to mitigating stress, is further underscored by choices required for measuring outcomes. The underlying assumption in all relocation research (as it is in most stress studies) is a homeostatic view of outcome. Failure is measured by departures in a negative direction from prior level of functioning; success is measured by absence of change. Outcome models based upon different principles (e.g., enhancement of functioning) have not pervaded this area of research. In a small test of the implications involved in using different outcome assumptions, Lieberman and Tobin (1983) utilized an enhancement model rather than a homeostatic model to reanalyze their data linking personality characteristics and outcome. Such an analysis yielded different personality characteristics linked to positive outcomes compared with those personality characteristics that predicted outcomes measured by a homeostatic framework. Thus, establishing careful linkages between outcome and risk factors associated with characteristics of the person prior to the stress condition may very well depend on the type of assumptions made about outcomes. Recent work by Yalom and Lieberman (1991) on reactions to bereavement by middle-age and elderly widows suggests a similar conclusion. Traditional measures of reactions to bereavement, level and intensity of grieving, mental health, and social functioning (a homeostatic model) were compared with a model based upon enhanced functioning (labeled *growth* by these investigators). It was found that these models of outcome were orthogonal and that the characteristics predicting one would not consistently predict the other.

Recommendations for Future Research

Despite the number of years gerontologists have invested in studying relocation, and despite the accrued knowledge represented by the collection of studies and conceptual analyses, simple, straightforward answers elude us as to what the effects of relocating the frail elderly are and what factors in the person or conditions of the relocation explain the observed effects. Explanations for this present state of affairs are many. Much of the early research was energized by investigators' concern with the human toll they believed relocation engendered. This preoccupation skewed the research toward an emphasis on the dramatic, which was usually translated into examinations of increased mortality rates. All too frequent was the absence of concern for adequate measurement and, perhaps even more important, measurement linked to and embedded within a theoretical framework.

Of necessity, much of the relocation research has been opportunistic in the sense that investigators have been required to take advantage of real-life situations that have occurred periodically and that have been frequently embedded in complex political circumstances. These constraints, which precluded the planning of a series of studies, almost always resulted in less-than-stellar experimental designs and made true randomization always beyond the investigators' grasp.

The history of this research, however, does provide a useful documentation of both the problems encountered and the solutions needed. To develop appropriate research, several steps need to be taken. A consistent framework for measuring the effects of relocation would go a long way toward making it possible to accumulate knowledge. The preoccupation with the field of excessive mortality rates has distorted the measurement of impact. Sensitive measures examining physical as well as mental health and social functioning based on individual scores is a viable and, in this investigator's view, more meaningful strategy. Indexing how much change takes place for individuals in both positive or negative directions based upon their prior functioning provides a much more sensitive indicator of what happens to people when they are relocated. Furthermore, reliance on mortality rates usually requires relatively larger samples compared with studies that cast a larger net of outcome measures. The all-too-necessary compromise involved in overcoming low base rates by increasing sample size for excessive mortality studies has often led to limitation of process measures and precision of control groups.

In the absence of random designs, more care must be given to the selection and assessment of contrast groups that can serve as control conditions. Matched groups in which the known characteristics are associated with subsequent physical, mental, and social behavior need to be constructed in order to assess, in precise ways, the effects of relocation.

Relocation effects and the processes linked to them can be fully understood only if we avoid the black-box strategy characteristic of so many relocation studies. Ample conceptual systems exist for the formation of a framework involving the impacts of relocation. Whether we see it in terms of cognitive characteristics of the person in interaction with the situations or in terms of environmental conditions, in any one particular relocation situation there will be variations in how stressed individuals are. Without attention to direct measurement of these variations, an accurate understanding of how process affects relocation cannot be constructed. To assume homogeneity based upon type of relocation without evidence for each individual involved is to make an unwarranted assumption in a given research context that rarely, if ever, permits true experimental variation.

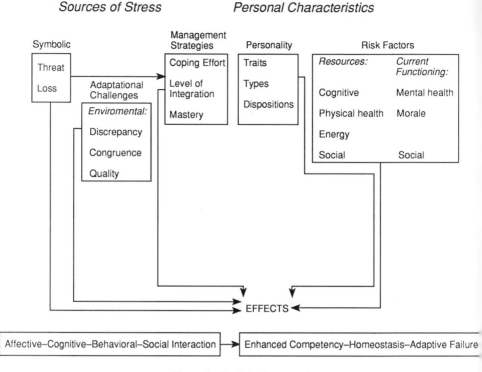

Figure 1 Predictor framework.

Lieberman and Tobin (1983) published a monograph on the series of relocation studies that presented a framework for such work. A modified version of this framework has been reproduced here. It is not assumed that this is the only, or even the best, framework, but rather it is intended to communicate that in order to understand relocation in all its ramifications, a relatively complex model is required. Empirical evidence reviewed in this chapter does exist to fill all of the categories portrayed in Figure 1, albeit often at a highly speculative level and in incomplete form.

References

Aldrich, C. K. (1964). Personality factors and mortality in the relocation of the aged. *The Gerontologist, 2,* 92–93.

Aldrich, C. K., & Mendkoff, E. (1963). Relocation of the aged and disabled: A mortality study. *Journal of the American Geriatrics Society, 11,* 185–193.

Aleksandrowicz, D. (1961). Fire and its aftermath on a geriatric ward. *Bulletin of Menninger Clinic, 25,* 23–32.

Anderson, N. N. (1967). Effects of institutionalization on self-esteem. *Journal of Gerontology, 22,* 313.

Beaver, M. L. (1979). The decision-making process and its relationship to relocation adjustment in old people. *The Gerontologist, 19,* 567–574.

Bennett, R., and Nahemov, L. D. (1965). The relation between social isolation, socialization, and adjustment in residents of a home for aged. In M. P. Lawton & F. G. Lawton, eds., *Mental impairment of the aged,* pp. 88–105. Philadelphia: Philadelphia Geriatric Center.

Blenkner, M. (1967). Environmental change and the aging individual. *The Gerontologist, 7,* 101–105.

Bortner, R. W. (1962). Test differences attributable to age, selection processes, and institutional effects. *Journal of Gerontology, 23,* 343.

Borup, J. H., Gallego, D. T., & Heffernan, P. G. (1979). Relocation and its effect on mortality. *The Gerontologist, 19,* 135–140.

Bourestom, N., & Pastalan, L. (1975). *Final report, forced relocation: Setting staff, and patient effects.* Manuscript, University of Michigan, Wayne State University, Institute of Gerontology. Ann Arbor, Michigan.

Bourestom, N., & Tars, S. (1974). Alterations in life patterns following nursing home relocation. *The Gerontologist, 14,* 506–510.

Brand, F., & Smith, R. (1974). Life adjustment and relocation of the elderly. *Journal of Gerontology, 29,* 336–340.

Brody, E., Kleban, M., & Moss, M. (1974). Measuring the impact of change. *The Gerontologist, 14,* 299–305.

Camargo, O., & Preston, G. H. (1945). What happens to patients who are hospitalized for the first time when over 65? *American Journal of Psychiatry, 102,* 168–173.

Carp, F. (1966). *A future for the aged.* Austin, Texas: University of Texas Press.

Carp, F. M. (1968a). Person-situation congruence in engagement. *The Gerontologist, 8,* 184.

Carp, F. M. (1968b). Effects of improved housing on the lives of older people. In B. Neugarten, ed., *Middle age and aging.* Chicago: University of Chicago Press.

Coffman, T. L. (1981). Relocation and survival of institutionalized aged: A reexamination of the evidence. *The Gerontologist, 21,* 483–500.

Cook, L. C., Dax, E. C., & Maclay, W. S. (1952). The geriatric problem in mental hospitals. *Lancet, 1,* 377.

Costello, J. P., & Tanaka, G. M. (1961). Mortality and morbidity in long-term institutional care of the aged. *Journal of the American Geriatrics Society, 9,* 959–966.

Csank, J. Z., & Zweig, J. P. (1980). Relative mortality of chronically ill geriatric patients with organic brain damage, before and after relocation. *Journal of the American Geriatrics Society, 28,* 76–83.

Dube, A. H. (1982). The impact of moving a geriatric population: Mortality and emotional aspects. *Journal of Chronic Diseases, 35,* 61–64.

Eckert, J. Kevin & Haug, Marie (1984). The impact of forced residential relocation on the health of the elderly hotel dweller. *Journal of Gerontology, 39*(6) 753–755.

Epstein, L. J., Robinson, B. C., & Simon, A. (1971). Predictors of survival of geriatric mental illness during the eleven years after initial hospital admission. *Journal of the American Geriatrics Society, 19,* 913–922.

Ferrari, N. A. (1963). Freedom of choice. *Social Work, 8,* 105.

Ferraro, K. F. (1983). The health consequences of relocation among the aged in the community. *Journal of Gerontology, 38*(1) 90–96.

Friedman, E. P. (1966). Spatial proximity and social interaction in a home for the aged. *Journal of Gerontology, 21,* 566.

Gelfand, D. E. (1968). Visiting patterns and social adjustment in an old age home. *The Gerontologist, 8,* 272.

Goldfarb, A. I. (1964). The evaluation of geriatric patients following treatment. In P. H. Hock & J. Zubin, eds., *The evaluation of psychiatric treatment,* pp. 271–308. New York: Grune and Stratton.

Goldfarb, A. I., Shahinian, S. P., & Burr, H. T. (1972). Death rate of relocated residents. In D. P. Kent, R. Kastenbaum, & S. Sherwood, eds., *Research planning and action for the elderly.* New York: Behavioral Publications.

Gutman, G. M., & Herbert, C. P. (1976). Mortality rates among relocated extended-care patients. *Journal of Gerontology, 31,* 352–357.

Haddad, L. B. (1981). Intra-institutional relocation: Measured impact on geriatric patients. *Journal of the American Geriatrics Society, 29,* 86–88.

Jasnau, K. F. (1967). Individualized versus mass transfer of nonpsychotic geriatric patients from mental hospitals to nursing homes, with special reference to death rate. *Journal of the American Geriatrics Society, 15,* 280–284.

Josephy, H. (1949). Analysis of mortality and causes of death in a mental hospital. *American Journal of Psychiatry, 106,* 185.

Kasl, S. (1972). Physical and mental health effects of involuntary relocation and institutionalization on the elderly—A review. *American Journal of Public Health, 62,* 377–383.

Kesteler, J., Gray, R., & Carruth, M. (1968). Involuntary relocation of the elderly. *The Gerontologist, 8,* 276–279.

Kay, D. W. K., Norris, Y., & Post, F. (1956). Prognosis in psychiatric disorders of the elderly. *Journal of Mental Sciences, 102,* 129.

Kent, E. A. (1963). Role of admission stress in adaptation of older persons in institutions. *Geriatrics, 16,* 515.

Killian, E. (1970). Effects of geriatric transfers on mortality rates. *Social Work, 15,* 19–26.

Kowalski, N. C. (1978). Fire at home for the aged: A study of short-term mortality following dislocation of elderly residents. *Journal of Gerontology, 33*(4) 601–602.

Kowalski, N. C. (1981). Institutional relocation: Current programs and applied approaches. *The Gerontologist, 21,* 512–519.

Kral, V. A., Grad, B., & Berenson, J. (1968). Stress reactions resulting from the relocation of an aged population. *Canadian Psychiatric Association Journal, 13,* 201–209.

Lawton, M. P., & Nahemow, L. (1973). Ecology and the aging process. In The psychology of adult development and aging. C. Eisdorfer and M. P. Lawton (eds.) p. 718. XIV. Washington, D.C.: American Psychology Association.

Lawton, M. P., & Cohen, J. (1974). The generality of housing impact on the well-being of older people. *Journal of Gerontology, 29,* 194–204.

Lawton, M. P., and Simon, B. (1968). The ecology of social relationships in housing for the elderly. *The Gerontologist, 8,* 108.

Lawton, M. P., & Yaffe, S. (1970). Mortality, morbidity, and voluntary change of residence by older people. *Journal of the American Geriatrics Society, 18,* 823–831.

Lieberman, M. A. (1961). Relationship of mortality rates to entrance to a home for the aged. *Geriatrics, 16,* 515–519.

Lieberman, M. A. (1966). Factors in environmental change. In F. M. Carp & W. M. Burnette, eds., *Patterns of living and housing of middle-aged and old people.* P.H.S. Publication 1496, pp. 117–125. Washington, D.C.: U.S. Dept. of Health, Education and Welfare.

Lieberman, M. A. (1969). Institutionalization of the aged: Effects on behavior. *Journal of Gerontology, 24,* 330–340.

Lieberman, M. A. (1974). Relocation research and social policy. *The Gerontologist, 16*(6), 494–501.

Lieberman, M. A., & Lakin, M. (1963). On becoming an institutionalized aged person. In R. H. Williams *et al.,* eds., *Process of aging, vol. 1, pp. 475–503.* New York: Atherton Press.

Lieberman, M. A., & Tobin, S. S. (1983). *The experience of old age: Stress, coping and survival.* New York: Basic Books.

Lieberman, M. A., Tobin, S., & Slover, D. (1971). *The effects of relocation on long-term geriatric patients.* (Final Rep. Proj. No. 17-1328). Illinois Dept. of Health & Committee on Human Development, University of Chicago.

Linn, M. W., & Gurel, L. (1969). Initial reactions to nursing home placement. *Journal of the American Geriatrics Society, 17,* 219.

Markson, E., & Cumming, J. (1974). A strategy of necessary mass transfer and its impact on patient mortality. *Journal of Gerontology, 29,* 315–321.

Markus, E. (1970). Post-relocation mortality among institutionalized aged. Mimeo. Cleveland: Benjamin Rose Institute.

Markus, E., Blenkner, M., Bloom, M., & Downs, T. (1970). Relocation stress and the aged. *Interdisciplinary Topics in Gerontology, 7,* 60–71.

Markus, E., Blenkner, M., Bloom, M., & Downs, T. (1971). The impact of relocation upon mortality rates of institutionalized aged persons. *Journal of Gerontology, 26,* 537–541.

Markus, E., Blenkner, M., Bloom, M., & Downs, T. (1972). Some factors and their association with post-relocation mortality among institutionalized aged persons. *Journal of Gerontology, 27,* 376–382.

Marlowe, R. A. (1974). When they closed the doors at Modesto. Paper presented at National Institute of Mental Health Conference on the closure of state hospitals, February 14–15. Scottsdale, Ariz.

Miller, D., & Lieberman, M. A. (1965). The relationship of affect state and adaptive capacity to reactions to stress. *Journal of Gerontology, 20,* 492–497.

Mirotznik, J., & Ruskin, A. P. (1984). Inter-institutional relocation and its effects on health. *The Gerontologist, 24,* 286–291.

Moose, R. H. (1974). *Evaluating treatment environments: A social ecological approach.* New York: John Wiley and Sons.

Nirenberg, T. D. (1983). Relocation of institutionalized elderly. *Journal of Consulting and Clinical Psychology, 52,* 693–701.

Novick, L. J. (1967). Easing the stress of moving day. *Hospitals, 41,* 64–74.

Ogren, E. H., & Linn, M. W. (1971). Male nursing home patients: Relocation and mortality. *Journal of the American Geriatrics Society, 19,* 229–239.

Pihkanen, T., & Lahdenpera, M. (1963). Observations of the effects produced by hospital transfer in a group of chronic neuropsychiatric and geriatric patients. *Acta Psychiatrica Scandinavica, 18,* 167–172.

Pino, C. J., Rosica, L. M., & Carter, T. J. (1978). The differential effects of relocation on nursing home patients. *The Gerontologist, 18,* 167–172.

Prock, V. N. (1965). Effects of institutionalization—A comparison of community, waiting list, and institutionalized aged persons. Doctoral diss., Chicago: University of Chicago.

Pruchno, R. A., & Resch, N. L. (1988). Institutional relocation: Mortality effects. *The Gerontologist, 28,* 311–317.

Rodstein, M., Savitsky, E., & Starkman, R. (1976). Initial adjustment to a long-term care institution: Medical and behavioral aspects. *Journal of the American Geriatrics Society, 24,* 65–71.

Schooler, K. K. (1969a). The relationship between social interaction and morale of the elderly as a function of environmental characteristics. *The Gerontologist, 9,* 25.

Schooler, K. K. (1969b). On the relation between characteristics of residential environment, social behavior, and the emotional and physical health of the elderly in the United States. Paper presented at the Eighth International Congress of Gerontology, Washington, D.C.

Schooler, K. K. (1976). Environmental change and the elderly. In I. Altman & J. F. Wohlwill, eds., *Human behavior and environment,* vol. 1. New York: Plenum Press.

Schulz, R. (1976). The effects of control and predictability on the physical and psychological well-being of the institutionalized age. *Journal of Personality and Social Psychology, 33,* 563–673.

Schulz, R., & Aderman, D. (1973). Effect of residential change on the temporal distance to death of terminal cancer patients. *Omega: Journal of Death and Dying, 4,* 157–162.

Schulz, R., & Brenner, G. (1977). Relocation of the aged: A review and theoretical analysis. *Journal of Gerontology, 32,* 323–333.

Shamian, J., Clarfield, A. M., & Maclean, J. (1984). A randomized trial of intra-hospital relocation of geriatric patients in a tertiary-care teaching hospital. *Journal of the American Geriatrics Society, 32,* 794–800.

Sherwood, S., Glassman, J., Sherwood, C., & Morris, J. N. (1974). Pre-institutional factors as predictors of adjustment to a long-term care facility. *International Journal of Aging and Human Development, 5,* 95–105.

Sherwood, S., Greer, D. S., Morris, J. N., Mor, V. (1981). *An alternative to institutionalization.* Cambridge, Mass.: Ballinger.

Silberstein, M. H. (1979). Moving a nursing home with minimal trauma. Paper presented at the meeting of the Gerontological Society. November, Washington, D.C.

Silverstone, B. M., & Kirschner, C. (1974). Elderly residents' reactions to enforced relocation during a hospital strike. *The Gerontologist, 14,* 71.

Storandt, M., & Wittels, I. (1975). Maintenance of function in relocation of community-dwelling older adults. *Journal of Gerontology, 30,* 608–612.

Stotsky, B. A. (1967). A controlled study of factors in successful adjustment of mental patients to nursing homes. *American Journal of Psychiatry, 123,* 1243–1251.

Tobin, S. S., & Lieberman, M. A. (1976). *Last home for the aged.* San Francisco: Jossey-Bass.

Triers, T. R. (1968). A study of change among elderly psychiatric inpatients during their first year of hospitalization. *Journal of Gerontology, 23,* 354.

Turner, B., Tobin, S., & Lieberman, M. (1972). Personality traits as predictors of institutional adaptation among the aged. *Journal of Gerontology, 27,* 61–68.

Wells, L. & MacDonald, G. (1981). Interpersonal networks & post-relocation adjustment of the institutionalized elderly. *Gerontologist, 21*(2) 177–183.

Whittier, J. R., & Williams, D. (1956). The coincidence and constancy of mortality figures for aged psychotic patients admitted to state hospitals. *Journal of Nervous and Mental Disorders, 124,* 618–620.

Wittels, I., & Botwinick, J. (1974). Survival in relocation. *Journal of Gerontology, 29,* 440–443.

Wolk, S. & Telleen, S. (1976). Psychological and social correlates of life satisfaction as a function of residential constraint. *Journal of Gerontology, 31*(1) 89–98.

Yalom, I. & Lieberman, M. A. (1991). Spousal bereavement and heightened existential awareness. *Psychiatry,* in press.

Zweig, J., & Csank, J. (1975). Effects of relocation on chronically ill geriatric patients of a medical unit: Mortality rates. *Journal of the American Geriatrics Society, 23,* 132–136.

7

Assistive Devices, Robotics, and Quality of Life in the Frail Elderly

GEOFF FERNIE[1]

Introduction

Quality of life in old age may be usefully defined with respect to two parameters:

1. Retention by the individual of the ability to make choices
2. Community standards

Many developers of technology and providers of service emphasize the independence of the elderly as the primary goal. However, many of us enjoy interdependent life-styles in which we are dependent on other members of the family or community for some functions and they are dependent on us for others. Such dependency relationships can often be viewed as positive. In many cultures, dependence in old age is viewed as an entitlement and the elders are accorded great respect. Perhaps choice is a better objective.

Technology should help enable the elderly person to choose whether to continue to live in the family home or move to a retirement resort, whether to continue to work or travel during retirement, and whether to remain fiercely independent or enjoy a more supportive environment. Frequently, there is no choice but to move into a long-term care facility when familial caregivers can no longer cope. Similarly, because of a high work load, nurses in long-term care facilities are often not able to spend the amount of time with the individual and provide the quality of care that they would otherwise choose. In order to facilitate choice, therefore, technology must also be designed to help the caregiver.

In order to retain as many options to choose from as possible, the primary role of technology must be to assist the individual to be self-regulating, with a particular emphasis on those routine activities of daily living that are burdensome

[1]Dr. Fernie is a National Health Scholar, supported by Health and Welfare, Canada.

142

Copyright © 1991 by Academic Press, Inc.
All rights of reproduction in any form reserved.

or unattractive to caregivers. Removal of a functional dependence for routine tasks such as bathing, toileting, and feeding is likely to increase social interaction by minimizing resentment and stress experienced by the disabled elderly person and the caregivers. Some of these tasks, such as lifting, may be impossible for familial caregivers and should receive a high priority for technical assistance. The notion that sense of control and quality of life are interconnected is supported by Abeles in Chapter 14.

It has been suggested that quality of life is primarily a subjective measure made by the individual on the basis of past experiences and on expectations for the future (see, for example, Svensson, Chapter 12). Such a definition avoids the risk of the evaluator claiming to know what constitutes a reasonable quality of life for another individual. However, such a limited definition is unrealistic and regressive, since it follows logically that an individual whose experience with life has been poor may consider his or her quality of life to be acceptable under circumstances of modest improvement that would be considered unacceptable by others from more fortunate backgrounds.

Readers who have worked directly with the elderly in the community and in institutions know that conditions are sometimes appalling; such readers are likely to regard a definition that does not include reference to a community standard as impractical. Examples of relevant community standards covering different aspects of the definition of an acceptable quality of life include legislation on nursing home design and operation. This second aspect of the suggested definition of quality of life is usually oriented to the setting of a baseline standard for an acceptable quality of life as defined by the community and as supplemented by the subjective opinion of the individual. This is in accordance with Lawton's definition of the quality of life, expressed in Chapter 1, as "the multidimensional evaluation, by both intrapersonal and social-normative criteria, of the person–environment system of an individual in time past, current, and anticipated." The focus of this chapter is on the potential contribution of technology to the person–environment interface, and thence to the quality of life.

The growing awareness of commercial opportunities resulting from the explosive growth of the elderly population has not always been beneficial to the quality of life (Dychtwald & Flower, 1988; Fernie & Fernie, 1990; Minkler, 1989). Many of the products that are marketed tend to highlight disabilities. The present author is of the opinion that the guiding principle for the development and design of products for senior citizens is that, wherever possible, these products should be useful to all of us. Everyone benefits from products that are attractive, safe, and easy to operate. Moreover, products that are designed to appeal to a broad sector of the population will tend to be affordable because of economies of scale. Such products will also be readily available and will not stigmatize the elderly who choose to use them. In contrast, products designed for the sole use of people with specific disabilities will tend to label the user as being different, with the likely consequence of a loss of self-esteem and a greater awareness by others of differences. These outcomes may tend to inhibit the integration of the disabled user. Family caregivers contemplating moving an elderly person into their homes may be deterred by the disruption and stigmatization caused by the presence of equipment that is perceived to be unattractive to guests or hazardous to children.

Environment

The environment for the elderly includes social, medical, spiritual, and physical components. The focus of most gerontological programs is on social gerontology. These programs have promoted recognition of broader social issues in the quality of life, such as incomes and housing, and have provided a balance to the study of aging from the medical perspective. The spiritual aspects of aging are personal and of varied importance, but there is no way of avoiding the fact that we live in a physical world where technology has a profound effect on every aspect of our lives. Surprisingly, engineering gerontology is not as familiar a term as social or medical gerontology. *Engineering gerontology* might be defined as the study of gerontology from the perspective of the engineering sciences. The field would encompass the effect of technology on the aging process as well as the application of technology to minimize handicaps resulting from physical and mental disabilities associated with aging.

The choices of environment range from macroscopic questions, such as whether it is wise to move to a rural community upon retirement, to microenvironmental questions, such as whether one should give up wearing fashionable shoes and place emphasis on less attractive but safer and more comfortable footwear.

Products for the elderly should be designed for rural as well as urban settings. Many people with mobility disabilities have benefited in recent years from powered wheelchairs that are often depicted in advertisements as traveling along rough country paths. Several all-terrain vehicles have been designed for disabled people and even include a high-speed, long-range snowmobile for use by amputees and paraplegics.

The disabled rights movements have improved the accessibility of urban environments, particularly through curb cuts, ramped accessways, and wheelchair-accessible toilets. However, a more concerted effort should be devoted to finding ways of increasing safety for elderly pedestrians on streets that are becoming busier every day. The length of time permitted for crossing at traffic lights is usually inadequate, and yet if that time is increased to allow for the slowest individual at every light change at every intersection, congestion will increase significantly. This particular example is unusual since it involves striking a balance between enhancing the quality of life of the elderly at the expense of inconveniencing others. This is not a common circumstance since most technological improvements for the elderly are beneficial to people of all ages. Should equipment be developed to sense the presence of slow ambulators and adjust the control signals appropriately? Although such devices would not be essential, they would presumably be helpful to drivers and pedestrians of all ages, including mothers with small children, by avoiding unnecessary delays but providing increased time when it is needed.

Microenvironmental issues include such technologies as clothing and footwear. Reduced vision and dexterity sometimes make it difficult to don clothing. Several companies, including the largest manufacturer of wheelchairs, are now marketing highly fashionable clothing that is adapted for easy wearing by people with disabilities. At least one researcher has been experimenting with providing custom-sized and adapted clothing using computer-aided design methods. The present author's laboratory (the Centre for Studies in Aging of Sunnybrook Health Science Centre in Toronto) has participated in a collaborative project to develop computer-aided design and computer-assisted manufacturing (CAD/CAM) techniques for the production of custom footwear.

Since four-fifths of elderly people report foot problems, accessibility to improved footwear is of high priority. Better footwear might be expected to relieve discomfort and minimize the progression of foot deformities. Unfortunately, although there are growing numbers of chiropodists and podiatrists treating foot problems and providing customized inserts for shoes, there are rapidly dwindling numbers of craftsmen capable of making customized shoes. The concept behind the CAD/CAM footwear project involves placing the foot into a measuring instrument that provides a high-speed, three-dimensional record of the shape using laser scanning methods, followed by input of the shape to a CAD system (see Figure 1). Critical measurements are taken from the digitized shape by the computer and are used to select the most appropriate shoe last from a range of shoe last shapes stored in the disc files. The selected last shape is then mathematically scaled (squeezed and stretched) to match more exactly the dimensions of the individual foot. An image of the foot and of the last shape is presented on the computer screen such that the CAD operator may make minor adjustments to shape to accommodate specific deformities before sending a file of machine control instructions to a numerically controlled machine tool that carves a custom last for use in the manufacture of the shoe.

It is conceivable that shoes, and clothing in general, will eventually be routinely designed and made by similar techniques. The purchaser would simply select the color and style of the product and hand over an optically encoded card similar in appearance to a credit card that would contain his or her personal shape files. The automated machines in the factory would then make the product, which would be supplied one or two days later. The additional costs of such a service might be outweighed, at least to some extent, by obviating the need for

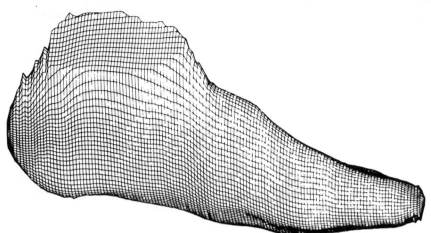

Figure 1   An example of a graphical representation of a foot (wearing a sock) produced using measurement data obtained by a high-speed foot-shape scanner. This scanner measures approximately 10,000 points on the surface of a foot in less than 3 sec and provides the input to a computer-aided custom-shoe design and manufacturing system.

large inventories of differently sized products and by providing the commercial advantage of being able to satisfy the customer by offering the latest fashion to order. Many elderly may be resistant to investigating the purchase of special footwear because of the stigma associated with the image of old-fashioned, rather bulky and ugly orthopedic shoes and boots. The availability of more attractive footwear through usual footwear stores is likely to influence more people to seek custom footwear as a preventive or treatment option.

Work

There are many issues associated with the ability of people in certain lines of work to continue to operate effectively and safely as they age. Even well before retirement age, arthritic and cardiovascular changes may make it difficult for a manual worker to continue with heavy tasks. It is not always easy to transfer that worker to light duties, since many of the more low-scaled clerical tasks have now been computerized. Ergonomists can recommend changes in workstation layout and equipment to reduce the physical stress; and simple biofeedback methods have been used to correct bad lifting techniques.

With the advent of robotics and automation, the physical demands of many jobs have decreased, but higher academic skills and levels of concentration are often required. Changes in aircraft cockpit design illustrate this trend. Pilots no longer need to touch the controls from takeoff to touchdown, but they must have the powers of concentration to identify quickly when the plane is malfunctioning and must have superior knowledge of the systems in order to correct the problem.

If an elderly person wishes to continue working at least part-time beyond retirement, he or she will find that the range of possible choices has increased because of the microcomputer, facsimile machine, and personal computer. In these days, when information is a valuable product, the simplicity and affordability of these electronic tools makes a part-time cottage industry a viable option. This may lead to increases in self-esteem, income, and motivation, with a consequent increase in the quality of life. Rehabilitation engineers have developed various assistive devices, such as robotic workstations for use by people with quadriplegia and voice synthesizers attached to word processors for use by the blind. These devices have become more reliable and affordable and now may sometimes be helpful for elderly with less severe degrees of disability.

However, elderly people have been found to be resistant to using computers. This may be attributed to the lack of familiarity with the newer technology as well as to other factors such as vision problems with computer screens. This reluctance may not extend to people who are motivated to use computers in a meaningful way in order to be able to continue to work from home, especially if the software and hardware are selected to provide a clear visual display and simple, menu- or icon-driven operation.

In the past, cottage industries were associated with low incomes. In the future, they may be associated with low overhead and high income. Word processing, accounting packages, and numerous other software tools make it possible for a resourceful individual to produce large volumes of work. The concept of a "factory in a box" is also becoming closer to reality. This concept implies a flexible machining system that adapts to making different products simply by the owner supplying different materials and files of computerized instructions. Small, tabletop, computer-controlled machining centers and molding machines already exist.

One particularly interesting new technology makes use of a laser to polymerize a resin. The machine consists of an elevating platform in a tank of circulating resin with a small laser mounted above on an x-y motion bed. The personal computer causes the laser to move and trace a cross section of an object in a fashion similar to a pen plotter. The resin polymerizes under the laser and the elevator advances. With successive cross sections being completed, a complex, three-dimensional form gradually grows. The technique is comparatively slow and its application is limited to certain prototypes manufactured presently, but one can envisage that similar technology will eventually make it practical to decentralize quite complex manufacturing processes. Although it would be far-fetched to suggest that such technology would be operated by the frail elderly, it is not, perhaps, unreasonable to envisage this technology reinforcing the ability of family members to provide care while continuing to earn income from home.

The development of cottage information processing and product manufacturing industries may reverse the trends whereby both partners in a marriage are usually working outside the home, making it impossible to care for elderly parents.

Recreation

Higher quality of life, increased positive socialization, and improved health are broadly accepted benefits of recreation (Mace, 1987; Needler & Baer, 1982). Various assistive devices have been engineered to enable the frail elderly to continue to participate to some degree in recreational activities that range from reading to active sports. Physical limitations may frequently be overcome by very simple devices. A very successful example is the bowling ramp. A bowling ball is placed on top of the ramp and the user helps, to the extent possible, aim the ramp and push the ball off the top. Another popular example is the adaptation of bingo cards. Frail elderly may not be able to place marks or objects on the numbers but may be able, through devices, to indicate that the number has been called. Cognitive dysfunction is usually addressed by simplifying the rules of the game.

Computer games are becoming more lifelike and familiar. This author recently had the experience of playing a computer golf game with an elderly individual who was once a professional golfer but who no longer has the physical ability to play golf. He was able to play at an expert level and was encouraged by the game to reminisce. These computer games also have the interesting possibility of allowing the user to play competitive games where the computer assumes the role of the other players.

Everyone has the right to choose recreation involving a reasonable degree of risk. For the very frail elderly, recreation may be limited to wandering. In the past, wandering was thought to be undesirable. Technology, in the form of restraints and barriers to movement, was used to limit activity and prevent the risk of creating a nuisance or becoming lost. The inappropriateness and ineffectiveness of restraints are recognized (Reisburg, Borenstein, Salob, Ferris, Franssen, & Georgolas, 1987; Risse & Barnes, 1986), and the advantages of the exercise and stimulation produced by wandering are accepted (Mace & Rabins, 1981; McGrowder-Lin & Bhatt, 1988). The level of risk may now be controlled by the use of electronic security devices. In the simplest form, these devices consist of door alarms that sound when the door is opened. More sophisticated devices make use of miniature circuits, often attached to wrist bands, that will sound an alarm and provide caregivers with the location of the exit and the identification of the individual. These systems have the advantage of allowing other individuals free passage without sounding alarms. Some wandering control devices include transmitters that are worn in a wristband or waistband and allow caregivers to find a wanderer who has left the building by using a tracking receiver to locate the transmitter signal.

It has been fashionable in long term-care institutions, at least in Ontario, to change the title of "social activities" programs to "activation" programs. However, elderly people may not always want to be "activated." It is important to accept leisure as a legitimate and healthy recreational activity. Technology should be developed to enable elderly people with disabilities to choose from their desires and not just from a restricted list of opportunities selected by someone else. Technology should empower people by facilitating choice from as wide a range of normal options available to nondisabled individuals as possible.

Activities of Daily Living

Although a degree of dependence may be acceptable, most people desire to be independent for essential, routine, daily activities. This independence enables individuals to preserve their dignity and ease the burdens of care giving.

Eating

Many needs can be met by careful selection of kitchen equipment and utensils for ergonomic features. Utensils with special handles suitable, for example, for arthritic hands are available from rehabilitation equipment suppliers. Many problems can be solved by rearranging storage and work surfaces. Nonslip mats and nonslip mixing bowls and plates can be useful for elderly who have lost the use of one arm through stroke. Although automatic feeding devices are rather inflexible and unattractive, some success has been achieved with robotic workstations for this purpose. Since some physical ability is required to prepare varied meals, and since it is desirable to eat in a social setting and to have assistance at hand in case of choking, personal feeding assistance is likely to be the most attractive option for the foreseeable future when neither hand is functional or when cognitive dysfunction is severe.

Cooking fires are the cause of 20% of domestic fires (Brodzka, 1985). These are particularly common with frail elderly who may forget that a pot has been left on the stove. Caregivers must sometimes respond by removing the fuses to disable the stove. Timers are now available that may be retrofitted and cause the stove to turn off if it is left on longer than a preset period without the timer being reset.

Toileting

One of the most effective technical solutions to incontinence would be the provision of more toilets so that the average distance to the closest toilet is reduced. In particular, care should be taken in the design of buildings to ensure that toilets are placed close to dining rooms. The accessibility of toilets can be improved by raising the height of the seat. This will enable ambulatory elderly to get on and off the toilet more easily. Care must be taken to be sure that the toilet will still accommodate a wheeled commode and an individual transferring laterally from a wheelchair. There are many opportunities for improvements in toilet design and in related hardware, such as back rests and grab rails. Toilets are available that provide an integral bidet function by spraying the perineum with a cleaning jet of water followed by drying with warm air.

Commodes offer an alternative in cases where the elderly person cannot walk as far as the toilet. Sometimes commodes are wheeled over the toilet and sometimes they are used with a potty in place. Generally these appliances are relatively unattractive and tend to be unstable, particularly with agitated individuals. In the case of the commodes with receptacles, it is necessary for someone to come and empty the receptacle. Chemical toilets, such as are used in camping trailers, may provide a useful alternative so long as an acceptable means is found for disposing of the contents in the home environment. Unfortunately, electrically incinerating toilets that burn and evaporate the waste cannot be used to solve this problem since the gases must be vented through a flue stack.

Bathing and Grooming

The roll-in shower has been popular, particularly in long-term care facilities, since it removes the need to transfer a resident in and out of the tub. Unfortunately, roll-in showers do not permit effective cleaning of the perineum. In recent years, many alternative tub designs have become available. The simplest of these employs a transfer seat that is operated by water pressure to lift the elderly person over the side of the tub and lower him or her into the bath. More complex baths now have doors that open and permit the bather to enter with an easy lateral transfer onto a seat inside the bath. The door is then shut and frequently a pneumatic seal is inflated. The bath then fills with water. The more successful designs of these systems have a tipping action so that the bath can be filled prior to entry. After entering, the bath tips, causing the water to surround the reclining individual. These are comfortable and reduce the time taken to bathe and the chance of the bather becoming chilled waiting for the bath to fill.

Dressing

Much can be done to increase independence through appropriate clothing design. A bilateral opening is helpful to accommodate individuals with left or right hemiplegia. Sometimes it is advantageous to have openings that are accessible only to a caregiver in cases where the confused elderly person is in the habit of publicly disrobing. Velcro® continues to be a popular fastening material, while zips and buttons require greater manual dexterity. However, its effectiveness does decrease as lint begins to accumulate through washing and wearing. Sometimes a reaching stick can be helpful to pull on clothing.

Housekeeping and Maintenance

There are many ways in which technical devices can help with housekeeping and maintenance tasks. Usually, the technology is very simple. For example, it can be difficult to reach a ceiling lighting fixture to change a light bulb. It is quite a good idea to make sure that all main room lights have at least two light bulbs so that if one fails the environment is still partially lit until someone can come and replace the used bulb. If possible, lamps should be at reaching height. Center room lights can be mounted so that they can be lowered for bulb changing and cleaning. Because of the risk of falling, it may not be appropriate to have a step ladder at hand. However, if a ladder is not present, the elderly person may be likely to resort to a less safe practice, such as climbing upon a kitchen stool. A stepping stool with a safety rail and a broad stable base may be useful.

The domestic robot capable of routine chores is foreseeable (see Figure 2).

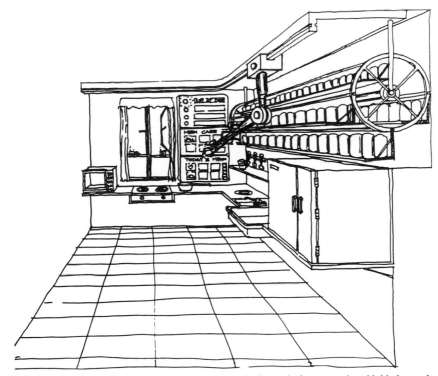

Figure 2   A conceptualization of a scheme to use a robotic manipulator to assist with kitchen tasks. Note the rotating storage system, the counters with unrestricted space underneath to increase wheelchair accessibility, and the electronic household systems monitoring panel, message center, and menu storage.

Presently, early versions of these systems are finding cost-effective applications distributing mail and various supplies within fairly large institutional buildings and acting as security watchmen patrolling corridors for signs of intruders and fire. These robots are essentially guided vehicles that follow a cable set in the floor or a line painted upon the floor and are equipped with various sensors to detect obstacles and activity. More sophisticated robots will use vision to chart a course through obstacles and to identify objects and position manipulators to grasp them. Most robots in industry actually perform repeated tasks that simply reproduce the motions of a human operator who accomplishes the task once manually while holding the manipulator arm and guiding it through the required movements. Autonomous, intelligent, manipulative robots are some way from being cost-effective in comparison with human homemaking assistants. It is interesting to note that robots are likely to face many of the accessibility problems of wheelchair users, requiring ramps and wider doorways.

Socialization

Technology can assist social interaction by bridging the distance between people either through improved accessible transportation or communication systems. In part, the degree of socialization of the elderly is influenced by the extent to which they are perceived to be normal and attractive in appearance. Assistive devices are still often characterized by shiny chrome and brightly colored, glossy vinyl upholstery. In recent years we have seen a rebellion against such institutional appearances. For example, brightly colored wheelchairs with racing stripes have become popular. Products may be expected to become available in more conservative but elegant styles that emphasize the normality and self-esteem of the elderly.

One of the common sights when visiting long-term care institutions is of residents slumped over or sliding out of wheelchairs and other seating. Properly designed and fitted seating will provide the user with the medical benefit of a corrected posture, which will improve respiratory function and better skin interface so that stress distribution will reduce the likelihood of decubitus ulcer formation. Correct positioning also has an important positive effect on social interaction. The elderly person is then able to view the world around him or her, rather than gaze at the floor or ceiling, and he or she thereby has a more normal and attractive stature.

Mobility

The Canadian Health and Activation Limitation Survey (1988) found that 39% of the noninstitutionalized Canadian population over the age of 65 reported a disability, with half describing their disability as moderate or major. The most common problems relate to reduced mobility as a consequence of strength, endurance, or pain limitations. Mobility involves many facets. As we age we spend increasing proportions of our time seated. The ability to rise from a chair is therefore an important part of mobility. For wheelchair users, the ability to transfer between the chair and other surfaces is as important as the ability to move through the environment in the chair.

Sitting and Seated Mobility

A fully adjustable seat-shape simulator was used in the laboratory at the Centre for Studies in Aging to attempt to determine the optimum shape for a lounge chair for the average elderly person (Holden & Fernie, 1989; Holden, Fernie, & Lunau, 1988). The most important finding was that the chair should be as high from the floor as possible in order to facilitate ingress and egress. Unfortunately, this means that the chair should also be equipped with some form of foot support. No satisfactory foot support has yet been devised that is an attractive part of the furniture and that does not create tripping or falling hazards, particularly when the user forgets that it is present when rising from the chair. It was found that the elderly preferred only mild lumbar support but greater lateral support in the backrest.

The major features of the ideal lounge chair contrast with many typical chairs designed for the elderly. In particular, most of those chairs have cushions that are too soft and seats that are too low for easy egress. Moreover, there is usually no space under the front of the chair to allow the user to place the feet back under the center of gravity when rising. The armrests are often inadequately broad and padded and do not extend forward sufficiently to assist with ingress and egress. Although the backrests often have distinguishing wings, these are usually of little functional value since they do not provide the lateral support required to maintain a comfortable upright posture.

The majority of wheelchairs that are sold now are lightweight aluminium or stainless steel tubular systems. They were initially developed for disabled sportspersons. There is probably more reason for an elderly person to have such a wheelchair, since that individual is less likely to be able to compensate for the extra weight of a heavier chair and since the spouse is very likely to be pleased to be lifting a lightweight chair in and out of the trunk of the car. The electric scooters have also provided improved mobility to many elderly. These devices are used by mailmen and security guards and have a less stigmatizing appearance. However, they do not provide as much postural support and are not as stable as powered wheelchairs.

There is much discussion in research groups at this time as to the amount of intelligence that the elderly might find useful in a powered wheelchair. It is generally agreed that collision avoidance and hazard detection might be two helpful features. Presently, the elderly are often discouraged from learning how to use powered chairs because of the hazards these chairs may present to themselves and to others. A simple collision-avoidance system would slow down or pause the wheelchair when an obstacle would come in its path. Many of the new powered wheelchair controllers already allow caregivers to set performance characteristics. For example, peak acceleration and maximum speed can be adjusted to reduce the chance of accident.

Transfer

The difficulty of lifting the frail elderly is frequently the cause for spouses having to admit that they can no longer manage to provide care at home. There are a number of mobile lifting aids available. Many of these resemble an engine block hoist with the person suspended in a sling hanging from the end of a boom. The major disadvantage of these designs is that they are cumbersome to wheel into place, occupy significant storage space, and require at least one operating attendant. For example, an elderly wife will find it very difficult if not impossible to maneuver a wheeled lifter on carpet with her husband suspended in the lifting sling. These lifters are not easily hidden and tend to give the room a hospital-like appearance. Hence, these devices are not used as frequently as they are needed.

An electric hoist installed on a ceiling track is a very attractive alternative. However, there is a higher cost because of the need to install these lifts in several locations. A novel solution has been developed by a designer at the Centre for Studies in Aging laboratory (see Figures 3 and 4), a portable, battery-operated

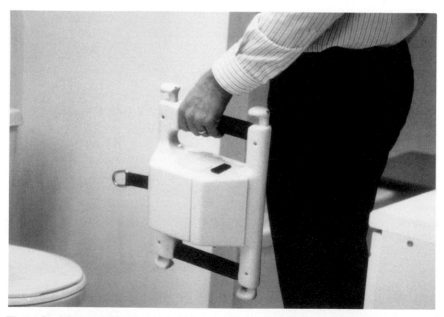

Figure 3   A battery-powered portable lifter weighing less than 10 lb that is extremely portable and occupies little storage space.

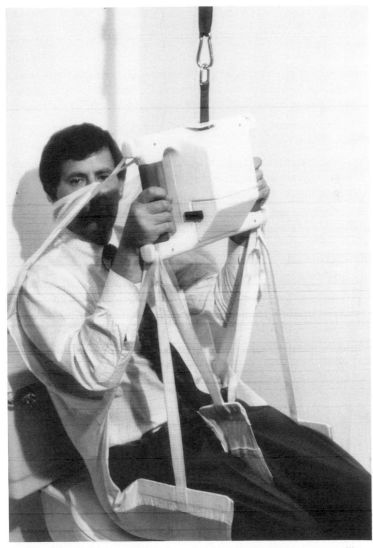

Figure 4   The portable lifter is clipped onto a strap attached to an inconspicuous, ceiling-mounted track. The harness is connected to the four hooks on the lifter and the user is gently lifted out of the bath or off the chair or bed. Once airborne, the user can be slid along the track with a very light touch and lowered onto the new surface. In most cases, the caregiver will operate the lifter from in front or from standing to either side. However, in this photograph the user is operating the device independently.

hoist that is easily carried in one hand and connected to a strap hanging from a simple, inexpensive ceiling track. The elderly person is lifted using a sling. The hoist can then be disconnected and taken to another site. The unit can be operated by the less frail elderly person. The ceiling track can be extended to allow for each person to be transferred directly without an intermediate transfer to a chair. The more able-bodied individuals can propel themselves by adjacent walls and furnishings, allowing themselves to glide along the length of the track.

Walking

The most interesting development in walking in recent years has been the popularity of shopping-cart walking frames. These are attractively finished walkers with an integral basket and often with a seat that permits the user to pause and rest. These carts resemble shopping "buggies" and have broad appeal. Consequently, they are less stigmatizing.

Driving

The ergonomics of car design has not improved greatly, except for much-improved seat and steering column positioning adjustability. With the advent of heads-up displays (HUDs) that have appeared on at least two models of cars, and with the increased use of microprocessors, there are possibilities for more efficient display of information to the driver. The HUD is a device that has been used by fighter pilots for many years to enable large quantities of information to be displayed visually in front of the pilot's eyes so that he or she does not have to look down at a console. Because there is so much information, a computer selects the most important parameters and represents them with appropriate graphical displays. This technology offers the same prospects for drivers by selectively displaying the most important and relevant information within the field of view of the driver.

A second area where the attention of researchers is deserved is the development of realistic driving simulators that can be used by elderly people for self-testing purposes. It may be envisaged that the elderly would volunteer to visit mobile testing facilities with the understanding that the results would be confidential. The realism of the computer simulation with displays of street scenes and with displays and information depicting the predicted consequences of errors made by the driver may be sufficient to prompt him or her to make appropriate voluntary adjustments to driving habits, including, if needed, abandoning driving or restricting driving to daytime.

Cognitive Function

It has been estimated that 10.3% of the elderly population over the age of 65 in the northeastern United States may have Alzheimer's disease and that the proportion rises to nearly half the population over 85 (Evans *et al.*, 1989). This condition and other etiologies, including vascular pathology, may result in decreased reasoning and deficits in short-term memory and orientation.

There is a growing trend toward the incorporation of artificial intelligence within consumer goods. Many appliances are now equipped with sensors that can detect different aspects of their current status and feed information to microprocessors to make appropriate decisions. For example, some cooking appliances contain menus of cooking instructions and will adjust temperature and time profiles appropriately.

The concept of linking household appliances with a common intercommunication system has attracted a great deal of interest amongst gerontologists. These systems are based on standard protocols for the exchange of information; the principle is that individual manufacturers would produce appliances that conform to these standards and that would be integrated within the intelligent household system simply by connection to the modified power outlet (Smart House, 1986; Uemura, 1985).

The principles of the intelligent house perhaps may be best explained by means of three examples: (1) One can envisage an intelligent communication protocol whereby there is only a low voltage supply to power outlets when they are not in use. This would minimize the possibilities for accidental electrocution. If an intelligent appliance were connected to the wall socket and turned on, it would send a message to the system describing its function and its power requirements. The system would acknowledge and would make power available at the full-supply voltage and would monitor the current being consumed. If the current rose above the specified level, the system would interrupt the supply and display a message to the user on the television, or by some other means, indicating that the particular appliance needed servicing attention. (2) A second example might be a dishwashing machine that, for efficient operation, requires higher-temperature water than is generally made available to the faucets in the house. This futuristic dishwasher would converse with the water heater, which would raise its temperature to supply sufficient water for the dishwasher's needs. (3) The third example is the person watching a favorite television program who receives a visual message from the stove informing him or her that baking of the cake is complete.

Many of these concepts would appear to have some utility, and others may simply be technological toys. The degree to which this technology may be helpful and accepted by the elderly is worthy of study. Adverse effects might include a sense of loss of control and disorientation because of the lack of familiarity of the systems.

The phrase "cognitive orthoses" has been coined to describe assistive devices for memory applications. Interesting research has been conducted using personal computers with software to guide an individual through a complex task step by step. This technology was developed for the American space program to help astronauts complete a complex series of tasks in operating various experiments. Earthbound demonstration applications have included a program to help an individual with severe memory impairment to bake a cake and a program to help a janitor perform his or her daily routines.

Many businesspeople now carry small, pocket-sized computing systems that provide a database of information, such as of addresses and phone numbers. Often, these systems also include an electronic dairy with alarm functions to remind the user of appointments. Possibilities of extending the application of these systems to elderly with short-term memory impairments are worthy of study. Such adaptive devices would need to be simple to use and have ergonomic displays that are suited to reduced levels of vision and dexterity. Elderly people often use reminding notes written by themselves or their caregivers. The difficulty is that it may be necessary to remember where to find the notes and to consult a given note at the appropriate time. Carefully designed electronic cognitive orthoses may therefore be useful in combination with simple strategies, such as removing cupboard doors so that the contents may be easily seen.

The most common issue with medication of the elderly is the problem of compliance because of poor understanding and short-term memory loss. Assistive devices have been developed in an attempt to reduce this difficulty. These range from simple, compartmentalized plastic boxes to very sophisticated, electronically controlled medication-dispensing units. The medication dispensers are usually programmed to provide an auditory and visual signal as a reminder of the need to take medication. Some of them have other systems to dispense the medication into a drawer (see Figure 5) and others indicate which compartment a medication should be taken from. At least one takes the form of an instrumented bottle cap that displays the last time it was removed and signals when the next dose is due.

The problem of drug interactions and multiple prescriptions with confused elderly may be addressed by means of shared computer databases. These allow a pharmacist to see all prescriptions filled for the individual by all pharmacists. Alternative technologies are based on a card carried by the consumer with prescription and medical information encoded. The pharmacist would insert this card into a reader/writer machine that causes the data to be displayed and allows information to be added. Optical recording systems allow several megabytes of data to be stored on a plastic card the size of a standard credit card. These various data storage and retrieval technologies may increase the safety of the elderly, but the pace of adoption is tempered by concerns related to privacy.

Cognitive function includes reasoning, memory, and orientation. There is a wealth of descriptive literature that discusses the topic of environmental cuing to assist with orientation to time and place. Orientation display boards are still used but are less favored since the messages attached to these boards contain information that may not be current. For example, the weather may have changed by the

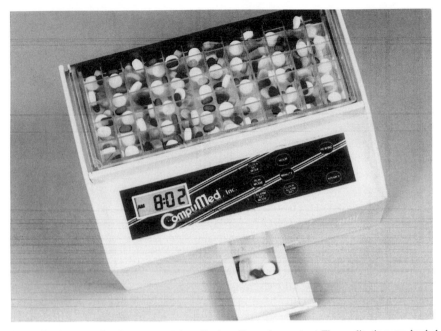

Figure 5 An example of an automated medication-dispensing system. The medications are loaded into the plastic compartmentalized tray that is seen on top of the instrument. When the time to take medication arrives the contents of the corresponding tray compartment drop into the dispensing drawer and an audible and visual alarm is triggered. The alarm is repeated at intervals until the patient removes the medications from the dispensing tray and resets it.

afternoon from the condition that was present in the morning, when the message describing the outside environment was attached to the board. It is particularly important to ensure that all clocks are carefully synchronized, since a clock reading the wrong time can be very disorienting. Centrally synchronized clocks are an option. Familiar objects and pictures of familiar things are particularly helpful for orientation to place.

Sensory Function

Approximately 8% of the elderly have significant visual impairment (National Center for Health Statistics, 1986). A variety of technical developments are relevant to blindness. These include laser canes to sense obstacles and texture, homing beacons to guide a blind person to his or her door, and audible road-crossing signals. The majority of visually impaired elderly have partial loss of vision. This loss causes problems, particularly with reading. Magnifiers with built-in illumination may be helpful. In extreme cases, low-vision aids that make use of television cameras to display written material in an enlarged form on a video screen may be appropriate.

Hearing aids help compensate for mechanical hearing loss and require no explanation. More recently, cochlear implants have become available. These implants convert sound to electrical signals that are applied via electrodes to the surface of the cochlea or directly to the auditory nerve. The sound is divided into a number of frequency bands, and the volume of signal within each band is presented to a different electrode. The signal is only a representation of some of the characteristics of the sound being received. Other aids for individuals with problem hearing include light strobes that can be attached to telephones and fire alarms as well as detectors that may be fitted to vehicles to indicate the proximity of emergency vehicles with sirens.

Designers' awareness of the need for facilitating the use of touch as a sensory input is increasing. Principles of good ergonomic design suggest that it should be possible for an individual to identify, for example, the help button on an emergency response system by its shape, size, and texture. Providing a notch a short distance from the end of all handrails is a second example of good design to optimize the use of this sensory modality.

As yet, there is little technology of practical value to augment the sense of smell. "Sniffer" devices are in use by law enforcement agencies to find drugs and explosives and by emergency services and utilities to detect gas leaks. It is reasonable to expect that devices may become economic and available in the future, particularly for homes supplied by gas or liquefied gas. Smoke detectors are now very sensitive and inexpensive and will often provide a warning signal of overheated cooking before a burning smell is detected.

Physical Health

The role of technology in acute care is undisputed. Imaging devices, cardiac monitors, defibrillators, and biochemical analyzers provide examples of the great array of equipment in use. Technology also has an important role to play in prevention, long-term care, and home care.

There is a growing awareness of the importance of indoor air quality. Problems have arisen with vapors given off by various building materials, insulation and carpet adhesives. Cigarette smoke and excessive carbon dioxide and radon gas buildup are hazards, especially in well-sealed buildings. A greater appreciation of these issues has led to improved standards of ventilation. Guidelines have recently been published for the prevention of hot-weather-related illnesses in the elderly. Technology to monitor and control the environment may become increasingly important if a global warming trend is realized.

Exercise has been accepted as an important health promotional activity. However, inappropriate vigorous exercise or excessive exercise may lead to medical complications. The value of low intensity exercise, such as walking, is reinforced. Bad weather, physical limitations, and security concerns may detract from this possibility. The design of exercise machines for elderly people may be worthy of attention. Such machines would emphasize low-intensity exercise and would provide incentives and interest. Rowing exercise machines now exist with a computer display showing boats in a race with one of the boats being propelled in response to the action of the person exercising. Elderly people with disabilities might enjoy the normalizing experience of using an exercise machine that simulates an activity that may no longer be within reach physically or financially. Perhaps this approach to motivation has some merit.

Accident Prevention

Falls are the leading cause of accidental death in the elderly and are a common cause of injury (Baker & Harvey, 1985). It is essential to provide handrails on stairways and helpful to provide them in corridor spaces. Biomechanical studies have demonstrated that handrails on stairs should be installed somewhat higher than is commonly practised in order to provide the optimum capability of resisting falls when descending (Maki, Bartlett, & Fernie, 1984). It also has been shown that rails should be circular, or near-circular, and of a diameter of approximately 1.5 in. so as to permit the hand to grasp around the rail. Larger rails, and particularly rails that are essentially planks on edge, must rely on the strength of a pinch grip and on the frictional forces that are generated. Such rails are therefore comparatively ineffective.

It is helpful to install grab bars wherever additional assistance or stability is needed. Unfortunately, if grab bars are to be installed everywhere they are needed, and if they are to be installed to allow for every size of person and every disability, then the predominant interior design feature would likely be grab bars. Furthermore, these installations require holes drilled in the walls and bars screwed into place. An alternative system has been developed in the laboratory at the Centre for Studies in Aging. This system consists of plastic components that clip together without tools and require no holes to be drilled in the building to support the structure. The basic component is a pole that is held in place by compression between the floor and the ceiling. Sometimes just one vertical pole will suffice. On other occasions, it may be more appropriate to install a horizontal grab bar, in which case two vertical poles are erected and are joined by a horizontal pole. More poles can be added to produce various layouts of grab configurations, and the system can be changed as the individual's needs change or when it is to be used by someone else. A broad range of accessories, including shelves, tabletops, and others, will soon be added to that product line. The system is designed to appeal to any user by having an attractive modern appearance that makes it suitable as an item of furniture for supporting bookshelves, lights, and so on (see Figure 6).

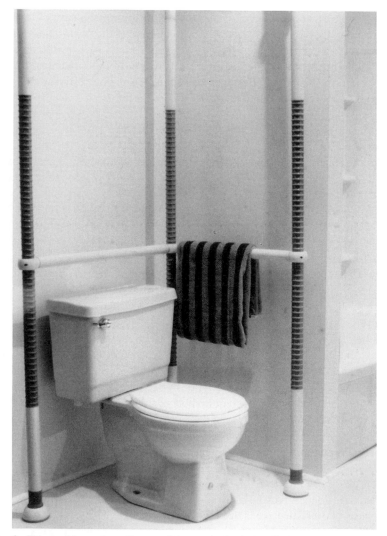

Figure 6 This modular system allows grab bars to be firmly installed in any location in a house without the use of tools and without having to fix anything to the walls. The vertical poles are held in place by spring compression between the floor and ceiling. They can be used singly or can be organized to support horizontal grab bars in various configurations. The layout can be easily changed or expanded as the needs of the user change or evolve.

Attention must be paid to the selection of floor surfaces. Carpeted floors have the advantages of providing a more homelike environment and of absorbing sound and preventing glare. However, they have disadvantages that include, perhaps, a greater tendency to induce tripping, greater rolling resistance for wheelchairs, and a tendency to retain odor. Laboratory studies have demonstrated that the peak load on a hip may be reduced by approximately 20% for the average person falling onto a carpeted as opposed to an uncarpeted floor (Maki & Fernie, 1990). However, this is likely to be offset by the disadvantages. Certainly, scatter rugs must be avoided and changes in coloring of floor surfaces and in the nature of floor surfaces may cause perception problems for elderly people with limited vision who may interpret them as changes in elevation. Very small changes in surface height may be expected to be sufficient to trip the elderly, particularly those with a typical shuffling Parkinsonian gait.

There are now many different lighting control units that may be substituted for ordinary light switches or may be plugged into power outlets. These controls consist of timers, motion detectors, and light-level detectors that will ensure that lights are turned on and off appropriately to provide safe illumination.

Emergency Response

Emergency response systems (ERSs) are gaining wider acceptance for seniors at risk (Downes, Severs, & Walden, 1988). These make use of the telephone system to place calls with monitoring stations when help is needed. The user usually wears a small portable transmitter and presses the button whenever there is a need to call for help. This activates the main unit, which dials a predetermined number to call the computerized assistance center. The operator responds, and a two-way voice communication is established. Information about the user is displayed on the operator's console. Once the operator has ascertained the nature of the difficulty, he or she is able to dial any of the listed preset help numbers by the touch of a single button. A typical scenario might involve the receipt of a call following a fall involving a hip fracture. The response center would immediately contact the ambulance service and provide them with a description of the problem and the address. The operator would then call to reassure the user that help was on the way and would follow any predetermined instructions, such as informing neighbors and relatives. The operator would also monitor the response to the call and be certain that help is provided.

ERSs also have monitoring capabilities that warn the operator if no activity has been detected in the house over a long period of time, which may be indicative of an incapacitating illness or loss of consciousness. Smoke detectors, intrusion alarms, and other devices may also be connected, and the operator may activate various devices such as a loud wailing siren to scare off an intruder or to waken the homeowner in the event of a smoke detector being activated.

Access to Health Care

Technology can assist with the trend away from hospital care and toward care in the community. A current project involving the development of a mobile seating clinic will be used to illustrate this point.

This seating clinic will employ computer-aided design and robot-assisted manufacturing (CAD/RAM) processes. The need for the system grew from the observation that elderly people in long-term care facilities in Ontario were frequently seen to be in need of better positioning. They were observed to be either sliding forward from the seats or slumping over the sides of seats. It was neither practical nor desirable to transfer these individuals to the few seating clinics that exist in major centers. Consequently, it was decided to develop a means of taking the technology to the long-term care facility and conducting the fitting on site.

The technology that has been chosen for this demonstration project employs a seating simulator. This seat is a very sophisticated system that can transform its shape under computer control. The computer will suggest an appropriate shape on the basis of a few questions posed to the operator concerning the characteristics and needs of the patient. If the operator is happy with this choice of starting seat shape, the simulator adopts that shape and the patient is transferred to the seat. The seat shape can then be changed interactively on the computer screen in response to the reactions of the patient and of caregivers, until the satisfactory shape is achieved. This shape will then be transferred to a central manufacturing plant where a robot manufactures an attractive and durable product that could be delivered the next day. If successful, this system will bring the benefits of a sophisticated design and manufacturing facility to the individual's home.

Psychological Health

Technology may be considered to offer positive advantages in promoting psychological health, but it also carries risks. Technological devices may be perceived as a threat and may lead to frustration and disorientation (Brickfield, 1984). They may also generate a feeling of helplessness and loss of control, particularly among those in whose earlier lives technology did not play a great role.

Improved mobility, transportation, and communication are possible with the help of technology. However, the degree to which the opportunities will decrease isolation depends on many factors. There is a risk that technology may be perceived as an alternative to personal service and that the elderly individual will become more isolated from direct personal contact. For example, an emergency response system may remove the priority that a relative would place on calling an elderly person to check on his or her status. The objective must be to encourage greater interpersonal contact by removing the dependency for instrumental tasks so that the dignity and privacy of the elderly person is reinforced and the opportunity is provided for a positive relationship with others that does not induce resentment of either party.

Many technological developments have tended to be adopted at the expense of self-esteem. The market for adult diapers has been estimated at $682 million per year; and there is evidence that a large proportion of these users could be more appropriately cared for by other, more dignified, means. Also, there are many examples of institutional furniture that may reduce the self-esteem of an individual simply because of appearance. Some products continue to be produced with institutional appearances. On the other hand, many products, particularly wheelchairs, are becoming very attractive. Some products increase self-esteem by enabling greater independence and by permitting esteem-building activities such as frequent bathing.

Security is one of the most commonly expressed anxieties. Intrusion alarms, emergency response systems, and more effective locks and surveillance systems contribute to overcoming some of these anxieties (Dibner & Dibner, 1985). Great care must be taken not to induce new anxieties because of the perception of a dependency on technology that is not understood.

Future Research Directions

Technology should become an important research focus for programs in gerontology. Care should be exercised to ensure that effort is directed at the less glamorous (but more common) problems of aging. These include falls, incontinence, and cognitive dysfunction. The temptation to focus on seductive high technology and search for applications should be resisted. Rather, the research effort should be driven by the problem, not by a technology.

It is particularly important to maintain a strong basic research commitment in support of product and service design. Technology itself can facilitate research by providing measurement tools to permit new observations to be made and to increase the power of controlled trials. A greater understanding of the etiology and nature of problems encountered by the elderly, combined with good market research on their desires, will provide a sound foundation for development.

Product designs should be attractive and, where possible, useful to a wide range of the public. If these conditions are satisfied, then the products are likely to be more affordable and will not stigmatize the user. Good technology has a powerful potential to provide frail elderly with greater choices and, therefore, improved quality of life.

In this author's experience, three elements are very helpful to the generation of useful innovations:

1. The involvement of an *excellent* engineer or industrial designer (preferably both)—This multidisciplinary field requires individuals with breadth of knowledge but who also have depth within their specialties. Products that

are to be depended upon by people with disabilities must be of the highest standard.

2. An open environment where engineers, designers, architects, and others come into close contact with elderly in need of assistance and with their caregivers.

3. An environment where the importance of basic research is respected, where technology is current, where lateral thinking and creative experimentation is encouraged, and where the leadership and resources exist to take the idea through all the stages to becoming a product or service on the market.

Universities could make an important contribution by involving engineers and industrial designers in collaborative programs at the graduate level with faculties of health and social sciences. Engineers should be as much a part of graduate programs in gerontology as are social or clinical scientists.

Conclusion

Technology has an important role to play in the prevention and management of disabilities affecting approximately 40% of people over age 65. However, biological systems are still a very long way ahead of engineering (ask an engineer to build an artificial insect!). The skills of engineers and designers must be challenged in order to develop devices and systems that compensate for the loss of biological function while being attractive, affordable, and nonstigmatizing. Thoughtfully designed technology has the potential of enhancing elderly people's sense of control and their perceptions of the quality of life. Technology may also raise the quality of life of the elderly, according to objective criteria, by improving the living environment and assisting both formal and informal caregivers.

References

Baker, S. P., & Harvey, A. H. (1985). Fall injuries in the elderly. In T. S. Radebaugh, E. Hadley, & R. Suzman, eds., *Symposium on falls in the elderly: Biologic and behavioural aspects*. Philadelphia: W. B. Saunders.

Brickfield, C. F. (1984). Attitudes and perceptions of older people toward technology. In P. K. Robinson, J. Livingston, J. E. Birren, eds., *Aging and technological advances*. New York: Plenum Press.

Brodzka, W. (1985). Burns: Causes and risk factors. *Archives of Physical Medicine and Rehabilitation, 66*, 746–752.

Dibner, S. S., & Dibner, A. S. (1985). Keeping in touch with Lifeline: An emergency response system. *Center Reports on Advances in Research, 8*, 1–5.

Downes, S., Severs, M., & Walden, D. (1988). The value of alarm systems and guidelines in their use. *Geriatric Medicine, February*, 71–77.

Dychtwald, K., & Flower, J. (1988). *Age wave: The challenges and opportunities of an aging North America*. Los Angeles: Jeremy P. Tarcher.

Evans, D. A., Funkenstein, H. H., Albert, M. S., Scherr, P. A., Cook, N. R., Chown, M. J., Hebert, L. E., Hennekenc, C. H., & Taylor, J. O. (1989). Prevalence of Alzheimer's disease in a community population of older persons. *Journal of the American Medical Association, 262,* 2551–2556.

Fernie, G. R., & Fernie, B. L. (1990). Technological innovations for individuals with Alzheimer's disease. *American Journal of Alzheimer's Care and Related Disorders and Research, 5,* 9–14.

Holden, J. M., & Fernie, G. R. (1989). Specifications for a mass producible static lounge chair for the elderly. *Applied Ergonomics, 20,* 39–45.

Holden, J. M., Fernie, G. R., & Lunau, K. R. (1988). Chairs for the elderly—Design considerations. *Applied Ergonomics, 19,* 281–288.

Mace, N. (1987). Principles of activities for persons with dementia. *Physical and Occupational Therapy in Geriatrics, 5,* 13–27.

Mace, N. L., & Rabins, P. V. (1981). *The 36-hour day.* Baltimore: Johns Hopkins University Press.

Maki, B. E., & Fernie, G. R. (1990). Experimental investigation of the impact attenuation provided by floor coverings in human falling accidents. *Applied Ergonomics, 21*(2), 107–114.

Maki, B., Bartlett, S., & Fernie, G. R. (1984). Influence of stairway handrail height in the ability to generate stabilizing forces and moments. *Human Factors, 26,* 705–714.

McGrowder-Lin, R., & Bhatt, A. (1988). A wanderer's lounge program for nursing home residents with Alzheimer's disease. *The Gerontologist, 28,* 607–609.

Minkler, M. (1989). Gold in grey: Reflections on business' discovery of the elderly market. *The Gerontologist, 29,* 17–22.

National Center for Health Statistics (1986). Aging in the eighties, impaired senses for sound and light in persons age 65 years and older. *Advancedata, 125,* 1–8.

Needler, W., & Baer, M. A. (1982). Movement, music and remotivation with regressed elderly. *Journal of Gerontological Nursing, 8,* 497–503.

Reisburg, B., Borenstein, J., Salob, S., Ferris, S., Franssen, E., & Georgolas, A. (1987). Behavioural symtoms in Alzheimer's disease: Phenomenology and treatment. *Journal of Clinical Psychology, 45,* 9–15.

Risse, S. C., & Barnes, R. (1986). Pharmacologic treatment of agitation associated with dementia. *Journal of the American Geriatrics Society, 34,* 368–376.

Smart House (1986). The smart house: Background information and technical update. *Building Standards, 55,* 15–18.

Uemura, K. (1985). A housekeeping system. *Mitsubishi Electric Advance, 32,* 8–10.

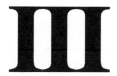

III

The Social World and Quality of Life in the Frail Elderly

8

The Role of Family and Friends in Quality of Life[1]

Neena L. Chappell

The present chapter focuses on informal support, that is, assistance provided by family and friends in the quality of life of frail elders. The major emphasis is on social support, sometimes used synonymously with social networks and social integration. The meaning of social support has evolved along with research in this area, so the definition will be discussed later in the paper.

It needs no reiteration here that the modified extended family, first elaborated by Litwak (1960), emphasizing mutual aid and close interpersonal ties among kin, is an important social institution in today's society. As Brody (1981) has articulated so well, present-day society is characterized by a continuation of the extended family, the strength of interpersonal ties, the continuity of responsible filial behavior, and the frequency of contact between the generations. What happens to this interaction when health (whether physical, mental, or both) deteriorates? The purpose of this chapter is to present a summary and integration of research on informal social support by categorizing it into three phases with different substantive foci.

While the phases are ordered chronologically, there is overlap with some current research being conducted in all three topic areas. Nevertheless, the three substantive areas help to bring order to a diverse and frequently unwieldy field. The first phase refers to a large amount of research that focuses on describing social support to elders. This research documents the amount and extent, the different types, and the varying sources of social support given to elders. This research, by and large, does not empirically examine the relationship between social support and quality of life but does frequently assume that the presence of social support has beneficial effects for quality of life. The second phase is

[1]Invited paper for the Anna and Harry Borun Center's conference, *The Concept of Measurement of Quality of Life and the Frail Elderly: A Research Conference*, Los Angeles, Calif., February 1990.

171

Copyright © 1991 by Academic Press, Inc. All rights of reproduction in any form reserved.

characterized by efforts to empirically examine the relationship between these two concepts. The literature is dominated by conceptual attempts to link the concepts, notably in the direct and indirect or buffering views of social support. It is out of the vast literature examining the relationship between these two concepts that researchers have come to recognize the tremendous complexity of the concept of social support itself, the concept of quality of life, and the underlying processes that may link the two concepts. Research is currently taking place in this third phase, which addresses many interesting and insightful questions to try to understand this complex area.

Phase 1: Documenting the Predominance of Assistance from Family and Friends

Early research in this area *assumed* the importance of interaction with others. The very existence of social support was accepted as beneficial for the recipient. This is evident in the definitions of social networks. As summarized by Sauer and Coward (1985), the definitions all refer to a common core of concepts. For example, Walker, MacBride, and Vachon (1977) define social networks as "that set of personal contact through which the individual maintains his social identity, and receives emotional support, material aid, services and information." Maguire (1980) refers to them as "preventive forces or buffers" that assist individuals in coping with transition, stress, physical problems, and social-emotional problems. Gottlieb (1983) states explicitly that such interaction is believed to have beneficial emotional or behavioral effects on the recipient.

Research in Phase 1 focused attention on documenting the types, the extent, and the sources of support that exist. This was an important research endeavor, which took place amid a belief in the isolated nuclear family who abandoned their elders to long-term care institutions. Social gerontologists documented the falsity of these assumptions and much was learned.

As Ward (1983) has indicated, when health deteriorates, it is family and friends who tend to provide care. The informal network is the "first resort" and the primary source of assistance for seniors in contemporary society. In the United States it has been estimated that approximately 80% of all care to elders comes from informal sources (Biaggi, 1980; Brody, 1981). Other American studies have shown that families provide the major caring function for most impaired and disabled individuals who do not require regular medical attention and who live in home settings. It is further estimated that 10% of those living in the community are as functionally impaired as those in institutions (Callahan, Diamond, Giele, & Morris, 1980). Canadian data (Chappell, 1985; Chappell & Havens, 1985) indicate that 94% of noninstitutionalized elders (i.e., those living in the community) receiving assistance do so from informal networks. In other words, it is well documented that care and assistance from family and friends is the dominant source of care to elders in our present-day society.

Such support can take a variety of forms. For example, it can involve assistance with instrumental activities of daily living, such as housework, preparing meals, household maintenance, transportation, shopping, and banking. Many elderly individuals have family or friends who assist in these matters. It frequently involves a reciprocal exchange and frequently is not defined as assistance. Functional difficulties in physical activities and those related to personal care—such as the ability to walk or to be personally mobile, to feed oneself, to wash or bathe, and to use the toilet—are more serious. They frequently lead to institutionalization. They are referred to as activities of daily living (ADLs) or basic ADLs and include activities necessary to survival. Fewer elders are impaired in these areas.

Emotional support is another area where assistance can be provided. Almost everyone requires companionship and intimacy (confidants). This is as true during old age as during the younger years. Chappell (1989a) indicates that 96% of community-living elderly persons have companions, and 84% have confidant relationships. The former refers to spending time with other people and sharing activities. The latter refers to relationships that include confiding in someone, being able to talk over personal matters and emotional issues. Frequently, the same person is both confidant and companion (50% in the study just noted name the same person as confidant and companion).

Information for effective decision making and use of resources is another area in which assistance can be provided by family and friends. Little is known about the informational needs of elders and their caregivers. There is, however, increasing recognition of the need for appropriate methods to convey relevant information about options and suitability of services (Binstock, 1987).

We also know there are a variety of sources of support. The vital role played by the spouse has been well documented. The spouse assists his or her partner during the marital career, including old age. Older couples tend to redistribute domestic and other chores when the health of either or both deteriorates. Because women tend to marry men older than themselves and have a greater life expectancy, they are more likely than their husbands to assume care-giving roles. Spouses, more so than anyone else, are more likely to provide more care for greater disability and illness, especially chronic conditions (Hess & Soldo, 1985; Shanas, 1981).

Children are second to the spouse in frequency as caregivers to elders, especially when a spouse is no longer available. Most seniors live close to at least one child (Hanson & Sauer, 1985; Marshall, Rosenthal, & Synge, 1981). Daughters provide hands-on and emotional care; sons are more likely to provide supervision of tasks and to provide money if and when needed. However, if a daughter is unavailable, either because none exists or because of distance, sons or daughters-in-law provide the care (Horowitz, 1981; Lipman & Longino, 1983). Some investigators (Lopata, 1978; Streib & Beck, 1980) report spouses and children as the sole informal caregivers to elders, with little or no extension to other kin or to non-kin. Others (Harvey & Harris, 1985; Matthews, 1987) report substantial support, especially from sisters. Chappell (1989b) reports siblings as the next most frequent source of support after spouses, children, and friends. We know the sister–sister bond is the closest of sibling bonds (Connidis, 1989), but we know virtually nothing about gender differences among siblings who provide care to frail elders.

Not as much is known about friendship ties, which social gerontologists characterize by voluntary involvement and affective bonds. Not only does one choose his or her friends, but one is chosen by them. Chappell (1987) found that friends were the next most frequent source of informal care after spouse and children. That is, caregiving to elders jumped outside of the kin network, rather than jumping another generation, after support from spouse, children, and siblings. Virtually nothing is known about gender differences among friends who assist one another.

The literature also suggests that in most cases there is one main helper, one person who provides most of the caregiving (Jones & Vetter, 1984; Tennstedt, McKinlay, & Sullivan, 1989). When others assist the main caregiver, these secondary caregivers provide less assistance than the primary one. When grandchildren provide care, it is as secondary caregivers to help their own parents provide care to grandparents.

This research documenting the extent, types, and sources of support debunked earlier assumptions about the isolation of elders, especially from their families. It recorded the wealth of exchanges that are commonplace in the lives of elders, including frail elders. Interaction with at least some members of the informal network, notably caregivers, can increase as health declines. Studies documenting and describing different aspects of support are still being conducted, but more are needed because of the many questions that remain unanswered. For example, some believe that the size of our social network decreases in old age, particularly among the old-old (Bould, Sanborn, & Reif, 1989) and that the variety of interactions also decreases (Sauer & Coward, 1985). This is due, among younger elders, to the empty nest and the exiting of social roles such as paid labor but also, particularly among the old-old, due to death. However, other investigators, for example, Minkler (1985), believe that despite contractions in their social worlds, most elders have the basic ingredients for social support. This is an important topic about which there is insufficient research to conclude what is correct and under what circumstances they are so.

Similarly, while some studies on secondary caregivers are starting to appear, we know very little about the role of these caregivers in the provision of assistance to frail elders. We do not know who they are or the circumstances that lead them to provide specific types of assistance. Cicirelli (1985) informs us that siblings stand in readiness to help; but aside from psychological help, few concrete forms of assistance are provided. We need much more research in this area.

Similarly, while much has been documented about the various sources of support, very little is known about the overlap of roles or role multiplicity (Peters & Kaiser, 1985). That is, a relative can also be a friend. A sibling can be a caregiver. A daughter can be a companion. We know very little about these types of interactions or the roles they play in the lives of frail elders. While some studies (Dobrof & Litwak, 1977; Smith & Bengtson, 1979) are available on the interaction and support provided by family and friends to institutionalized elders, insufficient evidence is available to even provide a profile of *who* it is that provides *what* types of interactions to these individuals.

In sum, this research has documented the wealth of assistance provided to elders as their health declines. It has helped debunk the myth of the isolated nuclear family and its abandonment of elderly members. However, much more research needs to be conducted in this area, and researchers are continuing to ask important questions that will further describe the social networks of frail elders and, thereby, increase our understanding of them.

Phase 2: Examining the Relationship between Social Support and Well-being

While research in Phase 1 assumed benefits accrued from social interaction, research in the second phase began empirically examining the relationship between the two concepts. These investigations sought to directly assess whether social support is, indeed, positively related to the quality of life of elders. These studies frequently fall into one of two camps. Both the direct and indirect effects models have received considerable attention in the examination of the relationship between social support and well-being. The direct effects view considers social support an ongoing part of everyday life. It is seen as important to meeting needs that require fulfillment on a more or less daily basis. Support enhances well-being irrespective of the stress experienced—when there is no stress, little stress, or much stress. Those assessing the adequacy of the direct effects view measure the direct relationship between social support and well-being (Lee, 1985; Liang, Dvorkin, Kahana, & Mazian, 1980). Some (Lowenthal & Haven, 1968; Ward, Sherman, & LaGory, 1984) argue that the effects of objective social support are mediated by the individual's perception of that support. That is, benefits are due to the perception that others are or will be supportive if necessary. When comparing specific studies, the research appears contradictory. For example, Thomas, Garry, Goodwin, and Goodwin (1985) report a positive relationship between social support and quality of life as measured in terms of good health and longevity among elders. However, Lin, Simeone, Ensel, & Kuo (1979) report a very weak relationship between social support and well-being. Similar contradictory findings between social interaction and well-being are apparent when quality of life is measured as life satisfaction (Bultena & Olyer, 1971; Graney, 1975; Mancini, Quinn, Gavigan, & Franklin, 1980).

Others have argued that the major relevance of social support for quality of life is not evidenced in day-to-day interactions but is reserved for crises or stress events. This view, known as the indirect model or the buffering hypothesis, suggests that social support mediates the effect of stressful experiences on quality of life. To examine this hypothesis, researchers examine the relationship between support and well-being only among those who are undergoing a crisis or experiencing stress. Much of this research examines stressful life events (such as widowhood, retirement, or illness), frequently adding the number of stresses experienced in a life event inventory. As such, it measures a buffer effect that cuts across several stressful situations rather than a specific stress situation. Kessler and McLeod (1985) argue that there can be little doubt of specific buffer effects in relation to particular stress episodes. Their review suggests that emotional support also has a pervasive buffer effect. Membership in affiliative networks does not. The evidence is inconsistent regarding perceived support.

More recently, research has begun examining chronic stresses and daily hassles (Kanner, Coyne, Schaefer, & Lazarus, 1981; Kessler & McLeod, 1985; Pearlin & Schooler, 1978). Some believe that buffering may be more pronounced for chronic than for acute strains. This possibility may explain marginal effects in studies of low stress and no stressful events. Chronic stress may be more important for emotional functioning than crisis events and can be studied in normal populations. The examination of chronic stresses and daily hassles for emotional well-being is an important area that will receive increasing attention in years to come.

Once again, contradictory findings are evident when examining this literature. For example, Badura and Waltz (1984) found that the relationship between serious illness, the quality of interpersonal relationships, and socioemotional support and psychological well-being was positive. Porritt (1979) examined quality versus quantity of social support and found that quality of reactions to a person in crisis were more important to outcome than quantity. However, Andrews, Tennant, Hewson, and Vaillant (1978) found that social support did not show a mediating effect on the relationship between life event stress and psychological impairment. Crisis support, though, did exert an independent effect on psychological impairment.

There is an abundance of studies that assess the relationship between social support and quality of life. Major difficulties in assessing this literature arise because of the tremendous diversity in the measures of social support (quality, quantity, and different types of support used), methodological differences in the studies (different samples, sample sizes, and methodological designs), and the measures used to tap quality of life (measures of illness and pathology, mental functioning, and psychological and emotional health). However, testament to both the interest in social support and the wealth of research appearing in the area, there have been several detailed reviews of the literature appearing recently. This literature generally confirms a relationship between the two concepts, although even the reviews do not always agree with one another.

Cohen and Syme (1985) conclude that direct effects generally occur when the support measure assesses the degree to which a person is integrated within a social network; but buffering effects occur when the support measure assesses the availability of resources that help the individual respond to stressful events. They conclude that there is fairly strong evidence for an association between support and mental health and for an association between support and mortality. The evidence is less convincing for a relationship between social support and physical illness.

Distinguishing between social network and social support measures, House and Kahn (1985) conclude that the only quantitative structural and interactional characteristic of networks that has consistently been reported to be associated with health and well-being is network size. In terms of functional measures, they conclude that emotional support has most clearly been linked to health both in terms of direct and buffering effects. Schulz and Rau (1985), however, argue that frequency of social interaction is a common correlate of life satisfaction throughout adulthood.

Kessler and McLeod (1985) reviewed the literature on social support and mental health in community samples and conclude that there is compelling evidence of a significant relationship between support and well-being. They further conclude that there can be little doubt that specific buffer effects exist and that certain types of support are more influential than others in certain types of situations. They go on to analyze whether there is a *pervasive* buffer effect and conclude that emotional support does have this type of effect but that membership in affiliative networks does not. The evidence for perceived availability of support is less conclusive.

In other words, there is general consensus that social support has both direct and indirect benefits for quality of life. Indeed, Cobb's (1976) conclusion over a decade ago is still valid:

> We have seen strong and often quite hard evidence repeated over a variety of transitions in the life cycle from birth to death, that social support is protective. The very great diversity of studies in terms of criteria of support, nature of sample and method of data collection is further convincing that we are dealing with a common phenomenon. We have, however, seen enough negative findings to make it clear that social support is not a panacea. (p. 310)

That is, a wealth of empirical studies have provided evidence for social support as beneficial to quality of life. However, this wealth has also led to a recognition of the tremendous complexity of the concepts and relationships that we are exploring. This leads to a discussion of the third phase of research on social support and quality of life, which characterizes current research efforts.

Phase 3: Recognizing the Complexity

Current research can be characterized by a recognition of the complexity of the concepts of support and quality of life and the relationship between the two. As Wortman and Conway (1985) note, investigators in the social support area agree it is time to move beyond demonstrations of a relationship between support and health outcomes to an investigation of the *processes* underlying support.

First, turning to the concept of social support, there has been increasing recognition of the conceptual distinctness of terms sometimes used synonymously, that is, social support is a multidimensional concept. For example, House and Kahn (1985) refer to the functional context of social support, such as the degree to which the relationships involve affection or emotional concern, instrumental or tangible aid, information, and so on. The term *social network* is used to refer to the structures among a set of relationships, for example, their density, their homogeneity, their range. *Social integration* or *isolation* refers to the existence or quantity of relationships. Berkman (1985), however, views social networks as combining both of the latter two definitions. In her use, it refers to the web of social relationships surrounding an individual and its characteristics, including its size, composition, geographic distribution, density, homogeneity, reciprocity, intimacy, and frequency of contact. She refers to social support as the aid (emotional, instrumental, and financial) transmitted between network members.

Cohen and Syme (1985) define social support quite simply as the resources provided by other persons. They then distinguish between the structure and the function of the network. The structure refers to the existence of the social network, such as its size, whereas its function refers to feelings of belonging or material aid. Cohen and Syme argue that structural measures are generally considered to be objective characteristics, whereas functional measures usually ask individuals about their perceptions of availability and adequacy. However, the provision, for example, of material aid can be an objective measure that is distinct from the individual's evaluation of its adequacy or desirability. Nevertheless, there is an important objective–subjective distinction. Even though aid may objectively be given, if the individual does not perceive it to be desired or adequate, it probably does not have the same effect. That is, both the objective–subjective and the social network–social support (sometimes referred to as structure–function) distinctions appear to be important.

Recent analyses conducted in Manitoba, Canada (Chappell & Badger, 1989), examined 10 common measures of social isolation and their relationship with decreased well-being. Multivariate analyses revealed that none of the network or structural characteristics (such as the size of the network, the number of children, whether they were married, and so on) were significantly related to psychological well-being when various control variables were included. The only two indicators that were significantly related to psychological well-being were having confidants and having companions. Such findings support Cohen and Syme's (1985) contention that functional measures are better predictors of health and health behavior than are structural measures. The important factor was the type of relationship and the function that it serves (i.e., providing emotional support and companionship), rather than the relationship per se (e.g., being married or having children).

As noted earlier, many studies have documented both emotional support and size of network as related to various aspects of well-being. Researchers are currently asking: What specific aspects of social support are related to what aspects of well-being, and what is the process by which this is achieved?

The issues of what support is, how we measure it, and what its various dimensions are are leading to new and exciting research questions for the future. Pearlin (1985) hypothesizes a specialization of support. In other words, different sources may be more effective for different problems. For example, support for a technical problem at work, of necessity, might come from a colleague rather than family. Support with child rearing may of necessity come from other parents rather than from friends or other children. Studies that confirm the buffering hypothesis of social support in specific stress situations add strength to the notion of the specialization of social support.

Pearlin (1985) refers to the changes in a problem as the natural history of the problem, which may call for different types of support at the beginning than at the end. Initially, one may require informational support; later on, one may require emotional support. Pearlin (1985) also recognizes that problems are seldom isolated from each other; individuals may suffer from a multiplicity of problems. Unfortunately, we know little about the specialization of supports, about the change in need for support as problems evolve, or about support in coping with a multiplicity of problems.

While most research on social support has examined its beneficial effects, it is increasingly recognized that there are potentially negative aspects to interactions involving social support. Some researchers have documented striking examples of negative support. Wortman and Conway (1985) report studies in which most healthy persons say that they will go out of their way to cheer up a person with cancer but in which the majority of cancer patients report the "unrelenting optimism" of others as unauthentic and disturbing. It is unhelpful when others minimize their problems. In a similar vein, women who have undergone mastectomy find that others think their major concern focuses on the loss of their breast, whereas the women involved are much more concerned about recurrence, death, and treatment side effects. In another example, patients generally report that when others prevent or discourage them from carrying out their usual chores, these others are forcing incapacitation on them.

The divergence of views between the support givers and the support receivers is striking. It is a reminder that different individuals may view similar situations in different ways. Wortman and Conway (1985) argue that because illness evokes negative feelings in others, most relationships with ill individuals will contain both negative and positive aspects. Far too little is known about negative aspects of social interaction and about the circumstances that help minimize their effects.

We also know very little about specific types of support. Kiesler (1985) argues that we must have a better theoretical understanding of the information aspect of social support. Is information provided from the informal network important because it is interpreted as a sign of concern and caring? Information provided from family and friends may be correct but may also be incorrect. Is there a role for objective information delivered through other channels that have been checked out as valid, and does this type of information have an independent effect on well-being, independent of social support?

The concept and measurement of reciprocity within social support is also in need of in-depth study. We understand little about its nature. Most of the caregiving literature focuses on assistance provided by caregivers to the elderly, with little focus on the reciprocity within this relationship. Equity or exchange theorists (Rook, 1987) argue that individuals seek to maintain balanced (reciprocal) or overbenefiting relationships in which more is received than given. Dowd (1986), however, is well known for his argument that elders in contemporary society cannot maintain reciprocity because age is correlated with losses in exchange commodities. Younger people provide support to elders based on their beneficence. Supporting the importance of reciprocity, Lee (1988) notes that the receipt of assistance has less effect on the morale of elders than does the inability to reciprocate. Similarly, Roberto (1989) reports that friendships are more satisfying if exchanges are equitable.

Added to the complexity of the concept of social support is the complexity of the concept of quality of life. This is the topic of other chapters (for a review, see Birren and Dieckmann, Chapter 17), but a quick perusal of the World Health Organization's definition of health as including physical, mental, and social well-being demonstrates difficulties in this area. Many studies examine well-being or quality of life in terms of mortality or in terms of specific morbidity. Other indicators of quality of life include: disability, days in bed or days in hospital, various indicators of psychological well-being, overall indicators of life satisfaction and morale, and a variety of mental impairment measures. The spectrum is broad, and we do not have a good understanding of whether certain types of social support are more important for particular aspects of well-being. Nor do we know which aspects of social support have which type of impact. Indeed, certain types of social support may be of benefit and others may be of harm.

The present chapter now turns to some of the current thinking on the relationship between social support and quality of life.

Looking Ahead

In terms of the relationship between social support and quality of life, there are exciting new questions being asked. Those examining the direct and indirect models of social support (which are linear models) are asking insightful questions concerning the process through which these models may work. For example, Berkman (1985) notes that if indeed social support does enhance quality of life, the process or mechanism through which this happens could include any number of possibilities. It may operate through the provision of advice, information, and services so that respondents have access to better care than others. Or perhaps the social support network actually provides services and tangible assistance to these individuals and that it is this tangible aid which leads to an increased quality of life.

It may be that social support works through social control and peer pressure. If social pressure forces individuals into healthy life-styles, this may affect their well-being, but if it pressures them into unhealthy life-styles, including excessive smoking, drinking, and so on, it would have the opposite effect. A fourth mechanism hypothesizes a direct physiological link. For example, it could be argued that social support may affect the individual psychologically in such a way that it affects one's physiological susceptibility to various illnesses through the neuroendocrine or immune system functioning (Jemmott & Locke, 1984). The process through which support and quality of life are related, if at all, is unknown. Any of the postulates put forward could be applied to either the direct or indirect model.

It must be recognized that any of these hypothesized relationships could hold for any particular source of social support but not hold for others and that they could hold in varying circumstances.

Another major question relates to the causal direction of the relationship. Not surprisingly, most studies are cross-sectional in nature. Most of the studies reporting a relationship between the two concepts are interpreted as evidence in favor of the hypothesis that social support strengthens well-being. Increasingly, however, it is recognized that illness, decreased mental functioning, or decreases in other aspects of well-being may lead to less involvement with others, that is, to less social support. They may lead to a loss of desire to be involved with others or to a decrease in social competence skills.

Investigators have argued (see Gore, 1985, for a discussion) that quality support is only forthcoming from spontaneous interactions. Those who engage in deliberate help-seeking behavior do so as a last resort because they have been unable to cope. Such a hypothesis does not argue for a reversal of causation but that the interpretation of the relationship between social support and quality of life is spurious. In this instance, some other factor, such as social competence, explains the relationship between social support and quality of life. Wortman and Conway (1985), for example, note that socially competent individuals may have easier access to social support and may be more effective at negotiating the health care system and thereby receive optimal treatment and care.

Another example relies on the individual's ability to cope. The respondent's ability to cope with an illness may be the causal factor that determines how much support he or she receives from others and his or her quality of life. How psychological coping intervenes between social support and quality of life, if at all, is not yet well understood (Bould *et al.*, 1989). Essex and Lohr (1986) find that an optimistic attitude is much more successful than a take-charge, direct action coping style, particularly for those with chronic physical pain and discomfort. Kahana, Kahana, and Young (1987) report that strategies such as complaining and keeping to oneself are effective in nursing homes but are ineffective in sustaining helping networks in the community.

Still others have argued that it is the absence of any supportive relationship which is the most deleterious; having any social support available enhances well-being (House, 1981; Kahn & Antonucci, 1980). This view argues that increases in relationships above a moderate number produces diminishing returns (Berkman & Syme, 1979; House & Kahn, 1985). Or, incorporating this idea into the buffer model, it is the lack of social support during stressful times that results in illness or a lessened well-being (Dean & Lin, 1977; Rook & Dooley, 1985). The hypothesis that no support leads to ill consequences argues for the effect of isolation on illness rather than the effect of support on better health.

Still others have argued that social support enhances well-being to a point but that there is an optimum level of social support beyond which the benefits diminish and can become negative, creating dependency. Krause (1987) hypothesized such a nonlinear relationship between social support and well-being, arguing that too much social support will diminish rather than increase feelings of control. Studying informational support, tangible assistance, emotional health, and integration (support provided by the respondent to others), it was concluded that social support is initially associated with moderate feelings of personal control; when approximately average levels are approached, the positive influence decreases. Additional emotional support beyond this point is related to decreased feelings of control. Similar findings are reported for integration but not for tangible assistance or informational support.

There are, in addition, many other questions concerning substantive sources of support. Only two examples will be discussed: the marital relationship and the relationship between elders and their friends.

As already noted, the marital relationship is taken as the primary relation within our society; and the support provided by the spouse is well documented.

As House and Kahn (1985) have noted, marital status is the most studied of social relationships and the most consistently related to health. Marriage appears to benefit men more than women. It has also been related to other measures of well-being and to mortality (Schulz & Rau, 1985).

One of the difficulties in studying the marital relationship is that most elderly who live with anyone live with a spouse. It is therefore difficult to empirically disentangle living arrangements from the marital relationship. However, recent research reported by Cafferata (1987) found that living arrangement rather than marital status was predictive of receiving informal support. Recent Manitoba research from a sample stratified by living arrangements, which allowed extensive analyses of those who live with nonspousal others, similarly reports that the structural characteristic of living with someone, rather than marital status, is the significant predictor for assistance with instrumental activities of daily living (Chappell, 1990). However, neither marital status nor living arrangement were predictive of emotional support. Such findings caution us to be wary of placing our own values and interpretations of particular relationships, such as marital status, before rigorous design in the examination of social support. These studies suggest that it is the quality of the relationship or its function, rather than the type of relationship or its structural characteristic, that is related to support.

Concerning the second example, interactions between elders and their friends, it is not unusual to find researchers who claim that poor health can curtail opportunities to service and develop friendships. There is a general belief that the older one becomes, the more vulnerable friendships are to erosion, through death but also through the ill health of participants (Babchuk, 1978–1979; Blieszner, 1989; Peters & Kaiser, 1985). However, as Allan and Adams (1989) point out, the effect of ill health on interactions with friends varies. Previous work by Adams (1986) found that in age-segregated buildings, helping the ill gave status and people wished to associate with those worse off. Opposite results are reported for age-integrated buildings.

Furthermore, a number of studies point out that interaction with friends is positively related to morale, life satisfaction, and happiness (in contrast with interaction with kin, Larson, 1978; Lee, 1979, 1985). This has been explained in terms of reciprocity and the element of choice within friendships. Researchers, however, have not integrated these two lines of thinking to examine whether interactions with friends decrease when one is ill, so as to explain why elders who interact more with their friends are happier (they are in better health). One of the major roles of friendship seems to be socialization. If one is ill, one may have neither the inclination nor the energy for such activities.

There are many other areas of social support and quality of life that have not been discussed here, including issues particular to minority and subcultural groups, care for caregivers, and rural–urban differences. The heterogeneity of the elderly population demands an awareness of these and many other issues.

Some questions for future research, arising from the issues discussed in this chapter, are outlined below.

Directions for Future Research

The argument being posed is that much has been accomplished in past research endeavors in the area of social support and quality of life for frail elders. Upon reflection, one can see a historical revolution of the types of questions that have been asked by researchers. If nothing else is clear, it should be obvious that the concept of social support and its relationship with other variables is complicated; it is not simple. While this means that we must be very cautious in drawing conclusions, it also means there are exciting new opportunities for research.

There are still many questions to be asked concerning the amount, type, and sources of social support. We know very little about companionship in old age—what it means to elders themselves and who is most likely to provide companionship and under what circumstances. We do not know the importance of pure companionship when one's health deteriorates or whether it is a secondary component of a care-giving relationship that provides more direct aid. We know very little about the type of social support that can be called "information for effective decision making." We know almost nothing about sources of different types of information for elders, about the effectiveness of various sources, or about elders' preferences among different types of sources.

We know very little about sources of support other than spouses and children. While more attention is being turned to siblings and friends, there is still little in this area; and almost nothing is known about relationships with nieces, nephews, aunts, uncles, cousins, in-laws, and so on. We know virtually nothing about the overlapping roles that are played by a particular individual in the lives of elders. For example, a sibling also can be a friend and a caregiver. Similarly, elders themselves can play multiple roles for other individuals in their lives. An elder can be a mother, friend, and adviser to her daughter. We know little about the role that support from family and friends play for the institutionalized.

The research directly examining the relationship between social support and quality of life has demonstrated the multidimensionality and complexity of the concept of social support itself. We do not know which aspects of social support are related to which aspects of quality of life, under which circumstances or for whom. How does our need for different types of social support change with the natural evolution of particular problems? What are the negative aspects of the different types of support, and when do these outweigh the positive aspects? How do people cope with negative aspects of support? What are the underlying processes linking social support and quality of life?

Finally, the present chapter has discussed the role of family and friends and the quality of life of frail elders. The focus has been on informal support rather than on quality of life or the concept of frailty. However, the latter two concepts have set the parameters for the discussion of social support. It is important to recognize that we know less about support to the cognitively impaired than we do about support to the physically impaired, especially its relevance for psychological and subjective quality of life. This is due in large part to the difficulty of measuring quality of life among the cognitively impaired. This dilemma points to the need to develop appropriate measures of quality of life for this special group of elders.

Conclusion

This chapter has sought to bring some coherence to the area of social support and quality of life for frail elders by categorizing the research in this area into three phases. The first phase focused primarily on documenting the amount and types of social support to elders. By and large, this research assumed that interaction with others was supportive. The literature is relatively vast and documents conclusively the amount of assistance from other people that is provided to elders as their health declines. Despite the amount of literature in this area, there is still much more to be documented.

The second phase saw empirical investigations of the relationship between social interaction and various indicators of quality of life. This research is also quite vast and generally supports a relationship between the two concepts. Many studies are available that find that various types of social interaction are related to different aspects of quality of life for the elderly. This research is still ongoing and has led to Phase 3, which characterizes current research efforts. Phase 3 sees a recognition of the complexity of the concepts of social support and quality of life and the relationship between the two. Many interesting and insightful research questions are being addressed.

There are no final answers in this intriguing area. It is clear that social gerontologists, like those in other disciplines, have a tremendous interest in the concepts and a belief that social support is important to quality of life. Indeed, there is an entire discipline (namely, sociology) based on the belief that interaction with others is essential and critical to the evolution of the self, that is, to the very creation of an individual's identity and its subsequent evolution. There are also applied schools (such as social work) based on the premise that interactions with others are helpful. The abundance of research that looks in particular at social support and quality of life among frail elders confirm these assumptions. However, the exact nature of the process and the circumstances under which it does and does not work have eluded the scientific researcher. The current state of research suggests that it would be premature to devise social policy in this area. One would anticipate, however, that in a decade from now, some firm conclusions might be drawn about the relationship between social support and quality of life as we are now able to make conclusive statements about the amount and extent of assistance to elders.

References

Adams, B. N. (1986). *The family: A sociological interpretation*, 4th ed. New York: Harcourt, Brace, Jovanovich.

Allan, G. A., & Adams, R. G. (1989). Aging and the structure of friendship. In R. G. Adams & R. Blieszner, ed., *Older adult friendship: Structure and process*, pp. 45–64. Newbury Park, Calif.: Sage.

Andrews, G., Tennant, G., Hewson, D., & Vaillant, G. (1978). Life event stress, social support, coping style, and risk of psychological impairment. *Journal of Nervous and Mental Disease, 166*, 307–316.

Babchuk, N. (1978–1979). Aging and primary relations. *International Journal of Aging and Human Development, 9*, 137–151.

Badura, B., & Waltz, M. (1984). Social support and quality of life following myocardial infarction. *Social Indicators Research, 14*, 295–311.

Berkman, L. F. (1985). The relationship of social networks and social support to morbidity and mortality. In S. Cohen and S. L. Syme, eds., *Social support and health*, pp. 241–262. Orlando, Fla.: Academic Press.

Berkman, L. F., & Syme, S. L. (1979). Social networks, host resistance, and mortality: A nine-year follow-up study of Alameda County residents. *American Journal of Epidemiology, 109*, 186–204.

Biaggi, M. (1980). *Testimony before the select committee on aging*. Washington, D.C.: House of Representatives, 96th Congress.

Binstock, R. H. (1987). Title III of the Older Americans Act: An analysis and proposal for the 1987 reauthorization. *The Gerontologist, 27*, 259–265.

Blieszner, R. (1989). Developmental processes of friendship. In R. G. Adams & R. Blieszner, eds., *Older adult friendship: Structure and process*, pp. 108–126. Newbury Park, Calif.: Sage.

Bould, S., Sanborn, B., & Reif, L. (1989). *Eighty-five plus: The oldest old*. Belmont, Calif.: Wadsworth.

Brody, E. M. (1981). Women in the middle and family help to older people. *The Gerontologist, 21*, 470–480.

Bultena, G., & Olyer, R. (1971). Effects of health on disengagement and morale. *Aging and Human Development, 2*, 142–148.

Cafferata, G. L. (1987). Marital status, living arrangements, and the use of health services by elderly persons. *Journal of Gerontology, 42*, 613–618.

Callahan, J. J., Jr., Diamond, L., Giele, J., & Morris, R. (1980). Responsibility of families caring for their severely disabled elders. *Health Care Financing Review, 1*, 29–48.

Chappell, N. L. (1985). Social support and the receipt of home care services. *The Gerontologist, 25*, 47–54.

Chappell, N. L. (1987). Living arrangements and sources of caregiving. Revision of paper presented at the annual meeting of the Canadian Sociology and Anthropology Association, Hamilton, Ontario.

Chappell, N. L. (1989a). Health and helping among the elderly, gender differences. *Journal of Aging and Health, 1,* 102–120.

Chappell, N. L. (1989b). Aging and gender. Invited address to the Department of Women's Studies, University of Waterloo, May. Waterloo, Ontario.

Chappell, N. L. (1990). Living arrangements and sources of caregiving. *Journal of Gerontology, Social Sciences, 46*(6), 51–58.

Chappell, N. L., & Badger, M. (1989). Social isolation and well-being. *Journal of Gerontology: Social Sciences, 44,* S169–S176.

Chappell, N. L., & Havens, B. (1985). Who helps the elderly person: A discussion of informal and formal care. In W. Peterson & J. Quadagno, eds., *Social bonds in later life,* pp. 211–227. Beverly Hills, Calif.: Sage.

Cicirelli, V. G. (1985). The role of siblings as family caregivers. In W. J. Sauer & R. T. Coward, eds., *Social support networks and the care of the elderly,* pp. 93–107. New York: Springer.

Cobb, S. (1976). Social support as a moderator of life stress. *Psychosomatic Medicine, 38,* 300–314.

Cohen, S., & Syme, S. L. (1985). Issues in the study and application of social support. In S. Cohen & S. L. Syme, eds., *Social support and health,* pp. 3–22. Orlando, Fla.: Academic Press.

Connidis, I. (1989). *Family ties and aging.* Toronto, Ontario: Butterworths.

Dean, A., & Lin, N. (1977). The stress-buffering role of social support. *Journal of Nervous and Mental Disease, 165,* 403–447.

Dobrof, R., & Litwak, E. (1977). *Maintenance of family ties of long-term care patients: Theory and guide to practice.* Washington, D.C.: U.S. Government Printing Office (DHHS Publication #81-400).

Dowd, J. J. (1986). The old person as a stranger. In V. W. Marshall, ed., *Later life: The social psychology of aging,* pp. 147–189. Beverly Hills, Calif.: Sage.

Essex, M. J., & Lohr, M. J. (1986). Chronic life strains and depression among older women. Paper presented at the annual meeting of the American Sociological Association, New York.

Gore, S. (1985). Social support and styles of coping with stress. In S. Cohen & S. L. Syme, eds., *Social support and health,* pp. 263–280. Orlando, Fla.: Academic Press.

Gottlieb, B. H. (1983). The contribution of natural support systems of primary prevention among four subgroups of adolescent males. *Adolescence, 10,* 207–220.

Graney, M. J. (1975). Happiness and social participation in aging. *Journal of Gerontology, 30,* 701–706.

Hanson, S. M., & Sauer, W. J. (1985). Children and their elderly parents. In W. J. Sauer & R. T. Coward, eds., *Social support networks and the care of the elderly,* pp. 41–66. New York: Springer.

Harvey, C., & Harris, M. (1985). Decision-making during widowhood: The beginning years. Paper presented at the Beatrice Paolucci Symposium, Michigan State University.

Hess, B. B., & Soldo, B. J. (1985). Husband and wife networks. In W. J. Sauer & R. T. Coward, eds., *Social support networks and care of the elderly,* pp. 67–92. New York: Springer.

Horowitz, A. (1981). Sons and daughters as caregivers to older parents: Differences in role performance and consequences. Paper presented at the annual meeting of the Gerontological Society of America, Toronto, Ontario.

House, J. S. (1981). *Work, stress and social support.* Reading, Mass.: Addison-Wesley.

House, J. S., & Kahn, R. L. (1985). Measures and concepts of social support. In S. Cohen & S. L. Syme, eds., *Social support and health,* pp. 83–108. Orlando, Fla.: Academic Press.

Jemmott, J. B., & Locke, S. E. (1984). Psychosocial factors, immunologic mediation, and human susceptibility to infectious diseases: How much do we know? *Psychological Bulletin, 95,* 78–108.

Jones, D. A., & Vetter, N. J. (1984). A survey of those who care for the elderly at home: Their problems and their needs. *Social Science and Medicine, 19,* 511–514.

Kahana, E., Kahana, B., & Young, R. (1987). Strategies of coping and postinstitutional outcomes. *Research on Aging, 9,* 182–199.

Kahn, R. L., & Antonucci, T. C. (1980). Convoys over the life course: Attachments, roles and social support. In P. B. Baltes & O. Brim, eds., *Life-span development and behavior,* vol. 3. New York: Academic Press.

Kanner, A. D., Coyne, J. C., Schaefer, C., & Lazarus, R. S. (1981). Comparison of two modes of stress measurement: Daily hassles and uplifts versus major life events. *Journal of Behavioral Medicine, 4,* 1–39.

Kessler, R. C., & McLeod, J. D. (1985). Social support and mental health in community samples. In S. Cohen & S. L. Syme, eds., *Social support and health,* pp. 219–240. Orlando, Fla.: Academic Press.

Kiesler, C. A. (1985). Policy implications of research on social support and health. In S. Cohen & S. L. Syme, eds., *Social support and health,* pp. 347–364. Orlando, Fla.: Academic Press.

Krause, N. (1987). Understanding the stress process: Linking social support with locus of control beliefs. *Journal of Gerontology, 42,* 589–593.

Larson, R. (1978). Thirty years of research on the subjective well-being of older Americans. *Journal of Gerontology, 33,* 109–125.

Lee, G. R. (1979). Children and the elderly: Interaction and moral. *Research on Aging, 1,* 335–360.

Lee, G. R. (1985). Theoretical perspectives on social networks. In W. J. Sauer & R. T. Coward, eds., *Social support networks and the care of the elderly,* pp. 21–37. New York: Springer.

Lee, G. R. (1988). Aging and intergenerational relations. *Journal of Family Issues, 8,* 448–450.

Liang, J., Dvorkin, L., Kahana, E., & Mazian, F. (1980). Social integration and morale: A re-examination. *Journal of Gerontology, 35,* 746–757.

Lin, N., Simeone, R. S., Ensel, W. M., & Kuo, W. (1979). Social support, stressful life events, and illness: A model and empirical test. *Journal of Health and Social Behavior, 20,* 108–119.

Lipman, A., & Longino, C. F. (1983). Mother is alone now: Sons and daughters of married and widowed mothers. Paper presented at the annual meeting of the Gerontological Society of America, San Francisco, Calif.

Litwak, E. (1960). Geographic mobility and extended family cohesion. *American Sociological Review, 25,* 385–394.

Lopata, H. (1978). Contributions of extended families to the support system of metropolitan area widows: Limitations of the modified kin network. *Journal of Marriage and the Family, 40,* 355–364.

Lowenthal, M. F., & Haven, C. (1968). Interaction and adaptation: Intimacy as a critical variable. In B. Neugarten, ed., *Middle age and aging,* pp. 390–400. Chicago, Ill.: University of Chicago Press.

Maguire, L. (1980). The interface of social workers with personal networks. *Social Work with Groups, 3,* 39–49.

Mancini, J. A., Quinn, W., Gavigan, M. A., & Franklin, H. (1980). Social network interaction among older adults: Implications for life satisfaction. *Human Relations, 33,* 543–554.

Marshall, V. W., Rosenthal, C. J., & Synge, J. (1981). The family as a health organization for the elderly. Paper presented at the annual meeting of the Society for the Study of Social Problems, Toronto, Ontario.

Matthews, A. M. (1987). Widowhood as an expectable life event. In V. W. Marshall, ed., *Aging in Canada,* 2nd ed., pp. 343–366. Markham, Ontario: Fitzhenry & Whiteside.

Minkler, M. (1985). Social support and health of the elderly. In S. Cohen & S. L. Syme, eds., *Social support and health,* pp. 199–218. Orlando, Fla.: Academic Press.

Pearlin, L. I. (1985). Social structure and processes of social support. In S. Cohen & S. L. Syme, eds., *Social support and health,* pp. 43–60. Orlando, Fla.: Academic Press.

Pearlin, L. I., & Schooler, C. (1978). The structure of coping. *Journal of Health and Social Behavior, 19,* 2–21.

Peters, G. R., & Kaiser, M. A. (1985). The role of friends and neighbors in providing social support. In W. J. Sauer & R. T. Coward, eds., *Social support networks and the care of the elderly,* pp. 123–158. New York: Springer.

Porritt, D. (1979). Social support in crisis: Quantity or quality? *Social Science and Medicine, 13A,* 715–721.

Roberto, K. A. (1989). Exchange and equity in friendships. In R. G. Adams & R. Blieszner, eds., *Older adult friendship: Structure and process,* pp. 147–165. Newbury Park, Calif.: Sage.

Rook, K. S. (1987). Reciprocity of social exchange and social satisfaction among older women. *Journal of Personality and Social Psychology, 52,* 145–154.

Rook, K. S., & Dooley, D. (1985). Applying social support research: Theoretical problems and future directions. *Journal of Social Issues, 41,* 5–28.

Sauer, W. J., & Coward, R. T., eds. (1985). *Social support network and the care of the elderly.* New York: Springer.

Schulz, R., & Rau, M. T. (1985). Social support through the life course. In S. Cohen & S. L. Syme, eds., *Social support and health,* pp. 129–150. Orlando, Fla.: Academic Press.

Shanas, E. (1981). The elderly: Family, bureaucracy, and family help. In W. M. Beattie, Jr., J. Piotrowski, & M. Marois, eds., *Aging: A challenge to science and society,* pp. 309–319. New York: Oxford University Press.

Smith, K. F., & Bengtson, V. L. (1979). Positive consequences of institutionalization: Solidarity between elderly parents and their middle-aged children. *The Gerontologist, 19,* 438–447.

Streib, G. F., & Beck, R. W. (1980). Older families: A decade review. *Journal of Marriage and the Family, 42,* 937–956.

Tennstedt, S. L., McKinlay, J. B., & Sullivan, L. M. (1989). Informal care for frail elders: The role of secondary caregivers. *The Gerontologist, 29,* 677–683.

Thomas, P. D., Garry, P. J., Goodwin, J. M., & Goodwin, J. S. (1985). Social bonds in a healthy elderly sample: Characteristics and associated variables. *Social Science and Medicine, 20,* 365–369.

Walker, K. N., MacBride, A., & Vachon, M. L. S. (1977). Social support networks and the crisis of bereavement. *Social Science and Medicine, 11,* 35–41.

Ward, R. A. (1983). Limitations of the family as a supportive institution in the lives of the aged. In D. B. Gutknecht, E. W. Butler, L. Criswell, & J. Meints, eds., *Family, self, and society: Emerging issues, alternatives, and interventions,* pp. 121–133. Lanham, Md.: University Press of America.

Ward, R. A., Sherman, S. R., & LaGory, M. (1984). Subjective network assessments and subjective well-being. *Journal of Gerontology, 39,* 93–101.

Wortman, C. B., & Conway, T. L. (1985). The role of social support in adaptation and recovery from physical illness. In S. Cohen & S. L. Syme, eds., *Social support and health,* pp. 281–302. Orlando, Fla.: Academic Press.

9

Minority Issues and Quality of Life in the Frail Elderly

E. PERCIL STANFORD

Introduction

The social world of the elderly is becoming much more heterogeneous as the number of older people in our society continues to burgeon. Currently, at least 10% of the population 65 and older is nonwhite. Recent census figures show that approximately 11% of the white population is 65 or over, while approximately 8% of African-Americans, 6% of Asian/Pacific Islanders, 5% of Latinos, and 5% of American Indians are in this age group. These figures are important in that the total minority population over 65 has reached a point where differences in language and other cultural distinctions must now be taken into consideration in greater detail. The shift in the percentage of minority elderly makes it necessary to focus on this population as a pivotal point for policy development and program implementation.

As we approach the 1990s and move into the twenty-first century, elderly from culturally diverse backgrounds, in many instances, will have been the marginal people able to bridge their native cultures and effectively survive in the mainstream. This distinction will be a tremendous asset. They will not only serve as interpreters for members of their particular groups but will also help to effectively provide leadership for the aging population as a whole. Their strength will be in their understanding of the needs and expectations of minority cultures as well as those of society at large.

Skeptics are apt to raise the question of the validity of viewing marginal minority older persons as interpreters for the needs of individuals from their cultural groups. It is true that many will have been living and generally operating on the fringes of the communities and cultures from which they originally came; however, there are very few who will have been completely divorced from the cultures that represent their backgrounds. Most will have grown up in areas

Copyright © 1991 by Academic Press, Inc.
All rights of reproduction in any form reserved.

where they were forced to experience segregation based on race, ethnicity, or religious belief.

Attention will be given to "minority" as a concept, in juxtaposition to the concept of "diversity." The discussion will be broadened to consider issues around education, training, research, health, long-term care, demographic concerns, quality of life, and the position and status of the frail elderly in our society.

It is imperative that distinctions are made regarding the utilization of terms such as *culture, race, ethnicity,* and *minority.* Green (1982) discussed several critical concepts in his book, *Cultural Awareness in the Human Services.* He pointed out that race is a social, rather than biological, concept and serves no purpose other than to highlight or justify differences between groups. On the other hand, the concept of culture is more important for understanding minorities and ethnicity. Barth (1969) suggested that culture is made up of elements relevant to communication across some type of social boundary. Culture takes into consideration significant events and situations that characterize the backgrounds and experiences of different individuals.

The concept of minority is difficult to explain in simple terms. A person of minority status may not necessarily be considered ethnically distinct or different. Minority does not necessarily mean that one is from a societal group that is a numerical minority; it is more closely related to influence and power rather than numbers, and may take into consideration the degree to which individuals have been denied access to available goods and services. In old age, from a numerical perspective, men are the true minority; however, in practice, older women are also designated as a minority, not because of numbers but as a consequence of their unfair and unequal treatment throughout life. Weaver (1977a) indicated that minorities can include communities of interest and may represent those who have similar sets of values or life-styles and expectations apart from the mainstream or the broader societal group. In general, as used in the literature, the term *minority* refers to social and economic disability and not necessarily to cultural differences.

In gerontology, minorities have been described as those individuals who are Asian or Pacific Islander, African-American, Latino, or American Indian. These are "groups of color" that have been identified in the Civil Rights Act as protected groups. These were the groups that received special attention as a result of the Civil Rights Act of 1964 with regard to the implementation of the Johnson administration's "Great Society Programs" (Manuel, 1982; Valle, 1989). The discussion in the present chapter will proceed from the standpoint of ethnic groups being defined as social groups distinguished on the basis of "race, religion, or national origin" (Gordon, 1964, 27). It is agreed that certain ethnic groups, such as blacks and American Indians, are distinguished by national origin and that other groups, such as Jewish Americans and Mormons, are distinguished by religion (Markides, Liang, & Jackson, 1990).

Bechill (1979) provided insights into the relevance of culture, race, and ethnicity in the public sector with regard to organizations that have responsibility for providing public services to older people. He made it clear that, in the early stages of its development, the Older Americans Act did not have a strong emphasis on issues related to "minoritiness," culture, or ethnicity. Bechill also indicated that it was pointed out by Professor Mary Wiley of the University of Wisconsin School of Social Work that public and private programs often fail to perform adequately, because they do not understand their beneficiaries' culturally determined attitudes, beliefs, and values. Further, programs designed for primarily Anglo, middle-class, urban populations are not necessarily adequate for implementation by agencies working with nonwhite populations. Therefore, when some of these programs are applied to the poor, the widowed, members of minority groups, residents of rural areas, or other groups, the results are often less than satisfactory.

Current Critical Issues

Recent history shows that while many social scientists have agreed that the "melting pot" concept was meaningful, the emerging consensus is that the idea is much less relevant for addressing cultural diversity. It has become clear that groups hold tenaciously to their particular values and normative structures. The pendulum is rapidly swinging in a direction clearly indicating that people of the world are comfortable with their differences. From the perspectives of research, service delivery, and social policy, one of the primary concerns regarding ethnic minority elderly and their differences and similarities is with determining the appropriate means of assessment and analysis.

Once the decision has been made to sanction diversity as a way of understanding minority older people, there will be less confusion about specific descriptors that must be taken into consideration. The quality of life of minority elderly as they become more dependent and frail, without doubt, will depend on their previous personal histories as well as on social and economic histories of specific ethnic groups. Theoretical constructs suitable for explaining the composition of the minority elderly are tremendously limited. One possible way of conceptually explaining this composition is through the "diverse life patterns" concept (Stanford, 1990). Diverse life patterns are a culmination of the cumulative effect of the experiences that have been unique to the minority older person. The primary component of the concept is that there is a distinctiveness and uniqueness about the minority experience that is not part of the social, economic, or political experience of other groups of older people.

Diverse life patterns offer an opportunity for researchers and others to examine the life circumstances of minority older persons without the burden of having to prove that there are significant differences between minority elders and their cohorts. This approach automatically assumes that the differences are acceptable based on who the older people are. Once there is a comfort level in accepting diversity, the next step is to consider the status of the minority older person within the context of his or her environment, without the need to justify whether life circumstances are better or worse than those for the majority elderly population. Diverse life patterns provide a pathway for explaining why many minority individuals indicate that their quality of life is good when compared with other older persons, even while it would appear to be of a much lower quality (Stanford, 1990).

Critical issues that impinge on the quality of life of minority elders as they become more frail are no different than those facing older people in the mainstream. Issues become identifiable as minority only when the solutions cannot be marketed or resolved without taking into consideration the traditions, culture, and normative structure of the older person, who in many instances may be frail. For example, meal programs that specify a minimum age limit may counter the expectations and traditions of some groups who believe that the young should have high priority in getting good nutrition, because they represent the group's future. In addition, communication processes and techniques should appropriately reflect the cultural specific needs of the elders.

More than a decade has passed since the Federal Council on Aging, with the assistance of the Human Resources Corporation (1978), identified some of the major barriers facing minority older people. Basic circumstances have not changed but, in most instances, have become more complex. Concerns have become more poignant because of an increase in the actual number of older people in the frail and minority ranks.

Accuracy of Data

The challenges to the accuracy of the census and the lack of adequate alternative data creates serious difficulties in assessing the scope of issues, problems, needs, and factors affecting minority elderly persons. The census continues to have flaws that make it problematic for use in accurately projecting for minority aging populations. Problems focus on areas such as (1) undercounting of minorities, (2) mislabeling, (3) gaps in time from collection to use, (4) sampling procedures based on the assumption that data can be collected via a random selection process, and (5) failure to break out the true heterogeneity of minority older subpopulations for specific analyses. This is a crucial problem since social service funding formulas and the allocation of other resources depend on the accuracy of the census.

Minority elderly are not located randomly throughout the country and are extremely heterogeneous. Planners, researchers, and service providers cannot take the position that a program, service, or research design can be developed to adequately service the wide range of minority older people in our society (Human Resources Corporation, 1978).

Life Expectancy

Life expectancy differs between minorities and nonminorities and has a profound effect on the "crossover effect" after age 75, which creates a problem for how policies regarding frail elderly are implemented in relationship to minority older people. It has been shown that after age 75 to 80, blacks, in particular, tend to show increased longevity in comparison with whites (Manton, 1982; Markides, 1983). The hypothesis surrounding the crossover effect is that genetic and environmental factors converge on a heterogeneous black population to bring about a hardier, older black cohort (Manton, 1982).

There continues to be a lack of data to adequately examine life expectancy and mortality rates for minority older persons. Available data clearly show that minority people will continue to live fewer years than Anglo elderly (Human Resources Corporation, 1978). The life expectancy factor should be considered in juxtaposition to social, cultural, and environmental factors. Serious consideration must continue to be given to lowering the eligibility age for minorities or combining age with functional and social assessment to better determine eligibility for a variety of programs and services.

Indigenous Support Systems

Natural support systems in many minority communities are generally overlooked, yet they need to be considered as a resource. Support systems in minority communities have a history of being reliable and accessible (Antonucci, 1985; Human Resources Corporation, 1978). Often, indigenous support systems have been overlooked by larger and more comprehensive service systems.

The family continues to emerge as the single most important element in ensuring that the older frail minority elderly have a good quality of life. There are also significant numbers of minority elderly who are living alone and often do not depend on family or kin for assistance (Antonucci, 1985). The major element provided by the family is an environment in which elders can continue to be involved in their cultural and belief systems without being questioned or ridiculed. The family environment is generally the place where the elderly can pursue their life patterns without considerable disruption. There are exceptions, though, for as minorities become more assimilated there are divergences from cultural practices to which many elderly do not adjust.

Consensus is that we must consider the existence of the modified extended family rather than the nuclear family in assessing the role of family in quality of life of minority elderly. Gelfand and Kutzik (1979) pointed out that adult children in many instances continue to assist older parents, and vice versa, after starting families of their own. Economics will generally dictate the extent to which the increasing frail minority older population will be supported by the modified extended family. The economic support needed to provide for the frail minority elder coincides with the increase in the number of minority older people needing support from family networks.

There are few institutions that provide outside of the home care within the community or in surrounding areas designed specifically for the minority frail older person. It is pointed out by Markides and Mindell (1987) that the family is the institution responsible for transmitting culture, important beliefs, values, and norms, both of the family and the ethnic group. It is within the family that roles and relationships are determined. The flexibility of family structures and roles will be affected noticeably by the duration, size, and influence of the intergenerational family. Bengtson, Rosenthal, and Barton (1990) discuss a variety of intergenerational structures, such as age-condensed, age-gapped, truncated, matrilineal, and step-family models, all of which have evolved because of the demographic revolution. As generations continue to live longer, the emphasis will begin to shift from youth to middle and older generations of elders. Older generations will be those who are more frail and in need of considerable care. More attention will be given to relationships between younger generations of older adults rather than focusing on youth and the larger categories of older people.

Perception of Needs

There are considerable inconsistencies between the perceptions of decision makers about the needs and problems of minority elderly and the perceptions of minority elderly themselves about their needs and problems. Depending on the degree to which this is true, the compatibility and utility of services and policies related to minority elderly are uncertain. More careful examination is needed to understand the extent to which misrepresentation of decision makers exists and how it can be corrected (Human Resources Corporation, 1978). Further attention must be paid not only to specific issues but also to "systems issues." Most services have not taken into consideration issues related to culture, language, and the perceived difficulties of access on the part of minority older persons. Very little research has been undertaken to assess the impact of federal policies and programs on minority elderly constituents (U.S. Commission on Civil Rights, 1982). The assumption that programs, once sanctioned by public bureaucracies, will automatically be implemented and utilized is a fallacy. It is at the local level that the intended resolution to service delivery will have a positive or negative impact on the minority elderly population.

Health

Health status is one of the most important issues for minority older people. It is more important for elderly who are frail and dependent upon effective health systems or extended family for meeting health needs (Cantor & Mayer, 1976). It has been noted that many ethnic groups reside in pockets or clusters within the larger community and remain somewhat isolated from the mainstream, which causes them to ignore or disassociate themselves from available health services. Once such pockets are located, it becomes necessary to determine the extent to which individuals utilize available health systems.

There are occasions when health needs and conditions are peculiar to, or disproportionately prevalent among, certain minority or ethnic groups. For example, African-Americans have been shown to be more susceptible to hypertension; Latinos have been reported to have greater incidents of tuberculosis than the rest of the population; and American Indians are reported to have 13 times greater incidents of pneumonia, influenza, and tuberculosis (Williams, 1980).

It is important to understand that having access to health programs and services is the key to a good quality of life for frail minority elders. The pivotal point for comprehensive health planning for minority elders is the integration of their needs with the mainstream (Williams, 1980). Health status is also multidimensional in nature and should be dealt with, measured, and interpreted from a multidimensional perspective. Therefore, it follows that the health status of minority elders cannot be considered or understood in terms of any single measurement but must be judged by a collective profile.

Kaplan (1988) discussed health as related to quality of life by referring to the impact of health conditions on function. He indicated that health often relates to quality of life independent of work, housing, air pollution, and other entities. Kaplan specified that many life measurement systems have come about during the past 20 years, some of which represent various traditions in measurement. There are two conceptual approaches indicated. One relates to the tradition of health status measurement that emerged during the 1960s and early 1970s. These measurements were guided by the World Health Organization definition of health status, which states that "health is the complete state of physical, mental, and social well-being and not merely the absence of disease." Kaplan (1988) pointed out that Croog et al., (1986) used a wide variety of outcome measures and collectively referred to them as quality of life. The measures included a patient's subjective evaluation of well-being, physical symptoms, sexual function, work performance and satisfaction, emotional status, cognitive function, social participation, and life satisfaction.

Pasick (1987) indicated that it is important to acknowledge and preserve diversity in pursuit of health and well-being. She also reminded us that recognition and protection of ethnic heterogeneity is not a revolutionary concept and has been a guiding principle in public health and health promotion policy, although it has not been carried out in practice. Pasick hastened to say that research from a health policy perspective that has been designed and implemented by non-minority professionals has not been adequate for minorities.

Access to health care by frail minority elders is a direct route to sustaining a good quality of life. It must be supported by family and community systems, and access channels should be sensitive culturally and provide the necessary outreach to encourage minority elders to become involved (Cuellar & Weeks, 1980; Mendoza, 1980). A high percentage of those providing outreach services should be indigenous to the community and understand that many older people will be venturing into the health system for the first time. Reasons for limited access consist of such things as high cost of medical services, lack of trust in medical doctors, language barriers, and transportation.

Overall, the elderly use their fair share of available resources. Brody (1980) pointed out that older people make up approximately 11% of the current population yet at the same time use approximately 30% of all the medical resources. He also pointed out that we do not know the differences between utilization that results from acute illness and that which results from chronic illness. These distinctions are critical when considering utilization patterns of minority frail older people, particularly with reference to the long-term care system. Utilization is influenced by the duration and severity of diseases. Diseases impact individuals and groups of individuals differently.

To enhance the quality of life of minority older people through service utilization, it is meaningful for providers to be able to predict utilization rates and patterns. Programs must not only be made accessible, attractive, and purposeful but should make every attempt to ensure cultural and ethnic relevance. For example, print material must be developed that describes the program in the language(s) and style that is familiar to participants or potential participants.

Quality Care and Significant Problems

There must be a commitment on the part of health care professionals to give high-quality care to minority elderly at all levels. The highest quality of care must come from those who are in control of health care programs. Secondarily, there must be well-trained and committed persons at the hands-on level. Weiler (1983) stated that successful treatment of disease in older people is essentially a tactical achievement no matter how great the treatment. There are two major considerations: the overall approach of the provider and the manner in which the older person is assessed and treated.

Each group of frail elderly minorities has special health issues that appear to be of particular concern or somewhat unique to them. There are many mitigating situations and circumstances that manifest these specific qualities. Distinctions between life-style differences and genetic tendencies are needed. African-American elderly have health problems and conditions that are often the same or similar to those of non–African-American frail elderly. Few, if any, are racially triggered or unique. Jackson (1978) said that those arguing the contrary usually have economically or politically vested interests, which are best served by unfairly categorizing elderly African-Americans monolithically. There is considerable credence given to the view that hypertension and heart disease are special diseases relegated to African-American older persons because of racial differences (Weaver, 1977b). Before ascribing these diseases to frail African-American elderly because of race, more attention must be given to the environmental and social conditions under which older African-Americans exist.

Older Asian and Pacific Islander elderly have special issues that determine their state of well-being and quality of life. One of the major issues is that the Asian elderly population over the age of 65 has a suicide rate that exceeds that for non-Asian elderly. Yee (1977) indicated that the Asian and American cultures are of two extremes with regard to how they treat older persons. In traditional Asian cultures, older persons are revered and have power. In the United States, older persons are often degraded, powerless, and helpless. In addressing suicide indirectly, Kamikawa (1982) indicated that such circumstances as denial of citizenship or of the right to own property and threats of deportation add to the explanation of how some elderly Asians feel about their well-being. The ethnic community provides a base for developing a sense of identity and well-being.

Life expectancy of the American Indian is somewhat uncertain. Figures range from 48 to 71 years of age (American Academy of Pediatrics, 1979). It is significant to note that American Indians are considered to be a young population, with approximately one-fourth of the total below age 20. Among the adult population of American Indians, alcohol continues to be a problem and takes on catastrophic dimensions. The Indian Health Service has indicated that approximately 75% of accidental deaths among American Indians are related to alcohol (National Institute on Alcohol Abuse and Alcoholism, 1985). The suicide rate among American Indians is twice the national rate. About 80% of American Indian suicide rates are estimated to be alcohol related (U.S. Department of Health and Human Services, 1980). Diabetes and tuberculosis are of higher incidence among the American Indian elderly than for other groups of minority older persons (U.S. Department of Health and Human Services, 1985, 1986). Each of these possible conditions or insults to the physical and psychosocial being of the elderly American Indian has made an indelible impression with regard to his or her quality of life and expectations for a high level of quality of life.

Many factors impinge on the level and quality of life of the frail elderly Latino (Anderson, Lewis, & Giachello, 1981). Pasick (1987) stated that among

Mexican-born Latinos aged 0 to 64, mortality rates for cardiovascular disease and cancer in both males and females were lower than those of Anglos. Excess incidence deaths also were found in areas such as diabetes, homicide (for both men and women), cirrhosis, and unintentional injuries (for males). As well, Latinos experience excess incidence of certain types of cancer, including cancer of the stomach, esophagus, pancreas, cervix, liver, and gall bladder. The conditions and circumstances surrounding health and its relationship to the quality of life of older Latinos is summarized in a study conducted by the Asociacion Nacional Pro Personas Mayores (1980).

Properly educating and training personnel will be the first step toward ensuring a reasonable quality of life for frail older people. Further, training and educational methods and procedures must take into consideration the diversity of the elderly population. Pritchard and Kitamura (1981) indicated that there must be a framework that assumes the importance of cultural pluralism and sociocultural differences. They reported that the integration of ethnic minority content would significantly improve all gerontological and geriatric curricula. Weiler (1983) asserted that: "In spite of the interest and success, the extent of training and education programs addressing the area of aging and wellness is limited." If the nonminority elderly are affected by the lack of interest in wellness of the elderly, the minority frail elderly are certainly at risk as well.

Social Policy

A strong social policy in aging will provide the underpinning necessary to ensure a good quality of life for frail minority older people. The phenomenon of a large number of long-lived minority elders is very new. The number of minority older people who are living long enough to reach the "frail stage of life" is recent enough for there to have been little or no planning. Morris's (1979) ideas regarding the role of the federal government continue to prevail. He indicated that whenever government has had to take a leadership role, it has taken the path of involving itself with industry and private citizens and not with state governments. If the concept of diverse life patterns is to be taken seriously, the federal sector cannot be expected to take full responsibility for shaping policies that will positively influence the quality of life of minority frail elders. States and their local counterparts have a deep and abiding responsibility to become more responsive to the burgeoning number of minority frail elders. Time is propitious in that minorities who are a part of the baby boom of the late 1940s are moving toward old age and will subsequently be included in the frail category. They will represent the first group of minority elders to experience frailty in large numbers.

A major policy issue concerns whether mainstreaming older people into services is a detriment. Consideration must be given to the fact that experiences of minority older persons trying to participate in mainstream programs have been relatively short; on the other hand, such experiences have been long enough for minority elderly to know that the feasibility of the mainstream approach being successful may not be reasonable.

Summary

Prior to the 1980s, little or no attention was given to the idea that minority older persons may be among the nation's frail in significant numbers. They have been virtually absent in major research studies of the last three decades. The paucity of ethnic minority research databases from which to build hypotheses and generate theoretical underpinnings has been a major oversight. Research with multiple groups will establish the degree to which independent variables assist in providing insights regarding the specific culture under review without having to make comparisons with similar or mainstream groups.

Quality education and training for minority scholars and others interested in minority aging continues to be a major need. It is fallacious to assume that meaningful research and theoretical advances will be made unless there are well-trained individuals to pursue scholarly work in ethnogerontology and geriatrics. The need is equally as great in service areas as it is in academia.

As the twenty-first century comes into focus, it is essential that policies determining the level and quality of service include clearly stated guidelines that will enhance services to minority elders. They will be most effective if they allow for minority older clients to be served by themselves, their families, or extended kin groups and/or institutions in the communities that normally serve them.

The ever-increasing multiple-generation ethnic minority family is a new phenomenon. As the number of minority elders increases, living arrangements will necessarily change. There will be more minority elders caring for each other, and, most likely, they will be living in communal situations in greater numbers than is currently the case. Without any major changes in income, a high percentage of minority elders will be living in high crime areas. Their activities will be geared more toward indoor rather than outside activities and will most likely take place in groups of two or more during daylight hours.

In general, the future outlook regarding the quality of life for minority frail individuals is that major economic, social, and behavioral changes must take place in order to keep pace with the burgeoning minority elderly population. Maintaining good health will continue to be a very high priority. To that extent, much more emphasis will be on prevention. In essence, there is no single cure that will suddenly ensure that minority older persons will experience a good quality of life. The only certainty is that, given the proper attention and input from a research, theoretical, and practice perspective, it is possible to move in a positive direction.

The plethora of issues that dominate and predict the life-styles of minority frail elders will continue to be exacerbated. The issues are complex and perplexing and will confuse those who do not take time to understand their uniqueness. Issues may appear to be the same in content; however, from an operational perspective there are severe differences.

There is a need to swiftly move away from the melting pot idea, which has stressed assimilation to a position of accepting diversity as a way of dealing with the uniqueness of different cultural and ethnic groups.

References

American Academy of Pediatrics (1979). California health care for children. California District.

Anderson, R., Lewis, S., & Giachello, A. L. (1981). Access to medical care among the Hispanic population of the southwest United States. *Journal of Health and Social Behavior, 22,* 78–89.

Antonucci, T. C. (1985). Personal characteristics, social support, and social behavior. In R. H. Binstock & E. Shanas, eds., *Handbook of aging and the social sciences,* 2nd ed., pp. 94–128. New York: Van Nostrand Reinhold.

Asociacion Nacional Pro Personas Mayores (1980). *A national study to access the service needs of the Hispanic elderly.* Los Angeles: A.N.P.P.M.

Barth, F. (1969). *Ethnic groups and boundaries.* Boston: Little, Brown & Company.

Bechill, W. (1979). Politics of aging and ethnicity. In D. E. Gelfand & A. J. Kutzik, eds., *Ethnicity and aging.* New York: Springer.

Bengtson, V., Rosenthal, C., & Barton, L. (1990). Families and aging: Diversity and heterogeneity. In R. H. Binstock & L. George, eds., *Handbook of aging and the social sciences.* San Diego, Calif.: Academic Press.

Brody, S. J. (1980). Toward a health policy for the elderly. *Generations, 5,* 4–5.

Cantor, M., & Mayer, M. (1976). Health and the inner-city elderly. *Gerontologist I, 16,* 17–25.

Croog, S. H., Levine, S., Testa, M., Brown, D., Bulpitt, C., Jenkins, C. D., Kleerman, G. L., & Williams, G. H. (1986). The effects of anti-hypertensive therapy on quality of life. *New England Journal of Medicine, 314,* 1657–1664.

Cuellar, J., & Weeks, J. (1980). *Minority elderly Americans: A prototype for area agencies on aging.* San Diego, Calif.: Allied Home Health Association.

Gelfand, D. E., & Kutzik, A. J., eds. (1979). *Ethnicity and aging theory, research, and policy.* New York: Springer.

Gordon, M. M. (1964). *Assimilation in American life.* New York: Oxford University Press.

Green, J. W. (1982). *Cultural awareness in the human services.* Englewood Cliffs, N.J.: Prentice-Hall.

Human Resources Corporation (1978). *Policy issues concerning the minority elderly: Final report.* San Francisco: Human Resources Corporation.

Jackson, J. (1978). *Special health problems of aged blacks in aging.* Washington, D.C.: U.S. Department of Health, Education, and Welfare, Office of Human Development Services, Administration on Aging.

Kamikawa, L. (1982). Expanding perceptions of aging: The Pacific/Asian elderly. *Generations, 6,* 26–27.

Kaplan, R. M. (1988). Health-related quality of life in cardiovascular disease. *Journal of Consulting and Clinical Psychology, 56,* 382–392.

Manton, K. G. (1982). Differential life expectancy: Possible explanations during later years. In R. C. Manuel, ed., *Minority aging: Sociological and social psychological issues,* pp. 63–70. Westport, Conn.: Greenwood.

Manton, K. G., Poss, S. S., & Wing, S. (1979). The black/white mortality crossover: Investigation from the perspective of the components of aging. *The Gerontologist, 19,* 91–229.

Manuel, R. C., ed. (1982). *Minority aging: Sociological and social psychological issues.* Westport, Conn.: Greenwood.

Markides, K. S. (1983). Mortality among minority populations: A review of recent patterns and trends. *Public Health Reports, 98,* 252–260.

Markides, K. S., & Mindell, C. H. (1987). *Aging and ethnicity.* Sage Library of Social Research, vol. 163, 97, Newbury Park, Calif.: Sage.

Markides, K., Liang, J., & Jackson, J. (1990). Race, ethnicity and aging: Conceptual and methodological issues. In R. H. Binstock & L. George, eds., *Handbook of aging and the social sciences.* San Diego, Calif.: Academic Press.

Mendoza, L. (1980). Health care access for minority elderly. *Generations, 5,* 32.

Morris, R. (1979). *Social policy of the American welfare state.* San Francisco: Harper & Row.

Nandi, P. K. (1980). *The quality of life of Asian Americans—An exploratory study in a middle-size community.* Chicago, Ill.: Pacific/Asian-American Mental Health Research Center.

National Institute on Alcohol Abuse and Alcoholism (1985). Alcohol and native Americans. *Alcohol topics: Research review.*

Pasick, R. J. (1987). *Health promotion for minorities in California.* Berkeley, Calif.: Western Consortium for Public Health.

Pritchard, D. C., & Kitamura, L. Y. (1981). Minority aging input in institutions of higher education. In E. P. Stanford & S. A. Lockery, eds., *Trends and status of minority aging.* San Diego, Calif.: University Center on Aging, Campanile Press.

Stanford, E. P. (1977). Perspective toward comprehensive services for minority elderly. In E. P. Stanford, ed., *Comprehensive service delivery systems for the minority aged.* San Diego, Calif.: Campanile Press.

Stanford, E. P. (1990). Diverse black aged. In Z. Harel, E. McKinney, & M. Williams, eds., *Black aged: Understanding diversity and service needs.* Berkeley, Calif.: Sage.

U.S. Commission on Civil Rights (1982). *Minority elderly services: New programs, old problems,* Part 1. Washington, D.C.: U.S. Government Printing Office.

U.S. Department of Health and Human Services (1980). *Facts in brief: Alcohol and American Indians.* Rockville, Md.: U.S. Government Printing Office.

U.S. Department of Health and Human Services (1985). *Health status of minorities and low income groups.* Washington, D.C.: U.S. Government Printing Office.

U.S. Department of Health and Human Services (1986). *Chemical dependency and diabetes.* Subcommittee on diabetes in report of the secretary's task force on black and minority health, vol. 7, January. Washington, D.C.: U.S. Government Printing Office.

Valle, R. (1989). U.S. ethnic minority group access to long-term care. In T. Schwab, ed., *Caring for an aging world: International models for long-term care, financing and delivery*. New York: McGraw Hill.

Weaver, J. L. (1977a). *National health policy and the underserved*. St. Louis: C.V. Mosby.

Weaver, J. L. (1977b). Personal health care: A major concern for minority aged. In E. P. Stanford, ed., *Comprehensive service delivery systems for the minority aged*. San Diego, Calif.: Campanile Press.

Weiler, P. G. (1983). Education and training in wellness for elders. *Generations, 7,* 34–36.

Williams, D. A. (1980). Consideration for comprehensive health planning for elderly minority populations. In E. P. Stanford, ed., *Minority aging: Policy issues for the 80s*. San Diego, Calif.: Campanile Press.

Yee, B. W. K. (1977). *Asian-American elderly: A life-span developmental approach to minorities and learned helplessness*. Paper presented at the American Psychological Association Convention, August. San Francisco, Calif.

IV

The World within Us and Quality of Life in the Frail Elderly

10

The Influence of Aging or Frailty on Perceptions and Expressions of the Self: Theoretical and Methodological Issues

ROBERT C. ATCHLEY

The self is an ancient concept with many meanings. Throughout the history of Western thought, poets, playwrights, and philosophers have devoted a great deal of time and attention to the self and its many facets. Indeed, to many, understanding the self is the greatest individual challenge. For contemporary scholars who study individuals, the self is seen as both a holistic, highly generalized concept as well as an organized collection of very specific ideas (Bengtson, Reedy, & Gordon, 1985; Breytspraak & George, 1982; Filipp & Klauer, 1986). Both general and specific ideas about the self are stored in memory. It is usually assumed that, as part of an individual's collected memories, the self is available for conscious reflection and retrieval from memory and that it can be directly studied empirically through self-reports and observations of behavior (Breytspraak & George, 1982) and indirectly through analysis of texts generated by the individual.

In his well-known theory of quality of life, Lawton (1983) identified four sectors of the good life: psychological well-being, behavioral competence, perceived quality of life, and objective environment. In Lawton's view, the most meaningful aspects of the good life are stored in the self:

> The exercise of behavioral competence builds perceived competence. The varieties of psychological well-being are reflections of the self. Perceived quality of life may be seen as the net of one's evaluation of the congruence between self and the external world. The objective environment is most distant from the self, but where it is salient to the person it may be the symbol of her competence and generativity, as in the long-occupied home. (p. 356)

In their landmark study on adjustment to entry into nursing homes, Lieberman and Tobin (1983) found that having a robust self increased a person's chances of

The Concept and Measurement of
Quality of Life in the Frail Elderly

Copyright © 1991 by Academic Press, Inc.
All rights of reproduction in any form reserved.

surviving the change. These are but two examples of work in gerontology that acknowledges the centrality of the self as an organizing concept in our attempts to understand both quality of life and individual aging. In addition, increasing quality of life is a major goal of most striving to perfect and maintain the self.

Despite the importance and the lengthy history of the self as a topic of social science scholarship, a great deal of conceptual and theoretical confusion still exists. After nearly 100 years of research, there is only modest agreement on the concepts and language that should be used to describe the various components of self. Theories about how the self is developed, maintained, defended, or changed are often incomplete; and research methods for the study of the self focus mainly on global self-esteem and on easily measured attributes of the self (Bengtson *et al.*, 1985).

Researchers and theorists have seldom looked at the self as a process; instead, most effort has dealt with structure and content. As a result, we have very little sense of the self as an entity that evolves in a particular direction, and very little knowledge of the dynamic processes through which this evolution takes place. Only recently has work on the self begun to include the notion that individuals might exert some influence over the development and maintenance of the self (Filipp & Klauer, 1986; Kaufman, 1986). In this latter view, we can begin to examine how an individual's motives and strategies are targeted toward the self and with what effects.

With the notable exception of locus of control (for a review, see Baltes & Baltes, 1986), there has been a relative neglect of research on the aging self. Most studies aimed specifically at aging and the self were done prior to 1975 (Bengtson *et al.*, 1985). The reason for this neglect is unclear, but it is probably related to increased reliance on available data sets (which seldom include data on the self) and a bias toward research topics that are amenable to quantitative research methods. In addition, some investigators are skeptical about the feasibility of measuring the self successfully (Lawton, 1983).

Recent literature reviews on aging and the self (Bengtson *et al.*, 1985; Breytspraak & George, 1982; Filipp & Klauer, 1986) all pointed out that measurement issues in the study of the self cannot be sufficiently resolved until at least a minimal level of conceptual and theoretical clarity is achieved. Most were not impressed with the level of conceptual development we have achieved to date. In addition, the reviewers concluded that there was no coherent theory on how either aging or frailty might be expected to affect the self.

This paper is an attempt to (1) organize existing concepts and theory about the self into a framework that can be used to inform research about aging and the self; (2) articulate a variety of theoretical relationships that might be expected between aging and the self; (3) explore theory with regard to how frailty interacts with the self; and (4) outline some of the methodological issues that must be resolved or at least taken into account in testing theories about aging, frailty, the self, and quality of life.

Concepts and Theory about the Self

Concepts and theory about the self can be separated into several categories: (1) ways in which the self is structured and in which the structural elements influence one another; (2) processes through which the self is developed, maintained, and changed; (3) the impact of social structural factors on self structures and processes; and (4) factors explaining the developmental direction that the evolution of self takes.

Structure of the Self

In the literature on the self, there is a fundamental distinction made between the self as awareness and the self as object in awareness. Mead (1934) called the self as awareness the "I" and the self as object the "me." As pure awareness, consciousness has no attributes and therefore no structure. It is the "objective self"—self as object of its own reflection—that has structure. The raw content of the self consists of a wide variety of self-referent conceptions—attitudes, values, beliefs, norms, and knowledge. This content is the result of a continuous process in which information about the self is sought, imposed, processed, perceived, evaluated, categorized, analyzed, enhanced, suppressed, and stored in that area of memory reserved for self conceptions (Filipp & Klauer, 1986). As Markus and Nurius (1986) pointed out,

> The individual's collection of self-conceptions . . . can include the good selves (the ones we remember fondly), the bad selves (the ones we would just as soon forget), the hoped-for selves, the feared selves, the not-me selves, the ideal selves, the ought-to selves. They also can vary dramatically in their degree of affective, cognitive, and behavioral elaboration. They also vary in valence. (p. 957)

Within this very large set of specific memories, scholars have traditionally differentiated self-knowledge into four categories: self-concept, ideal self, self-evaluation, and self-esteem (Atchley, 1982a). *Self-concept* is what we think we are like, *ideal self* is what we want to be like or think we ought to be like, *self-evaluation* is a moral assessment of how well we have lived up to what we think we ought to have done or been, and *self-esteem* is the degree to which we like or dislike ourselves. This typology is an elaboration of the traditional cognitive and affective dimensions of self (Rosenberg, 1979). Bengtson *et al.* (1985) also added a category they called the conative self, which referred to actions related to the self, to motivation and *self-striving*.

Traditional self theory asserts that self-esteem is a function of the comparison between the self-concept (what you are) and the ideal self (what you ought to be or want to be). Social role performances, social attributes such as gender, and qualities such as honesty are examples of ideas that are contained in the self-concept. The ideal self is what we expect of ourselves. If we have fallen short of our expectations, we are likely to assess that we have failed (evaluation) and to feel bad about it (lowered self-esteem). It is important to realize that, in this formulation, improved results can be produced either by lowering expectations or by improving the self-concept. Motivation and planning aimed at increasing self-esteem, and thereby improving quality of life, would be part of the conative self.

All these types of self-knowledge can exist at various levels of abstraction. For example, locus of control can exist in the self-concept as a generalized characteristic of the self across a variety of social roles and social situations. This is how it was initially used by Rotter (1966). In this sense, the concept is quite abstract. On the other hand, ideas about locus of control also can be specific to particular behavioral domains. This is the multidimensional and domain-specific approach advocated by Lachman (1986). Those who approach the study of the self from a more abstract perspective write about overarching self-schema (Filipp & Klauer, 1986) or self-themes (Kaufman, 1986). These abstractions are useful when or if it is necessary to come to long-range general conclusions about the self.

Specific dimensions of the self tend to be created by researchers to serve a particular purpose. For example, Markus and Nurius (1986) used diverse items such as sexiness, being in good shape, having wrinkled skin, and being paralyzed to indicate a domain they called *physical self-concept*. Markus and Nurius were interested not only in current self-concepts but also in what people saw as *potential future* self-concepts. Indeed, Markus and Nurius argued that instead of looking at the self-concept that is relatively stable, it may be more useful to deal with the *working self-concept*—the set of self-conceptions that are currently active in thought and memory. It may be that the working self-concept is more volatile and produces more day-to-day fluctuations in self-esteem than does the more stable historical self-concept, which tends to be tapped by social surveys. Temporal factors are certainly significant, and it is probably important to look not only at current self-concept but also at past and future selves as well.

Various social situations may also evoke different self-concepts in the individual. For example, in one person, being at work may activate a less competent self-concept, whereas being at church may activate a more competent self-concept, and for another person the result may be just the opposite. This process of selective evoking of various self-concepts occurs in part because of variations in the specific stimuli about the self that have primacy in various role contexts. It also occurs because the specific others with whom role negotiations take place are usually different across different roles. In urban life today, roles and social situations tend to be compartmentalized, with little overlap in roles or specific others.

It is difficult to develop scientific laws about how the self operates because there is wide variation in the extent to which individuals think about the self and store these thoughts away in memory as part of the self. As a result, much of what we know about the self is the result of studies of articulate, middle-class people. Even within this relatively narrow category, there are differences in amount of thought and depth of reflectiveness or the extent to which people engage in what Heidegger (1966) called "contemplative thinking." Those who frequently reflect on themselves are probably a minority in most walks of life; so we should be tentative about applying our concepts and theories about the self to other types of people without first exploring the possibility of as-yet undiscovered ways of thinking about or expressing the self.

Processes Affecting the Self

Processes that are used to develop, maintain, and modify the self include (1) sources of knowledge about the self, (2) personal/internal processes that occur mostly within the individual, and (3) social/interactive processes that involve interaction with others about the self or the use of culture to develop ideas about the self.

Sources of knowledge about the self include feedback from others, social comparisons with others or with the self at another time, observation of one's own states and behavior, and revisionist personal history (Filipp & Klauer, 1986). Also called reflected appraisals (Rosenberg, 1979), feedback from others about one's self has long been assumed to be a fundamental process for gaining knowledge of the self (Mead, 1934). In addition to direct feedback through the utterances and body language of others, there may be feedback from the individual's concept of the generalized other. The essence of feedback is the person's *perceptions* of how others actually respond to the presented self or *projected* responses to the presented self that could be expected from specific reference others or from the "generalized other" (Mead, 1934). Usually the concern is with some specific aspect or aspects of the self or specific portrayal of self, rather than with the self as a global construct.

Social comparisons involve comparing self with others. In general terms these comparisons may reveal that, in contrast to self, others are better off, worse off, or in about the same situation as the individual making the comparison. If others are seen as better off than the person, then feelings of relative deprivation may occur, which can result in negative self-assessment. If others are viewed as worse off, then positive self-assessment can result. If others are perceived as in about the same situation, there may be a feeling of kinship or belonging. A key aspect of this process is the specific others chosen for comparison. Most individuals are free to choose to compare themselves with others worse off than they are and, as a result, feel relative appreciation for themselves, yet some choose to compare themselves to others whose apparent successes make them seem superior.

Reference groups, groups whose members the individual wants to be like, probably play an important part in whether social comparisons result in feelings of relative appreciation or relative deprivation or belonging concerning the self. However, little or no research has been done on this topic.

Much of the traditional literature on the self leaves little room for individual initiative in the evolution of the self. However, most people are self-conscious to at least a modest degree. This self-consciousness means that over time the individual accumulates a large pool of his or her *own observations* of internal states, capabilities, and behavior. And unlike others, the individual evaluates the self not just in terms of the current self but in terms of probable future selves (Markus & Nurius, 1986) and past selves as well. Because others may not know about the past or future selves, the individual may discount feedback from them and put more stock in his or her own evaluations. This may be why Shrauger and Schoeneman (1979) concluded their review of over 50 studies with a statement that there was no clear evidence that feedback from others had much influence on self-evaluations.

Past personal history is an important part of the self for most people. Greenwald (1980) argued that people do not see their personal histories objectively. Instead, they fabricate and revise their personal histories through a set of processes that virtually guarantee a positive conception of the self throughout one's own history. First, the past is recalled as a drama in which the self is playing the lead part. Second, in the fabrication of this history, the self takes credit for successes and puts the blame for failures on outside forces. Finally, the self is a very conservative historian who insists that new information about the self must fit and support the prior view of the self. Of course, Greenwald's theory would not apply to people who take the opposite tack and construct a negative self by accepting no credit and seeking all available blame—the masochistic self (Atchley, 1982a). Filipp and Klauer (1986) pointed out that individuals reflect back on themselves in past actions and events and may create "new" information about the self by reinterpreting experiences, altering causal attributions, or changing the relative importance of the information. Kaufman (1986) also found that reinterpretation played a pivotal role in maintaining the self. These ideas point to an active role for the individual in constructing the past self.

In managing the self, the individual may use various forms of selection, such as selective perception, selective memory, and selective interaction. These techniques give the individual increased control over the flow of information about the self. The basis of these selection processes is a set of priorities for the self. The personal goals that make up the ideal self are arranged in a hierarchy—various personal goals are ranked in different positions in terms of relative desirability and capacity to motivate perception and behavior, including selection processes.

Motivation in relation to the self provides a sense of direction and can produce striving aimed at altering the self in specific ways. Markus and Nurius (1986) pointed out that the self-concept includes not only what we perceive ourselves to be but also what we hope to become or are afraid of becoming. Bengtson *et al.* (1985) used the concepts of valued and disvalued selves to capture this idea. In this formulation, the process of managing the self is not an aimless one. The individual perceives information and takes actions in such a way as to increase the chances of realizing the valued or hoped-for self and of avoiding the disvalued or feared self. Behavior is sometimes intended to test the feasibility of various possible selves. Markus and Nurius (1986) contended that individuals create probable future selves and then develop plans and strategies for making those selves happen.

Obviously, the individual is not entirely free to develop completely unrealistic conceptions of self. The self must be realistic enough to produce a modicum of predictability in responses from others, which allows the individual to trust his or her conceptions of self. Individuals probably seek a minimum degree of realism rather than going overboard. For example, if the person has a concept of self as relatively intelligent, he or she may confirm this with observations that others generally treat him or her as intelligent rather than by extensive IQ testing and precise ranking with regard to intelligence. The latter may provide more information than the person wants or needs.

Duration of various role relationships or group memberships has important results for the processes used to manage the self. At the beginning of new role relationships, people generally take on a ready-made self inherent in the role (Goffman, 1959). Within a short time, however, most people begin to attempt to personalize the roles they play by negotiating changes in role expectations to bring them more in line with the individual's definition of current or future self. Thus, role negotiations are an important tool people use to reduce conflict between role and self.

Social Structural Influences

Thus far, our discussion has implied that the structure and dynamics of the self are similar in all kinds of people. However, position in the social structure is an important variable that creates quite different situations for individuals. The ideal self is a composite of individual desires and social prescriptions, and both are influenced by subculture. For example, ideal selves differ substantially from one social class to another and from one ethnic group to another. In addition, social attributes influence the relevant ideal self even within social class or ethnic cultures. Gender and age are important individual attributes that influence social definitions of ideal self. However, social structural influences on variations in self across people have received relatively little study.

Developing, Maintaining, and Changing the Self

Much has been written about the initial development of self in childhood and adolescence. Information gathering, diagnosis, and behavioral experimentation are processes that dominate during this period. Once the individual achieves at least a working closure on some elements of the self, then processes aimed at conserving and maintaining the self and its sense of direction come into play. This often happens in young adulthood. Confirmation and reality-testing of the self are also important during this period. This working closure about the nature of the self is a necessary condition for self-confidence. In our individualistic society, with its belief in human perfectibility, notions of self-improvement are also common early in life. Here the individual is concerned with creating a new self more in line with the ideal self. In other words, self-improvement is about perfecting the self and thereby increasing self-esteem. This process involves specific efforts, goals, plans, and strategies.

The self can be changed through loss as well. For example, sudden disability can cause a fundamental upheaval in the self-concept, uncertainty with regard to the appropriate ideal self, and inconsistency in feedback from others. Coping skills are used to grapple with the problems associated with creating a new self-concept while at the same time carrying over as much of the old self-concept as possible (Atchley, 1989).

Theory about the Intersection of Normal Aging and the Self

Aging is often accompanied by developmental changes that improve subjective quality of life. *Normal aging* refers to usual, customary patterns of human aging (Atchley, 1989). It is characterized by a lack of mental or physical disability. Age changes usually slow people down but do not disable them. Both Breytspraak and George (1982) and Bengtson *et al.* (1985) contended that as yet there is no theoretical basis for assuming that aging per se influences the self. However, there are a number of aspects of normal aging that could be expected to affect the self, and they will be outlined in this section.

By definition, aging increases the individual's backlog of experience, including the results of testing various aspects of the self. Thus, compared to younger people, older people could be expected to have a more tested, stable set of processes for managing the self, as well as more robust self-concepts. By the time most normally aging people reach age 65, they have accumulated in memory a vast array of experiences of themselves in a wide variety of social roles and social situations. They have long since come to closure about what they are like and what is realistic for them to aspire to be like. A large majority have very positive self-esteem (Atchley, 1976). These outcomes result from the accumulation of time living with the adult self and the gradual refinements that come from decades of self-reflection and self-motivation and striving.

Because they have a large amount of data based on their own observations, older people are less likely than young adults to use reflected appraisals to maintain the self and more likely to use social comparisons with others, their own observations, and their own personal constructions of the past self as the bases of comparison in assessing or evaluating the self. This developmental change in the weight attached to various sources of information about the self explains how most older people are able to have a perception of self as competent and worthwhile in a society that bombards them with messages about the negative effects of aging. This feedback simply carries very little weight compared to the evidence the individual already has stored in memory. Satisfaction with the aging self is nowhere better illustrated than in the widespread perception among older people that even if they could know what they know now, they would not choose to go back to the insecurities of young adulthood (Atchley, 1982b).

Aging also increases self-acceptance, which usually results in a more realistic ideal self. Aging increases the number of times individuals have experienced ambiguities and contradictions in the self. The most common response to these experiences is to increase individual tolerance of ambiguity and contradiction, which means that the individual feels less pressure to resolve every ambiguity or contradiction within themselves. Part of this tolerance comes from decades of observing the results of attempting to change the self. As it becomes more apparent that the self is not perfectible, it may seem more reasonable to lower one's expectations, which puts the ideal self within closer reach. As aging increases the number of past successes that are stored in memory and as aging decreases expectations for the ideal self, self-denigration could be expected to decrease. Research results support this formulation (Pearlin & Schooler, 1978).

Another reason for greater acceptance of self with aging is the increasingly thematic way that individuals summarize the self. Young people tend to describe themselves in terms of their bodies, physical appearance, social roles, and attributes, with little content dealing with values, relationships, or successes. Older people, on the other hand, tend to summarize their lives in terms of recurring individualized themes that express their values and their sources of information about success, meaning, and self-esteem. In her extensive interviews with 60 older people, Kaufman (1986) found that her respondents attempted to "account" for their lives by constructing life stories that made their lives seem logical and coherent. These stories were not organized around social structural factors such as ethnic group membership or social class, or historical events such as the Great Depression or World War II. Instead, life stories were organized around themes such as "My whole life has been devoted to my law practice" or "My family is my life—I am nothing without them." These themes identified "the personal, idiosyncratic ways of experiencing and communicating meaning [and values] in the individual life—the ways in which people *interpret experience so as to give unique internal continuity and structure to the self*" (Kaufman, 1986, 115; emphasis added). This interpretive self can be constructed so as to be increasingly acceptable.

Aging gives people the opportunity to periodically reevaluate their values and to change them. Increased experience leads many aging people to shift their values, which are related to both self-concept and ideal self, away from achievement in the context of public social roles toward achievement in the context of private activities (Maehr & Kleiber, 1981). Even among people who are employed, Pearlin and Schooler (1978) found that adults in their 50s and 60s placed less value on money and found satisfactions in their work other than power, salaries, or promotions.

At all ages, some people have to deal with having a body that does not fit their ideal. However, a normally aging body exposes the person to a different kind of disvalued self, one that is more likely to activate negative reactions from strangers. Most young people make more of their own physical imperfections than other people do, but people in general make a bigger fuss over wrinkles and gray hair than do people who actually have them. Although there is every reason to suspect that body image might change with aging and have an impact on the self, this aspect has received little study.

Another potentially negative effect of aging on the self is the sense of a foreshortened future (Marshall, 1986). With the perception that life is finite and that the end, although perhaps still far in the distance, is in sight, the individual faces an existential problem of no longer seeing a limitless future in which to achieve the ideal self. In addition, future selves are more likely to be those that can be achieved in the short run. The potential negative result of the approaching end is often not death itself but dread of disability or dementia, which become more probable with each passing year. When increasing age changes disability from a remote to a more likely possibility, the results can be a concept of future self very much out of tune with the "ageless self" constructed by most normally aging people (Kaufman, 1986).

Aging also alters the social environment and how it influences the self (Atchley, 1982a, 1989). First, aging increases the duration of most role relationships, which in turn increases the probability that these relationships will be highly personalized and in tune with the self. This perspective applies mainly within the aging person's network of family and friends. Second, aging reduces the need to conform to externally imposed, nonnegotiable role demands. When people are freed from the demands of employment by retirement and from the responsibilities of child rearing by having launched their children into adulthood, two major sources of self-role conflict are removed. Third, aging puts the individual into a new social category—older person—a category that is socially disvalued. Most people age 65 or older reject the label "older person" as applying to them, but they cannot alter the fact that in both public opinion and public policy that is where they are placed. Although most aging people feel that the stereotypes applied to older people do not apply to them, they are bound to encounter situations in which others behave toward them as if the stereotypes of aging people as ugly, asexual, incompetent, aimless, and stupid (Comfort, 1976) do apply to them. Fortunately, most older people have adequate defenses for dealing with these messages, but it has important implications for the self that they are put on the defensive rather than made to feel at home. This often has subtle effects on self-confidence because older individuals cannot entirely predict when and where their own conceptions of themselves as worthy people will be called into question. We need to learn more about this.

It is also important to recognize that some aspects of aging have no systematic effect on the self. For example, life events associated with aging, such as retirement and the empty nest, apparently have little or no effect on the self (Atchley, 1982b; Troll, Miller, & Atchley, 1979).

As shown in this section, normal aging influences the self in many ways, mostly for the good. However, when aging reaches the point of frailty, then this positive picture changes.

Theory about the Intersection of Frailty and the Self

As a concept, *frailty* refers to physical or mental weakness, fragility, and vulnerability. Frail people may seem as if their bones would easily break; their physical reserve capacity may be extremely limited, their mental processes may be confused or slow, and it would not take much to make them disabled. Indeed, many frail people *are* disabled. In the absence of serious chronic illness, aging does not produce frailty until around the ninth decade. However, many aging people have chronic conditions that render them frail by age 65.

In contrast to aging, where there are as many, or more, potential advantages to the self as there are disadvantages, there are many reasons to expect that frailty would have more negative than positive effects on the self. These negative impacts include interrupted continuity of the self, much more need for defenses and coping with losses to the self, reduced capacity to use defenses such as selective interaction, difficulty identifying possible selves, depersonalization of the social environment, changes in reference groups, and rusty skills in using feedback to reconstitute the self.

Frailty often comes on gradually, and the individual has time to adjust, including incorporation of new information into the self. However, at the point where frailty becomes disability, more than fine-tuning is required and the individual usually must redefine the meaning of competence and self-reliance. Lawton (1978) pointed out that as they age, people increasingly rely for evidence of competence on mundane activities such as housework. When one can no longer cook waffles in a toaster, put on shoes, or open a dresser drawer, it probably becomes more and more difficult to maintain a definition of current self as instrumentally competent. Instead, the locus of one's concept of competence might shift to qualitative aspects of self such as warmth, humor, or interpersonal skills. As one retired teacher told me, "As you become more like a prune on the outside, you have to become more like a peach on the inside."

People want to maintain continuity of self as an abstraction. The details may change a great deal, but people continue to see themselves as the same general type of person (Atchley, 1989). They want to see inner change as connected to their past and to see their past as sustaining, supporting, and justifying the new self (Lieberman & Tobin, 1983). Kaufman (1986) found that older people reinterpreted their current experiences "so that old values could take on new meanings appropriate to present circumstances." Lieberman and Tobin (1983) found similar processes at work among the participants in their study of institutionalization. However, the new definition of self must be realistic enough to allow the individual to anticipate accurately the responses of others (Lieberman & Tobin, 1983). This requires that frailty be acknowledged as a reality and not be denied.

Whereas aging stimulates processes that focus on maintaining and affirming the self, frailty and disability stimulate defensive processes that focus on coping with losses. Dependence on others is a socially disvalued role for adults. In social comparisons, frail or disabled people are more likely to feel relative deprivation than relative appreciation. They are more likely to see feared or disvalued selves as becoming reality rather than valued or hoped-for selves. Potential for self-denigration may increase with degree of frailty or disability. In order to maintain a positive sense of self, many frail people use the past to reinforce a concept of themselves as having competence and worth. Unfortunately, with age, frailty often is accompanied by attrition through death in the circle of family and friends who could affirm this past self. In addition, able-bodied aging people may no longer seem to be an appropriate reference group, but exactly what group should replace them may be unclear. Their skills in using feedback from others to fashion new self-conceptions may be rusty because for many years they have had stable self-conceptions that did not require change and they have been operating in social environments that continuously affirmed those conceptions.

In addition, frail people sometimes must interact with service providers who have no sense of them as people with worthwhile pasts. However well-meaning, service providers sometimes impose stereotypes of helplessness on their frail clients and subtly pressure them to accede to these images as a condition for getting service. In these cases, because they need the services, clients are unable to use selective interaction to avoid people who will not affirm their conceptions of self. Nevertheless, clients often pass numerous messages to service providers about themselves in the past. These messages are an attempt to personalize the interaction as well as to give the worker a sense of the client's self-image. Unfortunately, service providers too often ignore these messages as being irrelevant to the client's current condition. Such problems are sometimes compounded by the fact that service providers are of a gender, social class, or ethnic background that is itself an assault on the client's sense of dignity. To be forced by circumstances to allow yourself to be bathed by a person you define as inappropriate for this task has great potential impact on self-respect. For example, an older woman I know is very unhappy about the fact that in the facility where she lives, certain private "bed and body" tasks are done by men, which never ceases to embarrass and demean her.

Larson, Boyle, and Boaz (1984) found that the person's level of disability had direct negative effects on self-esteem. Part of the problem here is related to difficulty in conceiving of a positive self that is disabled. In cases of paralysis due to neck injuries, for example, I have seen peer counseling have good results in getting disabled young people to the point where they can conceive of a worthwhile future self. Perhaps similar efforts with frail older people could help them develop the concepts needed to see the possibility of a worthwhile frail self.

The possibility of a positive experience of self among frail older people was suggested by Gadow (1983), who in the written work of Scott-Maxwell (1979) and Blythe (1979) found indications that when the body no longer will allow the individual to act on thoughts, energy may be turned inward to produce a vital inner life totally unseen by the outside world. This possibility needs to be investigated systematically.

Obviously, frailty has many potential intersections with an individual's self-conceptions. It is difficult to conceive of an adequate examination of frailty and psychological quality of life that would not include self-conceptions. The research agenda here is extremely open because very little work has been done in this area to date. This chapter provides some hypothetical relationships and concepts that could be used to inform such an effort.

Methodological Issues

There is no question that much more research is needed on aging and frailty and the self. In order to pursue these topics, more attention needs to be paid to methodological issues. At an abstract, conceptual level, consideration needs to be given to the limits of scientific research and the value of alternative methodologies, as well as on achieving balance between differentiation and integration, putting greater emphasis on self as process, and dramatically increasing the sheer volume of research on the self. At a more mundane level, studies of aging

and the self suffer from many of the problems that plague other areas of gerontology research: research design problems, sampling problems, and measurement
problems.

At the outset, it may be important to understand that some aspects of the self
are more amenable to scientific investigation than others. For example, people
can rate themselves on various physical, mental, and social attributes and social
role performances. They can also reveal how these various characteristics rank in
their personal hierarchy of relative desirability. They can identify general pictures
of both possible and probable future selves. They can rate themselves in terms of
the stability of their self-conceptions. They can identify their strategies and plans
for self-improvement. They can identify disvalued and feared aspects of self.
Their responses to questionnaires appear to show a social desirability bias, but
socially desirable is an accurate representation of the way they see themselves
(Breytspraak & George, 1982). Any one of these dimensions of self can be
studied scientifically, provided it is broken down enough for operational definition. The limits of science are seen most often when people try to take the results
of scientific investigations and put them together into some sort of whole.
Bengtson *et al.* (1985), for example, did a wonderful job of summarizing dozens
of studies on just a few dimensions of self, but at the end, they achieved only a
very limited degree of integration.

Self-reports and clinical observations are by far the most common ways that
scientific data on self-conceptions are collected. There is a conspicuous absence
of studies of self-referent behavior, such as concrete plans and social support
activities aimed at self-improvement or self-acceptance. Observations of interactions of older people reveal an appreciable volume of stories about self. Analysis
of the content of these stories could reveal a great deal about the self and its
dynamics. On these and many other topics, more qualitative research is needed
(Bengtson *et al.*, 1985).

In comparison with the scientific approach, the average individual with good
intellectual training and modest reflective skills is much better able to integrate a
large array of incomplete and contradictory information into a holistic view of
the self and how it operates. In this sense, there is much to be learned from
looking at autobiographical accounts, life reviews, and artistic portrayals of
sensitive novelists or poets in terms of how the various dimensions of the self are
integrated into a stable but ever-changing whole.

By the same token, structure of the self is much easier to define operationally
than self as process, partly because in everyday life most of us learn more about
how to articulate the outcome than how we get there. Aside from psycho-
therapists, people seldom ask, "How did you come to think about yourself the
way you do?" Instead, they say, "Tell me about yourself." They want to know
about the outcome, not the process.

Part of the reason that our theories are heavy on differentiating and defining the structure of the self and light on the processes that create and transform the self is that there has been very little research on self-reflective processes. When people want research funding, they propose to study self-esteem because there are agreed-upon concepts and measures of this dimension and there are existing studies that can be used to justify a new one. If one wants to study self as process, one must propose the ever-unpopular "fishing expedition." We tend to forget that *all* fields of knowledge must begin with exploration of uncharted territory and that a certain amount of charting—descriptive work—is a necessary condition for later scientific work. To encourage studies of self as process, we must create specific initiatives. New areas of research seldom succeed in unrestricted competition with areas already having a strong empirical base, well-developed theory, and agreed-upon quantitative methods.

Because science tends to look at small slices of reality, to get a balanced view of the self as affected by aging or frailty will require a substantial increase in the sheer volume of research being done. We need large numbers of bits and pieces, not a bit here and a piece there.

Studies of aging and the self suffer from a lack of longitudinal studies of age changes (Bengtson *et al.*, 1985; Breytspraak & George, 1982). Most studies infer age changes from cross-sectional data. In most areas of aging research this practice is problematic, but it is downright wrong in an area dominated by personal constructions. No self can serve as an adequate baseline for a given individual's current self except that individual's earlier self.

Sampling problems occur because most of the studies, especially those with qualitative data, are from samples of white, middle-class, educated people. Most of the longitudinal studies come from people in the San Francisco Bay Area. As we begin to sample from more diverse populations, dealing with variations in measurement and meaning will become an even greater challenge.

Adequate measurement revolves around issues of validity and reliability. Studies of self have persistently suffered from problems in both areas (Wylie, 1961, 1974, 1978), and studies of aging and the self have not been exceptions (Bengtson *et al.*, 1985; Breytspraak & George, 1982). For an excellent review of existing measures of self, including evaluations of validity and reliability, see Breytspraak and George (1982).

From the point of view of analytical concerns, a major issue in the study of the self is the relative amount of stability and change in various dimensions of self over the adult life course. Bengtson *et al.* (1985) pointed out that there are no conventions concerning the level of correlation that constitutes "stability" or the lack of it that constitutes "change." Generally, if measures are corrected for unreliability, then the correlation in measures of self over time tends to be higher, and in rating scale measurements, there tends to be more stability than change. In open-ended measures, stability is still a major theme, but more change with age is observed (Bengtson *et al.*, 1985; Breytspraak & George, 1982).

There are also several types of stability. Structural stability refers to the persistence of factor structures or latent structures over time. These are typically measured by factor analysis and LISREL, and large rating-scale inventories are usually the source of raw data. With regard to stability within components of self, assessments can be made of stability over time of the degree or level within particular self-conceptions such as temperament or physical abilities. Comparative stability deals with the degree of stability over time in rankings of different aspects of self in terms of importance to the individual or comparisons in levels of stability across individuals. As usual, the more we try to deal with the issue of stability versus change, the more difficulties and complexities we uncover in arriving at an answer (Filipp & Klauer, 1986).

Future Research Directions

This paper lays out an ambitious agenda for future research on aging and frailty and how they affect the self and quality of life. In the area of aging and the self, how does aging change the reference points used in social comparisons? How is the past actively reconstructed to provide a perception of continuity of self in the face of age changes in both the individual and his or her circumstances? How do aging individuals cope with changing body images? How does a perception that disability is near influence conceptions of the future self? How does ageism influence self-confidence?

In the area of frailty and the self, as frailty increases do people shift the focus of the ideal self from instrumental competence to qualitative competence? What effect does the prospect of a feared, disvalued self (dependency) have on self-concept and self-esteem? Are there interventions that can enable frail older people to conceive of a positive future self? Does disability increase the vitality of a person's inner life? How is it that some people are able to cope positively with frailty in a way that does not diminish their self-esteem?

To study these and other questions about the self and how it is influenced by aging or frailty, we need to broaden our approach to research on the self. More study is needed of spontaneous messages about the self that are generated by aging and frail people in everyday situations, of plans people make for changes in the self, of strategies people use to manage the self, of the stories people tell about themselves, and of how people synthesize the complex array of information about the self into a whole that has historical integrity. More emphasis is needed on study of the self as process, using concepts such as the interpretive self, the managed self, the intentional self, or self-striving. There is a strong need for more descriptive mapping of the structure and processes of the self in aging or frail people from a diversity of populations. Specific initiatives are needed in order to increase the volume of research on aging and frailty and the self.

Conclusion

The self will always be a crucial but difficult topic to study. Cognitively, the self is a "fuzzy set" made up of a very large number of specific memories. Existentially, the self-reflective ideas that seem relevant to the individual probably fluctuate to some extent from one social situation to another. Conceptually, general structural dimensions of the self have been identified, and the relations among self-concept, ideal self, self-evaluation, and self-esteem have been specified. However, concepts and theory about the processes through which the self is established, maintained, and changed over the life course are less well developed.

I have outlined a basic set of theoretical scenarios in which various aspects of aging might be expected to influence the self. Most of the processes could be expected to result in greater self-acceptance and a more tested, stable self. On the other hand, frailty is not as amenable to positive personal construction, and many of the implications of frailty for the self are negative. Nevertheless, there are people who cope positively with frailty, and we need to learn more about how this is done.

I have argued that many of the more abstract, holistic aspects of self do not lend themselves easily to scientific study. To achieve the balanced understanding that is needed, we may want to broaden the base of information sources that are used to include material coming from the analysis of texts generated by aging people, such as stories people tell about themselves and autobiographical writings, as well as material coming from more traditional social scientific sources. We also could make more use of qualitative approaches such as content analysis and observational methods.

Because of the relative neglect of the concept of self in aging research, we need solid descriptive studies to chart the territory of the aging self. The research that has been done clearly shows that many of the concepts and theories about the self aimed at understanding the structure and dynamics of the self among children and adolescents have little application in the study of a long-standing adult self. In addition, there is need for special incentives to increase the volume of research on aging and frailty as they influence the self.

References

Atchley, R. C. (1976). Selected social and psychological differences between men and women in later life. *Journal of Gerontology, 31,* 204–211.

Atchley, R. C. (1982a). The aging self. *Psychotherapy: Theory, Research and Practice,* 19, 388–396.

Atchley, R. C. (1982b). Retirement: Leaving the world of work. *Annals of the American Academy of Political and Social Sciences, 464,* 120–131.

Atchley, R. C. (1989). A continuity theory of normal aging. *The Gerontologist, 29,* 183–190.

Baltes, M. M., & Baltes, P. B., eds. (1986). *The psychology of control and aging.* Hillsdale, N.J.: Lawrence Erlbaum.

Bengtson, V. L., Reedy, M. N., & Gordon, C. (1985). Aging and self-conceptions: Personality processes and social contexts. In J. E. Birren and K. W. Schaie, eds., *Handbook of the psychology of aging,* 2nd ed., pp. 544–593. New York: Van Nostrand Reinhold.

Blythe, R. (1979). *The view in winter: Reflections on old age.* New York: Penguin.

Breytspraak, L. M., & George, L. K. (1982). Self-concept and self-esteem. In D. J. Mangen & W. A. Peterson, eds., *Research instruments in social gerontology. 1. Clinical and social psychology,* pp. 241–302. Minneapolis: University of Minnesota Press.

Comfort, A. (1976). Age prejudice in America. *Social Policy, 7,* 3–8.

Filipp, S., & Klauer, T. (1986). Conceptions of self over the life span: Reflections on the dialectics of change. In M. M. Baltes & P. B. Baltes, eds., *The psychology of control and aging.* Hillsdale, N.J.: Lawrence Erlbaum.

Gadow, S. (1983). Frailty and strength: The dialectic in aging. *The Gerontologist, 23,* 144–147.

Goffman, E. (1959). *The presentation of self in everyday life.* New York: Anchor Books.

Greenwald, A. (1980). The totalitarian ego: Fabrication and revision of personal history. *American Psychologist, 35,* 603–618.

Heidegger, M. (1966). *Discourse on thinking.* New York: Harper & Row.

Kaufman, S. R. (1986). *The ageless self: Sources of meaning in late life.* Madison, Wis.: University of Wisconsin Press.

Lachman, M. E. (1986). Locus of control in aging research: A case for multidimensional and domain-specific assessment. *Psychology and Aging, 1,* 34–40.

Larson, P. C., Boyle, E. S., & Boaz, M. E. (1984). Relationship of self-concept to age, disability, and institutional residency. *The Gerontologist, 24,* 401–407.

Lawton, M. P. (1978). Leisure activities for the aged. *Annals of the American Academy of Political and Social Sciences, 438,* 71–80.

Lawton, M. P. (1983). Environment and other determinants of well-being in older people. *The Gerontologist, 23,* 349–357.

Lieberman, M. A., & Tobin, S. S. (1983). *The experience of old age: Stress, coping, and survival.* New York: Basic Books.

Maehr, M. L., & Kleiber, D. A. (1981). The graying of achievement motivation. *American Psychologist, 36,* 787–793.

Markus, H., & Nurius, P. (1986). Possible selves. *American Psychologist, 41,* 954–969.

Marshall, V. W. (1986). A sociological perspective on aging and dying. In V. W. Marshall, ed., *Later life: The social psychology of aging,* pp. 125–146. Beverly Hills, Calif.: Sage Publications.

Mead, G. H. (1934). *Mind, self and society.* Chicago: University of Chicago Press.

Pearlin, L. I., & Schooler, C. (1978). The structure of coping. *Journal of Health and Social Behavior, 19,* 2–21.

Rosenberg, M. (1979). *Conceiving the self.* New York: Basic Books.

Rotter, J. B. (1966). Generalized expectancies for internal versus external control of reinforcement. *Psychological Monographs, 80,* 1–609.

Scott-Maxwell, F. (1979). *The measure of my days.* New York: Penguin.

Shrauger, J. S., & Schoeneman, T. J. (1979). Symbolic interactionist view of self-concept: Through the looking glass darkly. *Psychological Bulletin, 86,* 549–573.

Troll, L. E., Miller, S. J., & Atchley, R. C. (1979). *Families in later life.* Belmont, Calif.: Wadsworth.

Wylie, R. C. (1961). *The self-concept.* Lincoln, Nebr.: University of Nebraska Press.

Wylie, R. C. (1974). *The self-concept,* rev. ed., vol. 1. Lincoln, Nebr.: University of Nebraska Press.

Wylie, R. C. (1978). *The self-concept,* rev. ed., vol. 2. Lincoln, Nebr.: University of Nebraska Press.

11

Physical Activity and Quality of Life in the Frail Elderly

WANEEN W. SPIRDUSO

AND

PRISCILLA GILLIAM-MACRAE

The Meaning of Movement in the Quality of Life

From the moment we are born, movement and physical capacity are as much a part of our personality and self-concept as our intelligence, race, and culture. Unless we have some control over our lips, throat, and extremities, we cannot communicate so much as one thought to anyone else. Our posture, locomotive patterns, and gestures are so integrated into ourselves that they become as much a part of our identity as our facial characteristics, the color of our hair, and the tone of our voice. We can recognize our friend in the blurry black-and-white photograph by the way he leans against the car, and we can tell by her walk which of our friends is coming down the dimly lit hall before we see her face.

Our physical capacities empower us to enrich our souls, to climb to mountain peaks and view the incredible beauty that awaits. All of the physical accompaniments of the climb—our hair whipping in the wind, our heart pounding and our lungs heaving, and the tingling sense of fatigue in our muscles—contribute to the exhilaration of the moment. Moments like these allow us to experience awesome beauty, to understand our capacities, to relish our sense of accomplishment.

Physical mobility and endurance enable us to spend long, uninterrupted, and attentive hours in intellectual analysis and study and allow us to go to the theater or the symphony to refresh our human spirit. At every age our physical capacity delimits our human experiences, determining in part the size of the windows that we open to the world. Perhaps more so in the early and late periods of life, our physical activities and abilities greatly determine the quality of our life. The loss of physical mobility is more than just the inability to transport our brain from one place to another. The losses may involve diminished communica-

Copyright © 1991 by Academic Press, Inc.
All rights of reproduction in any form reserved.

tion, changes in self-identity, deteriorated mood states, and limitations in self-actualization.

Physical Activity: What People Choose to Do

Physical activity level varies among cohorts and may be dramatically different among individuals within a cohort. Many individuals in our society are quite sedentary even in youth, preferring to watch others move rather than be physically active themselves. The majority are relatively physically active in the first two decades but participate in less and less physical activity with each ensuing decade. In the eighth and ninth decade, only 14% of men and 13% of women report that they participate in some type of systematic exercise program four or more times per week (Cullen & Weeks, 1978). It remains to be seen whether the larger numbers of physically active individuals who are now in their 40s and 50s will remain active through their 70s and 80s. Those individuals who have been chronically sedentary and those who have grown sedentary with increasing age have a high probability of becoming what gerontologists describe as the "frail elderly." A much smaller percentage of individuals in our society are active in vigorous physical activity all of their lives, and it is more accurate to describe them as the "robust elderly." Another life-style group is composed of sedentary individuals who are driven in their middle age to change their life-style and become physically active. We do not know how close they can come to attaining the status of robustness.

The Third Dimension of Human Frailty: Disuse

Bortz (1983) has pointed out that human frailty has three dimensions. The first dimension, time, is an insidious and relentless thief of energy and vitality. Inevitably, the passage of time results in death. The second dimension, disease, is due to internal errors or external agents that damage body systems and lead to weakness, system fatigue, frailty, and, eventually, death. The third dimension, disuse, although less well understood, is also significant in the transformation from robustness to frailty. We have no control over the passage of time and limited control over disease prevention but almost total control over the extent to which we use our mental, physical, and social capacities.

Testimonial evidence that disuse of the physical system accelerates aging is abundant. The following is Bortz's (1983) description of his experience following a skiing injury:

> When the cast was removed, I found my leg giving all the appearance of the limb of a person forty or fifty years older. It was withered, discolored, stiff, painful. I could not believe this leg belonged to me.

> *The similarity of changes due to enforced inactivity to those commonly attributed to aging was striking.*
>
> And, in fact, if one were to go to all the standard textbooks of geriatrics and write down all the changes which seem to accompany aging, set the list aside, and then go to the textbooks of work physiology and write down all the changes subsequent to inactivity—and then compare the two lists, one would see that they are virtually identical.
>
> The coincidence is not random. It is intense. It forces the conclusion that *at least part of what passes as change due to age is not caused by age at all but by disuse.* (p. 2)

More scientific evidence regarding the debilitating effects of disuse is available from research on bed rest and water immersion and, more recently, from space research on weightlessness. What all of these conditions have in common is that they drastically alter three classes of stimuli that humans experience: hydrostatic pressure, compression force on long bones, and level of physical exercise (Greenleaf, 1984). The consequences of disuse alterations are detrimental to human health, and the more our life-style approximates these conditions, the more negatively affected we are. Prolonged periods of sitting in recliners or on couches simulates bed rest, and transient bed rest effects have been readily observed. When many older people stand up from prolonged sitting or lying, for example, the relatively sudden changes in fluid compartment volumes lowers blood pressure so that they experience a light-headed sensation. If the fall in blood pressure is significant, they will faint (Convertino, Montgomery, & Greenleaf, 1984). Exercising the lower limbs greatly aids the blood flow and pressure that maintains adequate perfusion of the brain by assisting in the venous return process and by maintaining the important reflexes that compensate for changes in posture.

The complete inactivity that occurs in bed rest predisposes the body to hypertension, deterioration of the neuromuscular system, and osteoporosis. It is well established, especially in the elderly, that three major problems that can develop from bed rest in healthy people, as well as those confined for medical reasons, are (1) lung edema, (2) venous and arterial thrombi, and (3) hydrostatic pneumonia (Booth, 1982; Greenleaf, 1984). Other symptoms associated with bed rest include bed sores, foot drop, general muscular weakness and atrophy, muscle shortening, knee-joint stiffness, restriction of joint motion, loss of appetite, minor dyspepsias and heartburn, constipation and occasional intestinal obstruction, increased tendency for urinary calculi, and accentuation of symptoms during the course of multiple sclerosis and tabes dorsalis (Greenleaf, 1984). Certainly, one would have to agree that amelioration of any or all of these symptoms would increase the quality of life. As will be discussed later in this chapter, physical activity has been shown to make significant contributions to the prevention and reversal of most of these inactivity-induced ailments, which are far too prevalent in the elderly.

Why Disuse?

The list of health problems that can be attributed at least in part to physical inactivity is so long and the problems so debilitating that it is hard to account on rational grounds for the extent to which humans disuse their bodies. Why do people, especially as they age, become less and less physically active? Many explanations have been proposed: general biological tendency to slow down with age, lack of time, lack of social network with whom to exercise, and inadequate facilities and equipment. Conrad (1976) has proposed that older individuals also have undue fears about participating in vigorous exercise, underestimate their own physical capacities, and tend to overestimate the benefits of light, sporadic exercise. Older adults also perceive their work load to be greater than young adults perceive it (Bar-Or, 1977; Sidney & Shephard, 1977). Two factors that substantially discourage very old adults from participating in exercise, however, are ageism and the imposition of frailty.

Ageism

Ageism refers to the use of chronological age to define capability and roles of individuals; an ageist is an individual who expects and/or tries to force others into particular behaviors based upon the number of years they have lived. The process of social-psychological "age grading" and learning to "act your age" begins very early in life (Berger, 1988) and may be more obvious in our physical domain than in other life domains. We learn at a very early age that some physical activities are "appropriate" for older people and some are not (Ostrow, Keener, & Perry, 1987). These expectations and biases are present in college students (Ostrow, Jones, & Spiker, 1981) and probably remain for the rest of our lives. Individuals older than 65, when asked to evaluate the appropriateness of several activities for ages ranging from 20 to 80, based their judgments on perceptions of age appropriateness (Ostrow & Dzewaltowski, 1986). The reports of Ostrow's work with preschool children, college students, and older adults collectively are compelling evidence that ageism regarding physical activity participation is pervasive, not just a cohort phenomenon.

We are conditioned to believe that sports injuries and exercise soreness is natural for young adults but a sign of deterioration and risk for the older adult. In one study, 90% of young individuals agreed that a regular exercise program was important to maintain health, but that percentage dropped to 77% for 55- to 64-year-olds, and only 70% of those older than 65 agreed (Shephard, 1987). The ravages of a hypokinetic life-style and ageism lead almost everyone in our society to have low expectations for our own physical capacities and abilities. R. N. Butler, the first director of the National Institute on Aging, took his fellow physicians to task regarding the promotion of ageism in physical activity:

> Doctors have to go beyond the simple prescriptions they give to older people, such as 'Take it easy' or 'Once in awhile go out and exercise,' or perhaps the most common of all, 'What do you expect at your age?' The following story concerns a volunteer in our human aging studies at NIH in the 1950s, Morris Rocklin.
>
> I first saw Morris when he was 94 and I last saw him when he was 101. He died at 102. He told me when he was 101 about a recent visit he'd had with his physician, complaining about pain in his right knee. And his doctor said, 'Morris, what do you expect at your age?' At which point Morris jumped out of his chair—feisty character that he was, unintimidated by doctors—pounded on the table and said, 'Now, look here. My left knee is also 101 and how come it doesn't hurt?' The point of the story is that regardless of age, every older person deserves a thoughtful, comprehensive diagnostic evaluation and not a casual write-off on the basis of age, or even worse, senility. (Butler, 1981, p. 39)

Society has always viewed extremely common syndromes such as falling, loss of mobility, fainting, urinary incontinence, confusion or delirium, and dementia as normal signs of aging. Medical science has been slow to try to prevent or cure what are perceived to be normal symptoms of aging (Rowe, 1989). But we should ask the questions, "Is it normal to feel fatigued after the slightest exertion, to have muscle contractures, and to fall?" "Is it normal to feel stiffness in the joints after physical activity?" *"How much frailty is imposed by ageism?"* If an octogenarian is told day after day that he or she is frail and incapacitated and should take it easy and stay out of the way, why wouldn't he or she internalize this belief? And further, why not exacerbate the situation and act that way? Why not reap the benefits of extra service, sympathy, attention, and social support that are provided to those who are immobile? In short, why not let the system take care of him or her?

Imposed Frailty

Institutional life, as exists in most long-term care centers, is an extremely sedentary existence. Submissive patients who do little are considered "good patients." Many nursing homes and alternative care centers are not prepared to carry out activities that the more physically fit and mobile occupants could perform. Most have not provided trained personnel nor facilities for even the most rudimentary and minimal of physical activities.

Two practices that occur in some institutions for the aged that would certainly curtail physical movement and mobility are the extensive use of medication and physical restraint. The results from a national survey of nursing facilities (U.S.P.H.S., 1976), which indicated that hypnotic/sedative drugs were prescribed for more than a third of institutionalized clients, sparked a controversy in the gerontology community as to whether hypnotic/sedative drugs were being overly prescribed to control patient behavior. Since the appearance of that report, several studies supported these findings and several failed to find excessive medication patterns. A national pattern of extensive use of hypnotic/sedative drugs has not been documented, but, conversely, many incidences of it have certainly been reported. It should be recognized, however, that medications such as insulin, levodopa, diuretics, hypnotics/sedatives, and benzodiazepines that are prescribed for many types of illness may lower blood pressure and alter motor function. Lower blood pressure and minimal to no physical activity increases the probability of orthostatic hypotension, a risk factor for falling (Wells, Middleton, Lawrence, Lillard, & Safarik, 1985). In addition, tricyclic antidepressants, antipsychotics, and hypnotics/sedatives can act directly to lower blood pressure or may interact with antihypertensive agents to exacerbate hypotension, increase orthostatic hypotension, and thus increase the risk for falling. Antihypertensive agents may also have a sedative effect due to their increased central nervous system effects in the elderly. Thus, heavily or overmedicated older individuals find themselves in a vicious downward spiral. The illness, which has already disrupted health and decreased physical activity, is treated with drugs that further decrease older persons' mobility and physical capacity, pushing them more toward a simulated bed-rest condition, which in turn weakens and exacerbates the illness, increasing the likelihood for prescription of more medication. Because so many drugs impair or discourage motor function, their use should be cautiously prescribed. The case of Eula Weaver, described later in this chapter, suggests that in many cases physical activity and dietary changes may complement, and in some cases even eliminate, the need for medication.

It is easy to understand why a medicated population would be easier for a long-term care center to handle. Schedules are easier to maintain for a medicated, passive, and inactive population. A more highly trained staff is required to deal with more active people. People who are more active may not want to go to bed at 8:00—some may want to go to bed at 11:00. Some may want day trips, some may want entertainment imported to the institution, some may want sexual activity. Many institutional administrators assume that a passive clientele is a safer clientele and that the risk of injuries, and subsequently of lawsuits, is less. They argue that the high cost of hiring trained personnel prevents the implementation of physical activity programs for the frail elderly. However, this is a false perception of financial savings, as a physically stronger, more independent clientele will ultimately be less expensive to maintain. An institutional exercise program that prevents even one hip-fracturing fall by increasing the leg strength and balance of residents will result in substantial financial savings to the institution.

A second practice of some long-term care centers that could have dire health consequences is the use of routine physical restraint, for reasons of safety, protection, and facilitation of treatment. Evans and Strumpf (1989, 221A) suggest that "the practice appears to have increased and become entrenched in North American health care institutions, especially in contrast to other countries." Certainly, the health and physical consequences of physical restraint should be carefully examined in each instance in which it is used. No better example of imposed frailty can be imagined than the practice of routine physical restraint. Blakeslee (1988) cited her observations of older, newly admitted residents of a nursing center:

> The restraint policy's effects on them [older people] were apparent. People who had walked into the facility on admission could barely walk to the bathroom with the assistance of two caregivers one month later. Remove their restraints? No! They might fall, break a hip, and we would be sued. We had rendered them helpless in 30 days and crippled them safely. (p. 833)

Bed rest, or any state of physical disuse that approaches it, does not just decrease the quality of life, it is a death sentence. Experts in the medical profession generally agree that the most effective way to accelerate the aging process is to do nothing (Wiswell, 1980).

Benefits of Physical Activity

The benefits of physical activity certainly include improved physical function, but physical activity also has some modifying effects on mental and emotional function and on individual self-esteem.

Physical Function

Although some variation is present, the senescence of many of our physical systems after reaching maturity is linear, about 1% per year, or 10% per decade. Age-related decrements in oxygen capacity, muscular strength, flexibility, and motor skills are well documented from approximately 20 to 75 years of age. Much rarer are studies in which these systems are analyzed in individuals from the age of 70 to 100. The majority of studies include categories of young (20–30 years), middle-aged (30–50 years), and old (60+ years). The "60+" category usually includes subjects ranging in age from 60 to 90, with group numbers that diminish as the age category increases, until the 80s and 90s may be represented by only two or three subjects. Individual data are not generally published in these studies, and, because of the wide discrepancy between the performance of 60-year-olds and 90-year-olds, the group statistics are generally useless as a basis for understanding the physical competencies of the very old. However, even though research data are scarce for these older ages, informal observation provides ample evidence that these systems continue to decline.

The cumulative effects of time, disease, and disuse inevitably force those who survive to very old ages to experience several different functional health states. Individuals who live to their seventh, eighth, and ninth decade range from those who are in a state of excellent health to those who are in a state of morbidity. Figure 1 illustrates several points with regard to the contribution of systematic physical activity and good health habits to the physical, mental, and emotional capacities of the very old. This model is a schematic representation of how the functional capacity of three hypothetical groups, all of whom reach 90 years of age, may differ as a function of living very different life-styles with regard to physical activity.

The "sedentary" line represents average Americans: sedentary individuals who pay little attention to their health until it is threatened and who never participate in any type of physical activity. These individuals may begin operating

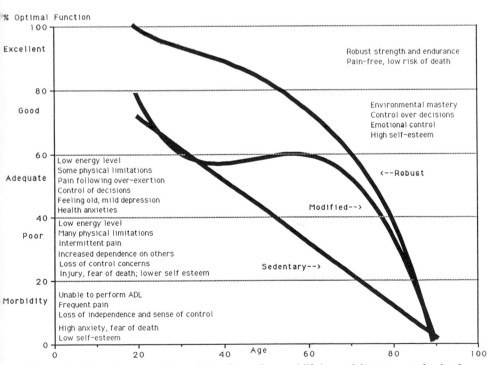

Figure 1 Schematic representation of the effects of age and lifetime activity pattern on levels of functioning. Adapted from Fries (1988).

at very low levels of capacity as early as their sixth or seventh decade, experiencing severe limitations in their activities of daily living and becoming dependent on others. Negative psychological changes may also accompany these limitations.

The "modified" line represents similar sedentary individuals, who, at approximately the age of 40, initiate a physical activity program and improve their health habits. Recent epidemiological studies have shown that health habit interventions significantly reduce risks of disease such as coronary heart disease and cancer (Paffenbarger, Hyde, Wing, & Hsieh, 1986). Fries, Green, and Levine (1989) point out that the cessation of cigarette smoking returns the risk of heart attack to normal in two years and returns the risk of lung cancer to normal in ten years. A two-year program of exercise in older individuals produces stronger bones, and atherosclerotic lesions can be reversed by diet and exercise. Intervention strategies such as exercise (Buskirk, 1985), good nutrition (Roe, 1983), and the adoption of a healthy life-style (Avorn, 1986) have been shown to delay senescent decline. Most investigators who have studied the effects of physical training intervention longitudinally have shown that exercise programs undertaken by relatively healthy older adults later in life, *even if these adults had been completely sedentary,* can produce benefits in cardiovascular, musculoskeletal, and nervous system function. These studies and others like them suggest that it is probable that the *rate* of decline in some systems can be slowed with interventions, but the extent to which the rate can be changed and the optimal intervention for each age remain to be clarified. A change in health habits and physical activity in midlife that moves individuals in the direction of their optimum capacity is represented by a displacement to the right of the "modified" line shown in Figure 1. A "family" of health- and exercise-induced displacement curves could be drawn for each age group, which would describe the type and intensity of exercise at each age, as well as the amount of improvement that might be expected in moving individuals toward their maximum potential. The nature and shape of these curves are involved in the research questions of critical importance to the future. In fact, intervention results have been so promising that Fries *et al.* (1989) have suggested that public policy emphasis in educational health promotion programs should be redirected from the young to the old, because the old are so much closer in time to the potential onset of morbidity.

The "robust" line in Figure 1 represents individuals who, through a physical training program, achieve 100% of their optimal physical capacity at an early age and continue a life-style of physical activity and good health. This line was estimated by averaging the percentage of decline in the national age records for cyclists, swimmers, and runners. These individuals begin the inevitable age-related physical decline at the highest point of physical efficiency possible. If an individual maintains good health habits and an exercise program, is not genetically predisposed to a debilitating chronic disease, and is lucky enough to avoid accidents, the evidence is persuasive that the onset of cardiovascular disease (Topp *et al.*, 1989) and other conditions of morbidity (Fries, 1988) can be substantially postponed.

The crucial factor with regard to the quality of life is *how long* an individual spends in each of the functional states. In the hypothetical cases shown in Figure 1, sedentary individuals could live for 20 years in poor functional health and for 15 years in a state that has been described by Fries (1988) as morbidity. In sharp contrast, physically fit individuals could live in a state of poor functional health only five years and spend little or no time at all in the morbidity state.

Cardiovascular Function

The evidence that regular aerobic exercise can bring about positive changes in many aspects of circulatory function in the older adult is compelling. Changes in circulatory functions with exercise include increases in maximal oxygen consumption, decreases in resting blood pressure and heart rate, and improvements in blood lipid levels and glucose tolerance (Adams & deVries, 1973; deVries, 1970; Hagberg *et al.*, 1989; Niinimaa & Shephard, 1978; Seals *et al.*, 1984; Seals, Hagberg, Hurley, Ehsani, & Holloszy, 1984). The one aspect of aging circulatory function that is not modified with exercise training is the decline in maximal heart rate, a decline which prevents physical endurance from being maintained throughout life at youthful peak levels. Nevertheless, great benefits can be accrued through training at even advanced ages. The American College of Sports Medicine has summarized this in a position statement: "Age in itself does not appear to be a deterrent to endurance training" (1978, p. viii).

Maximal oxygen consumption, a measure that defines the functional limits of the cardiovascular system, declines at a faster rate when measured longitudinally than when measured cross-sectionally. Because most studies of maximal oxygen consumption age differences are cross-sectional studies, the decline in this system has been underestimated for sedentary men. However, the rate of decline in maximal oxygen consumption has been shown to be substantially less for physically active men (Bortz, 1982; Kasch, Boyer, Van Camp, Verity, & Wallace, 1990; Pollock, Foster, Knapp, Rod, & Schmidt, 1987), as is reflected by the much more gradual decline of the upper line in Figure 1. In one of the few longitudinal studies in this area, Kasch *et al.* (1990) reported a decline in maximal oxygen consumption of only 13% in a group of older men (age 45 to 68) who maintained their exercise training over an 18-year period. This decline was much less than the 41% decline in maximal oxygen consumption of the older men (age 52 to 70) who had not exercised over a similar time period.

Physical training can produce, in a reasonably healthy individual at any age, improvements of 10 to 25% in maximal oxygen consumption (Shephard, 1987). In a classic study, deVries (1970) pointed out that older individuals do not achieve the same absolute gains in maximal oxygen consumption as young people, but their relative gains are very similar. Hagberg *et al.* (1989) have reported significant improvements in maximal oxygen consumption and other measures of cardiovascular function even in 70- to 79-year-old men and women who had never exercised before.

Exercise program intervention can also provide significant benefits even for those with chronic disease. Morey *et al.* (1989) found that an exercise program which included stationary cycling, stretching, weight training, and walking produced significant improvement in submaximal physical work capacity, submaximal heart rate, resting heart rate, hamstring flexibility, and abdominal strength in an elderly population of men that included chronically ill individuals. Only quadricep strength failed to improve significantly in their study. Of the participants who began the program, 49 (71%) completed the program. The mean age of the men was 70 years, and 76% had at least one chronic disease, such as arthritis, hypertension, or heart disease.

A dramatic example of potential exercise effects in octogenarians was provided by Biegel (1984):

> Only five feet three inches tall and weighing 100 pounds for the past 40 years, Eula Weaver had developed cardiovascular disease and was treated for angina at age 67. At age 75 she was hospitalized with a severe heart attack; by age 81, she had developed an arthritic limp and had congestive heart failure, hypertension, and angina. When she began a regimen of dieting and walking at age 81, her limp limited her walking to 100 feet; the circulation in her hands was so impaired that she wore gloves in the summer to keep her hands warm. Gradually increasing her walking, she was able, by age 82, to be free of drugs and her previous symptoms. After four years of increased activity, she participated in the Senior Olympics in Irvine, California, where she won gold medals in the half mile and mile running events. The following year, age 86½, she repeated those runs for another two gold medals. Each morning she runs a mile and rides her stationary bicycle 10–15 miles; three times weekly she works out in a gymnasium; and she follows her diet strictly. (p. 31)

Finally, although reports of exercise interventions with demented patients are almost nonexistent, Ingebretsen (1982) suggested that physical training and movement exercises might be useful in working with patients who have lost important cues of contact both with themselves and with the environment. Movement lessons could contribute to reality orientation therapy and training in self-help. Movement training might provide some pleasure from self-mastery, from which even severely demented patients might benefit (Paraspiropoutos *et al.,* 1979).

Muscular Strength, Endurance, Flexibility, and Mobility
The severe age- and disuse-related decline in muscular strength and endurance that are seen in the frail elderly can be a major delimiting factor in their quality of

life. Not only is muscular atrophy and weakness delimiting in terms of traveling and participating in social activities that require minimal physical strength, but it is frequently so debilitating that it precludes or substantially alters daily activities such as walking, stair climbing, and carrying objects. Muscular strength and endurance also play a role in preventing falls and accidents, particularly in older adults.

It is well established that strength can be increased through resistive exercises in older adults (Moritani & deVries, 1980; Orlander & Aniansson, 1980). Older adults have been shown to increase their maximal arm strength the same percentage (20%) as young adults after eight weeks of progressive strength training (Moritani & deVries, 1980). In a more recent study, Frontera, Meredith, O'Reilly, Knuttgen, and Evans (1988) examined the effects of a strength-training program on skeletal muscle function and muscle mass in older men, 60 to 72 years of age. After a 12-week strength-training program, they reported significant strength increases of 107% for knee extensors and 227% for knee flexors. An increase of 10 to 20% in isokinetic peak torque of the knee extensors and flexors was also found. This increase in strength was accompanied by significant muscle hypertrophy, due to an increase of approximately 30% in both types of muscle fibers. Findings of this type were recently extended to men 86 to 96 years old by Fiatarone *et al.* (1990), who studied strength gains in a group of frail, institutionalized individuals. Mean increases in knee extensor strength of 174% after eight weeks of high-intensity weight training were obtained. This increase in strength was associated with a 9% increase in midthigh muscle mass and an improved tandem gait speed of 48%.

The report of Fiatarone *et al.* (1990) provides objective support for claims that have emanated from Pavel Dobrev's weight training school in Bulgaria. For years Dobrev has astonished most of the biologists, doctors, weight-lifting experts and rehabilitation experts from around the world who have visited the school. Dobrev claims that his

longitudinal observations and research from 1960 show without any doubt that the systematic and purposeful practicing with weights have a big preventive, rehabilitation and remedial effect even with totally untrained persons over 70–80 years of age, including those suffering from high blood pressure, arterosclerosis or after a myocardial infarction or brain apoplexy. (Dobrev, 1980, p. 28)

Though not as dramatic as the performances discussed above, substantial gains can be made in strength, flexibility, and mobility with low-impact and light exercise programs (Gillett, 1989), even those that begin with minimal movements of participants while seated in chairs (Reynolds & Garrett, 1989). Sager (1984), who has conducted exercise classes for over 2000 seniors, finds that her participants report increases in strength, flexibility, and mobility.

The effect of exercise on the maintenance and improvement of strength, mobility, and flexibility is particularly important because impairment in these factors has been associated with an increased risk of falling (Tobis, Friis, & Reinsch, 1989). The rate of falls is reported to be at least 40% for those over the age of 80 who live in the community (Prudham & Grimley-Evans, 1981) but much higher for those in institutions (61%; Tinetti, 1987). The causes of falls are usually multifactorial in origin, but they include decreases in strength and balance, impaired gait, declines in sensory function, medications, and cognitive impairments (Tinetti & Speechley, 1989). Strength seems to play an important role in the prevention of falling by enabling an individual to correct momentary losses of balance in time to prevent catastrophic falling events. Flexibility of joints, which enhances mobility and thereby decreases the risk of falling, can be improved in shoulder, knee, and hip joints with 10 weeks of nonstrenuous exercise (Holm & Kirchoff, 1984).

Physical Performance Testing

A more comprehensive understanding of the role that systematic physical activity can play in the improvement of mobility and prevention of falls and of how it can lead to an improvement in quality of life will be contingent, however, on the development and *standardization* of a measure of the physical and motor function of individuals who can successfully complete all items on an activities of daily living inventory such as the ADL (Katz, Downs, Cash, & Grotz, 1970) and the PADL (Kuriansky & Gurland, 1976) but who cannot complete the least-demanding protocol of an aerobics work capacity test or produce minimal amounts of torque on standardized strength tests. At present, it is difficult, if not impossible, to determine physical benefits that might accrue to the frail elderly who participate in an exercise program, because pre-exercise functional capacity cannot be determined. A functional fitness test battery for adults over the age of 60 was developed by the American Association for Health, Physical Education, Recreation, and Dance (Osness, 1987). It is composed of a one-half-mile walk, a sit-and-reach test of flexibility, a sit-and-stand test for strength/endurance, a chair test for body agility, a motor control test, and a one-foot stand for balance. It would be too physically demanding for many institutionalized individuals. The timed "up and go" test—which times a patient rising from an armchair, walking 3 meters, turning, walking back, and sitting down again—has been reported to be a reliable and valid screening test for functional mobility (Podsiadlo & Richardson, 1989). Reuben & Siu (in press) have developed two versions of a physical performance test (PPT) that can discriminate among a wider range of abilities at the lowest end of the physical function spectrum, but these tests are so new that they have not been used. To make progress in determining the benefits of exercise programs for the frail elderly, one or more hierarchical tests of physical and motor function must be developed and standardized to assess physical capacity, ranging from the ability to pass the ADL to the ability to complete existing standard tests of aerobic capacity, strength, and flexibility.

Sleep

Daily exercise has always been a component in the cluster of good health habits that are presumed to enhance sleep, but the evidence regarding the association of health and fitness to sleep patterns is very sparse. Some investigators, using a measure of the increase in slow wave sleep (SWS; a marker of sound sleep that seems to have a restorative function), have found increases in SWS following daytime exercise (Shapiro, Bortz, Mitchell, Bartel, & Jooste, 1981); other investigators have not. Griffen and Trindler (1978) found that SWS was greater overall in physically fit individuals. A daytime exercise bout seemed to increase SWS in the fit individuals but decreased it in unfit individuals. They acknowledged that the higher overall levels of SWS in the fit subjects could be attributed to several factors: a chronic exercise-induced adaptation of SWS, a residual effect of each day's exercise bout, genetic differences, and exercise-related nutritional patterns. They suggested that the reason a decrease in SWS was seen in the unfit group was that the exercise bout was a stress-evoking disruption in their daily schedule, whereas for the physically fit, it was a part of their daily routine. This led the investigators to conclude that in order for exercise to have a facilitative effect on SWS, the level of exercise must be matched to the level of fitness. These studies were focused primarily on young subjects and on the acute effects of an exercise bout. Even fewer investigators have attempted to analyze long-term effects of an exercise program on sleep. Reiter (1981), whose study was focused on exercise and mood states, has observed that participants of an exercise program reported enhanced sleep. Also, Vitiello, Schwartz, Abrass, Bradbury, and Stratton (1989) administered a retrospective sleep quality questionnaire to 13 healthy elderly men (69.0± 5.1 years), who completed a six-month, five-day/week training program that resulted in a 21% increase in their maximum oxygen consumption. They found that the general sleep quality was enhanced, with the soundness and depth of sleep being greater and with a greater sense of morning refreshment. Their subjects also reported decreases in the length of time necessary to go to sleep and decreases in the length of nighttime awakenings and periods of daytime sleepiness.

Disease

The effects of exercise on the prevention or rehabilitation of acute or chronic diseases in the frail elderly has become of increasing interest. The four chronic diseases that cause the greatest physical disability in the elderly include cardiovascular disease (including hypertension), diabetes mellitus, chronic lung diseases, and arthritis. Aside from the well-known effects of exercise on the prevention and rehabilitation of cardiovascular disease and diabetes mellitus (see Shephard, 1987, for a review), there is increasing evidence that exercise is important in the prevention of osteoporosis (see Martin & Brown, 1989; Smith, 1988, for reviews). The role of exercise in the treatment of arthritis remains unclear, but there is preliminary evidence that individuals with rheumatoid arthritis and osteoarthritis can benefit from regular systematic exercise (Panush, 1989). Clearly, more research is needed to clarify the "dose–response" relationship between exercise and disease prevention or rehabilitation in the frail elderly.

Mental Function

Cognitive

The benefits that exercise might have on older adult cognitive function seem intuitive and are probably based on the belief in *mens sana in corpore sano* (a sound mind in a sound body). Indeed, results from an increasing number of studies support the hypothesis that, especially in older adults, systematic and habitual exercise appears to be related to some types of cognitive function. The nature and strength of that relationship, the cognitive functions involved, the intensity of physical activity necessary to modulate mental function, and the amplitude of effects that physical activity might have on the mental function and functional operation of adults older than 75 remain to be determined. An association between habitual physical activity and several types of mental function has been reported for information-processing speed, such as simple and choice reaction time (Chodzko-Zajko & Ringel, 1987; Milligan, Powell, Harley, & Furchtgott, 1984; for review see Spirduso, 1986; Spirduso & Gilliam-MacRae, 1990); event-related potentials (Bashore, in press); and fluid intelligence (Elsayed, Ismail, & Young, 1980). The subjects of these cross-sectional investigations have been older adults who have been habitually physically active most of their lives. Other investigators have failed to find a relationship between fitness and fluid intelligence (Powell & Pohndorf, 1971) and crystalized intelligence (Elsayed *et al.*, 1980).

A few investigators have pursued the study of the exercise-cognitive function relationship hypothesis by using an experimental or longitudinal design in which older adults who present a sedentary life history are enrolled in a physical activity or a social control program. Of these, Dustman *et al.* (1984) found improved speed of information processing (measured by simple reaction time and the digit-symbol substitution test) in the aerobic exercise group but not in the control groups. The conclusion of Stones and Kozma (1989, 315), based upon a thorough review of the literature on the subject of exercise and cognitive function, as well as their own extensive and theoretically based research, was that "the effects of an aerobic exercise intervention were of simultaneous benefit to endurance fitness and cognitive performance. . . . The effects of chronic exercise were both predicted and found to be generalized across interrelated domains of physical and psychological function." Elsayed, Ismail, and Young (1980) found improvement in the fluid intelligence scores of middle-aged men who exercised for four months. Memory and intellectual abilities of older institutionalized persons were improved with an exercise program (Powell, 1975); and Stamford, Hambacher, and Fallica (1974) reported that the memory functions of geriatric institutionalized mental patients were improved with physical activity. Even very light exercise programs in older adults who could not exercise vigorously significantly improved a measure of memory within 30 minutes after the exercise bout (Diesfeldt & Diesfeldt-Groenendijk, 1977).

Several mechanisms have been proposed by which physical activity and exercise might modulate mental function: maintained use of neurons facilitates their health and maintains their function; increased cardiovascular efficiency increases oxygen transport and thus reduces brain hypoxia in active brain regions; control of blood pressure enhances mental function; physical activity enhances the balance and function of brain neurotransmitters; and neural activation and stimulation of the reticular activating system influences attentional processes. These mechanisms are discussed in review papers of Spirduso (1980). An excellent review paper in which various models of the effects of exercise on mental function are examined is that of Stones and Kozma (in press).

Not all reports from exercise program intervention studies are positive. Emery and Gatz (1990) found only limited support for a relationship between physiological improvement and enhanced fluid intelligence, and the crystallized intelligence of middle-aged men did not appear to be improved by a four-month exercise program (Elsayed et al., 1980). Blumenthal and Madden (1988), using the Sternberg memory search paradigm, found a fitness relationship in middle-aged adults only with parameters that are associated with peripheral response factors; Blumenthal's group (1988) later failed to find exercise-enhanced performance in neuropsychological tests of memory function and psychomotor function. Perri and Templer (1985) also found no change in memory following an exercise program intervention. A pioneering effort to measure the effects of a three-month exercise program on neuropsychological function in very old institutionalized patients failed, probably because the exercises, which were designed to improve balance, coordination, and muscle strength, did not evoke increased heart rates of more than 10–20 beats per minute above resting levels for any length of time (Molloy, Richardson, & Crilly, 1988).

Finally, although reports of exercise interventions with demented patients are almost nonexistent, Ingebretsen (1982) suggested that physical training and movement exercises might be useful in working with patients who have lost important cues of contact both with themselves and with the environment. Movement lessons could contribute to reality orientation therapy and training in self-help. Movement training might provide some pleasure from self-mastery, from which even severely demented patients might benefit (Paraspiropoutos et al., 1979).

Emotional Function

Many studies have been conducted to identify the relationship between exercise and psychological improvement in nonelderly populations (see Hughes, 1984, for a review). Only a few of these studies have focused on the role of habitual exercise in fostering psychological benefits in older persons, and none has focused on the frail elderly (see Hird & Williams, 1989, for a review). Conclusions from this general field of research have been obscured by methodological defects such as poor choices of psychological measures, experimenter/subject biases, and inadequate descriptions of methods. It is suggested that older adults may in fact exhibit more psychological and physiological benefits from exercise since they may be in poorer physical and emotional health compared with their younger counterparts.

Exercise has long been proposed as a therapeutic modality to alleviate depression, stress, and anxiety in young and middle-aged adults, and the few investigators who studied older adults found that exercise programs seemed to provide positive benefits (see Berger, 1988, for review; see also Gillett, 1989; Reiter, 1981; Tredway, 1978). However, the effects of exercise and fitness on anxiety and depression are far from clear, since factors such as the nature of anxiety or depression, the fitness level of the subject, and the intensity and length of the exercise program confuse the issue. Hughes (1984) concluded after an extensive review that almost all studies of the psychological benefits of aerobic exercise have methodological problems that render their findings open to severe criticism.

Self-efficacy, as defined by Bandura (1977), refers to an individual's perception of his or her capability to successfully execute a certain behavior (e.g., "I think I can walk four blocks"). It might be considered a "situational specific" measure of self-confidence. Self-efficacy is not concerned with the skills an individual possesses, but rather with individuals' perceived confidence. It is affected by performance accomplishments, vicarious experiences, verbal persuasion (social expectations), and physiological arousal (Bandura, 1977). The strongest source of efficacy information is performance accomplishments. Older adults who have never exercised or have exercised only in their youth are likely to have low efficacy with respect to performing exercises. However, participation in exercise can provide experiences that enhance their perceived physical abilities and thereby enhance self-efficacy. Observing other very old people performing exercise may increase the observer's perceptions of his or her own ability to exercise. Currently, few such role models exist for the oldest adults.

Many frail elderly have misconceptions about their physical capability. On the basis of these misconceptions, they limit their behavior by avoiding desirable activities they perceived to be beyond their physical abilities. These are the very individuals who may benefit most from an exercise program designed to develop competence and overcome misconceptions about their physical abilities. Older adults' participation in an exercise program could enhance their self-efficacy with respect to the specific exercises performed, and this enhancement may generalize to other performance-related situations such as completing chores, learning a new skill, or going on a travel tour (Hogan & Santomier, 1984; Ray, Gissal, & Smith, 1982).

Self-Esteem and Feelings of Well-Being

Confidence in our physical capacity and the knowledge that we can take care of ourselves and go where we want when we want are major contributing factors to our self-esteem. As we age, and as we realize that physical capabilities are diminishing, the importance of health, physical mobility, and endurance becomes more and more prominent in our sense of control and, consequently, the way we feel about ourselves. The relation between health and a sense of control grows stronger with increasing age (Rodin, 1986). Based on a review of 30 years of research on the subjective well-being of people over 60 years of age, Larson (1978) concluded: "Among all the elements of an older person's life situation, health is the most strongly related to subjective well-being." Not only is good health, which provides freedom from physical pain, in and of itself extremely important, but it is also associated with other indicants of well-being, such as the ability to manage one's own living environment, to be transported, to travel, and to engage in social activities. The loss of control over physical ability may very well result in feelings of a loss of control over all of life's events, making it difficult to maintain a sense of internal locus of control. In one study, subjects (average age 80) who rated their health as poor tended to have an external locus of control, whereas those who perceived their health to be "acceptable to good" were able to maintain an internal locus of control (Brothen & Detzner, 1983). Both an internal locus of control and a high self-concept were significantly related to an excellent self-rated health and excellent self-rated appetite (Bonds, 1980). Stated another way, people who are physically active and perceive themselves as being healthy feel more confident that they control their own destiny.

For many older individuals who live independently, maintaining muscle tone, strength, endurance, and physique through daily physical exercise enhances self-esteem. Participation in exercise programs enables people to become realistic about their physical ability, gives them self-confidence, and facilitates positive changes in life-style (Ray, Gissal, & Smith, 1982). Participants generally report an enhanced feeling of well-being at the conclusion of the programs (Gillett, 1989; Perri & Templer, 1985; Reynolds & Garrett, 1989). These individuals tend to eat better, sleep better (Reiter, 1981), and take better care of themselves. The incorporation of these good health habits also further increases their self-esteem. Conversely, older physically inactive individuals, especially women, have been shown to have a distorted body image (Kreitler & Kreitler, 1970). Organized exercise programs, on the other hand, have improved the body image of older subjects and consequently have enhanced self-esteem (Shephard, 1987).

The feelings of "well-being" experienced by individuals who exercise are very difficult to quantify experimentally. But even in exercise-intervention studies in which no significant effects of exercise were found on other types of psychological factors—such as perceived quality of life, indices of basic mental health, or activity level—the subjects reported an improved sense of well-being (e.g., Blumenthal & Madden, 1988; Gitlin *et al.*, in press; Windsor *et al.*, 1989).

Because physical activity is a very quantifiable activity, it provides immediate feedback with regard to accomplishment and change. Healthy older adults who exercised on a bicycle reported a significantly higher sense of accomplishment than did controls (Windsor *et al.*, 1989). In general, individuals who succeed in physical tasks that they could not complete a few weeks before feel a sense of accomplishment and satisfaction, whether the task is running 5 miles instead of 4 or walking 50 yards instead of 10. Physical accomplishment is relative to the capacity available, and changes in these capacities with training mean that a goal has been reached, self-discipline has been confirmed, and beneficial change has occurred.

Health, Quality of Life, and Life Satisfaction

Researchers who have studied the literature over the past four decades have generally concluded that subjective health status plays a very large role in feelings of life satisfaction of older adults (e.g., Larson, 1978; Okun *et al.*, 1984). Recently, Willits and Crider (1988) reported that this relationship apparently also exists in middle-aged adults, as they found that a personal health rating was the best single predictor of overall life satisfaction. Moreover, it did not interact with gender or other life satisfaction measures such as education, income level, and marital status. Lohr, Essex, and Klein (1988), however, remind us that life satisfaction is a very complex issue in which coping patterns, at least in women, buffer the relationship between perceived health and life satisfaction. In the study from Lohr, Essex, and Klein (1988), women who had objectively assessed poor health but strong positive coping behaviors did not appear to allow physical health problems to reduce their feelings of life satisfaction. But they also suggested that at all levels of health, women who have a coping strategy of passively accepting their incapacities were more likely to perceive themselves as impaired and subjectively judge their health more negatively. It is self-reported health, not objectively assessed health, that has appeared to be highly related to feelings of life satisfaction and judgments of quality of life. Optimizing life satisfaction, therefore, may depend upon doing as much as possible to enhance perceived health while at the same time developing positive coping strategies for the inevitable losses that occur in all individuals who live to a very old age.

The direct or indirect effects of mild exercise or limited physical activity have apparently been so beneficial, at least to many older adults age 50 to 70, that it would seem that it should also have potential to contribute to the quality of life of many individuals in nursing homes and alternative care facilities. Even a minimal degree of movement and activity by those who have physical limitations could produce many of the contributions mentioned above, only at a lower level. An exercise opportunity in a nursing home is also an opportunity for decision making, for providing some control over the day's activities. A walk alone along the corridors or outdoors on the grounds of the facility can provide an opportunity to those who profoundly miss their privacy. Physical activity-related stimulation can play a role in preventing unnecessary and premature resignation and apathy (Lindsley, 1964; Melin & Steen, 1975). Physical activity can provide an opportunity to be alone, for those who are able, at their own discretion. An opportunity to exercise may also provide some relief from the severe and crushing regimentation of institutional schedules.

The extent to which increased activation and exercise in the very old institutionalized population will be of benefit to cognitive and emotional function; the degree to which it might improve the daily living conditions of individuals, however, is almost unknown. Most professionals who have initiated activity programs for very old institutionalized patients have reported multidimensional beneficial results (Ingebretsen, 1982), but the physical activity programs in these studies were not isolated from other aspects of institutional programming and the physiological changes that might have occurred in these programs were not measured.

Some investigators also have reported negative results, such as no change in irritability (Powell, 1975); and at the conclusion of one program designed to stimulate and reactivate the patients, the patients were assessed as being more restless and "strange." Those who stopped playing a passive patient's role were regarded as "difficult." Yet in all cases where physical activity programs have been implemented, they have been readily accepted and appreciated by the patients. Documenting beneficial effects of relatively short-term exercise program interventions on psychological constructs such as life satisfaction and self-esteem is particularly challenging, since quantification of these constructs is not yet reliable, and the constructs themselves are built upon a long lifetime of experiences and are probably extremely stable. Weiss and Kayser-Jones (1989) reported that considerable differences existed between what residents of a nursing home valued and what physicians valued in terms of the residents' quality of life: "Physicians . . . tend to emphasize mental competence and the ability to communicate, while residents value simple day-to-day activities such as reading, taking a walk, and listening to music."

The Upper Limits of Physical Function in the Elderly: What Is Possible?

The contribution of physical activity to the quality of life will be as different for each older individual as every other aspect of the aging process is. But the limitations of those contributions should be a matter of individual choice—based upon the physical, psychological, and emotional constraints that are present—and made within a full range of opportunities. Expectations for older individuals should always remain optimistic, and all professionals should be aware of the upper limits of physical performance in older adults. These upper limits, which can be documented by personal testimonies and record-book examples, demonstrate the capabilities of older adults to perform outstanding physical feats. The photographs in Figures 2, 3, and 4 are of people who admittedly are exceptional, but they provide some indication of the upper limit of physical performance in older adults. More importantly, the dramatic reversals from poor health and debilitation to good health and outstanding physical performance are inspirational and should modify our expectations for older adults.

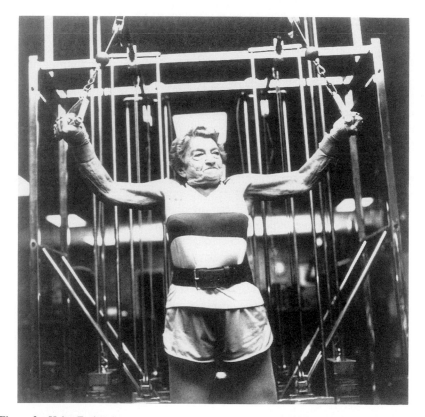

Figure 2 Helen Zechmeister, age 81, holds eight national age-group power lifting records (deadlift, 245 lb; benchpress, 94.5 lb; squat, 148 lb). She once competed in a men's 35-years-and-older bracket because there were no other women entrants. She won (Clark, 1987, 2).

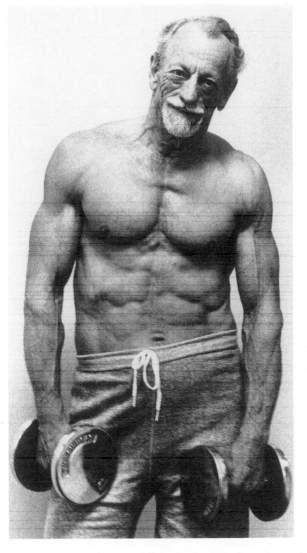

Figure 3   John Turner, age 67, is a psychiatrist who leads a sedentary professional life. He compensates by weight-lifting, jogging, and taking long walks (Clark, 1987, 14).

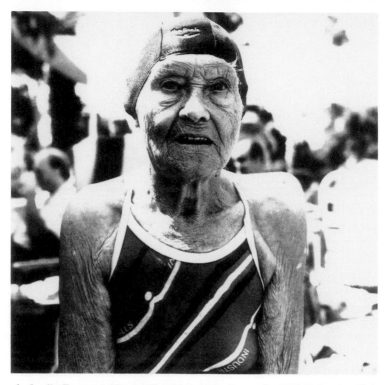

Figure 4 Luella Tyra, age 92, was the oldest competitor at the 1984 Swimming Nationals in Mission Viejo. An observer saw Luella bundled up, waiting for her races, and thought, "How frail she is!" When it was time to race, Luella stepped up and dove in. The observer said, "I saw her do the backstroke, the breaststroke, the butterfly and freestyle. The frail lady I first saw became a tiger in the water" (Clark, 1987, 107).

Recommendations for Future Research

A cardinal goal in gerontology is to compress the morbidity period of the very old, thus extending the active life expectancy of all aging individuals and greatly reducing medical costs associated with aging. Based upon existing knowledge, reasonable objectives for exercise programs for the frail elderly include the maintenance of function (activities of daily living), the prevention of disease (osteoporosis, cardiovascular disease, diabetes mellitus), and the treatment of conditions such as arthritis, injurious falls, strokes, and depression. In addition, exercise in this population may also be important in the prevention of the secondary consequences of demantia such as immobilization, falls, pneumonia, anorexia, pressure sores, anxiety, insomnia, and depression.

Research is needed, however, in several areas:

1. The types of physical activity and the quantity and quality of physical movement needed to improve the disease or functional status of very old individuals should be determined. It is important to discover not only the exact nature of the physical, mental, and social benefits of exercise but how these benefits affect the ultimate goals of compressing morbidity, decreasing the use of health care resources, and uplifting life satisfaction for the very old.

2. At all ages, exercise must be undertaken sensibly to avoid pain and injury, but assessing and controlling the risks involved for exercising septuagenarians and octogenarians should have a priority in gerontological research. Cost–benefit ratios can be calculated to determine the financial ramifications of an exercise program. Strategies that could reduce costs and motivate patients to be more mobile, such as training older adult volunteers in institutions to be the leaders of the exercise programs, should be explored and evaluated.

3. The question "Why isn't exercise integrated into the life-style of so many of the very old?" must be answered. What factors serve as barriers to participation in physical activity? For example, how potent is ageism as a barrier to participation in physical activity? What are the attitudes of the frail elderly and their caregivers toward exercise? Do exercise-related attitudes of the elderly or society's view of age-appropriate exercise deter implementation of exercise programs in institutions? Can these attitudes be changed? If so, how can this best be accomplished?

4. In parallel to the pragmatic and applied questions that demand an answer as quickly as possible, basic questions regarding the mechanisms of biological and psychological adaptations to exercise in the older organism need to be developed. The dramatic improvements in function that sometimes follow participation in an exercise program might be described as reversibility (albeit temporary) of aging processes. Understanding the mechanisms of reversibility should provide greater insights into the process of aging itself.

    The extreme difficulties of behavioral and physical measurement of the frail elderly, the heterogeneity of aging humans, and the fact that the relationship of physical health status to life satisfaction is an extremely complex issue (Lohr et al., 1988), has contributed to less rigor than we would desire in the research on the role of health and fitness in the quality of life for the frail elderly. But the converging evidence from research is that individuals who pursue and maintain a healthy and physically active life-style will remain involved in society in personally satisfying and socially useful ways and are more likely to experience the highest possible functioning and quality of life in their waning years.

References

Adams, G. M., & deVries, H. A. (1973). Physiological effects of an exercise training regimen upon women aged 52–79. *Journal of Gerontology, 28,* 50–55.

American College of Sports Medicine (1978). Position statement on the recommended quantity and quality of exercise for developing and maintaining fitness in healthy adults. *Medicine and Science in Sports, 10,* 7–10.

Avorn, J. L. (1986). Medicine, health and the geriatric transformation. *Daedalus, 115,* 211–225.

Bandura, A. (1977). Self-efficacy: Toward a unifying theory of behavioral change. *Psychological Review, 84,* 191–215.

Bar-Or, O. (1977). Age-related changes in exercise perception. In G. Borg, ed., *Physical work and effort.* New York: Pergamon Press.

Bashore, T. R. (in press). Age-related changes in mental processing revealed by analysis of event-related brain potentials. In J. W. Rohrbaugh, R. Johnson, & R. Parasuraman, eds., *Event related potentials of the brain.* New York: Oxford University Press.

Berger, B. (1988). The role of physical activity in the life quality of older adults. In W. W. Spirduso & H. Eckert, eds., *The academy papers: Physical activity and aging,* pp. 42–58. Champaign, Ill.: Human Kinetics Publishers.

Biegel, L. (1984). *Physical fitness and the older person.* Rockville, Md.: Aspen Systems Corporation.

Blakeslee, J. A. (1988). Untie the elderly. *American Journal of Nursing, 88,* 833–834.

Blumenthal, J. A., & Madden, D. J. (1988). Effects of aerobic exercise training, age, and physical fitness on memory search performance. *Psychology and Aging, 3,* 280–285.

Bonds, A. G. (1980). The relationship between self-concept and locus of control and patterns of eating, exercise, and social participation in older adults. *Dissertation Abstracts International, 41,* 1397-A.

Booth, F. W. (1982). Effect of limb immobilization on skeletal muscle. *Journal of Applied Physiology: Respiration, Environment, and Exercise Physiology, 52,* 1113–1118.

Bortz, W. M., II (1982). Disuse and aging. *Journal of the American Medical Association, 248,* 1203.

Bortz, W. M., II (1983). On disease . . . aging . . . and disuse. *Executive Health, 20,* 1–5.

Brothen, T., & Detzner, D. (1983). Perceived health and locus of control in the aged. *Perceptual and Motor Skills, 56,* 946.

Buskirk, E. R. (1985). Health maintenance and longevity: Exercise. In C. E. Finch & E. L. Schneider, eds., *Handbook of the biology of aging.* New York: Van Nostrand Reinhold.

Butler, R. N. (1981). The "E" in elderly: Exercise, Synopsis of the National Conference on Fitness and Aging. President's Council on Physical Fitness & Sports, September 10–11. Washington, D.C.

Chodzko-Zajko, W. J., & Ringel, R. L. (1987). Physiological fitness measures and sensory and motor performance in aging. *Experimental Gerontology, 22,* 317–328.

Clark, E. (1987). *Growing old is not for sissies: Portraits of senior athletes.* Corte Madera, Calif.: Pomegranate Calenders and Books.

Conrad, C. C. (1976). When you're young at heart. *Aging, 258,* 11–13.

Convertino, V. A., Montgomery, L. D., & Greenleaf, J. E. (1984). Cardiovascular responses during orthostasis: Effect of an increase in VO_2 max. *Aviation Space and Environmental Medicine, 55,* 702–708.

Cullen, K. J., & Weeks, P. J. (1978). Sporting activities and exercise habits of the 1975 Bussleton population. *Medical Journal of Australia, 1,* 69–71.

de Vries, H. A. (1970). Physiological effects of an exercise training regimen upon men aged 52 to 88. *Journal of Gerontology, 25,* 325–336.

Diesfeldt, H. F. A., & Diesfeldt-Groenendijk, H. (1977). Improving cognitive performance in psychogeriatric patients: The influence of physical exercise. *Age and Aging, 6,* 58–64.

Dobrev, P. A. (1980). Complex experimental investigations of the influence of weight training on persons in middle, advanced and old age. *Scientific Methodical Bulletin, 3,* 27–28.

Dustman, R. E., Ruhling, R. O., Russell, E. M., Shearer, D. E., Bonekat, H. W., Shigeoka, J. W., Wood, J. W., & Bradford, D. C. (1984). Aerobic exercise training and improved neuropsychological function of older individuals. *Neurobiology of Aging, 5,* 35–42.

Elsayed, M., Ismail, A. H., & Young, R. J. (1980). Intellectual differences of adult men related to age and physical fitness before and after an exercise program. *Journal of Gerontology, 35,* 383–387.

Emery, C. F., & Gatz, M. (1990). Psychological and cognitive effects of an exercise program for community-residing older adults. *The Gerontologist, 30,* 184–188.

Evans, L., & Strumpf, N. (1989). Routine physical restraint: Historical context and reexamination of the practice in hospitals and nursing homes. *The Gerontologist, 29,* 221A.

Fiatarone, M. A., Marks, E. C., Ryan, N. D., Meredith, C. N., Lipsitz, L. A., & Evans, W. J. (1990). High-intensity strength training in nonagenarians. *Journal of the American Medical Association, 263,* 3029–3034.

Fries, J. F. (1988). Aging, illness, and health policy: Implications of the compression of morbidity. *Perspectives in Biology and Medicine, 31,* 407–428.

Fries, J. F., Green, L. W., & Levine, S. (1989). Health promotion and the compression of morbidity. *The Lancet, 8636,* 481–483.

Frontera, W. R., Meredith, C. N., O'Reilly, K. P., Knuttgen, H. G., & Evans, W. J. (1988). Strength conditioning in older men: Skeletal muscle hypertrophy and improved function. *Journal of Applied Physiology, 64,* 1038–1044.

Gillett, P. (1989). Aerobic and muscle fitness in high risk and overweight senior women. *The Gerontologist, 29,* 258A.

Gitlin, L. N., Lawton, M. P., Windsor, L. A., Kleban, M. H., Sands, L. P., & Posner, J. (in press). *In search of psychological benefits: Exercise in healthy older adults.* Philadelphia, Penn.: Philadelphia Geriatric Center.

Greenleaf, J. E. (1984). Physiological responses to prolonged bed rest and fluid immersion in humans. *Journal of Applied Physiology: Respiration, Environment, and Exercise Physiology, 57,* 619–633.

Griffen, S. J., & Trinder, J. (1978). Physical fitness, exercise, and human sleep. *Psychophysiology, 15,* 447–450.

Hagberg, J. M., Graves, J. E., Limacher, M., Woods, D. R., Leggett, S. H., Cononie, C., Gruber, J. J., & Pollock, M. L. (1989). Cardiovascular responses of 70–79 year old men and women to exercise training. *Journal of Applied Physiology, 66,* 2589–2594.

Hird, J. S., & Williams, J. M. (1989). The psychological effects of chronic exercise in the elderly. In A. C. Ostrow, ed., *Aging and motor behavior,* pp. 173–200. Indianapolis, Ind.: Benchmark Press, Inc.

Hogan, P. I., & Santomier, J. P. (1984). Effect of mastering swim skills on older adults' self-efficacy. *Research Quarterly for Exercise and Sport, 55,* 294–296.

Holm, K., & Kirchoff, K. T. (1984). Perspectives on exercise and aging. *Heart and Lung, 5,* 519–524.

Hughes, J. R. (1984). Psychological effects of habitual aerobic exercise: A critical review. *Preventive Medicine, 13,* 66–78.

Ingebretsen, R. (1982). The relationship between physical activity and mental factors in the elderly. *Scandinavian Journal of the Society of Medicine, 29* (Suppl.), 153–159.

Kasch, F. W., Boyer, J. L., Van Camp, S. P., Verity, L. S., & Wallace, J. P. (1990). The effects of physical activity and inactivity on aerobic power in older men: A longitudinal study. *The Physician and Sportsmedicine, 18,* 73–83.

Katz, S., Downs, T. D., Cash, H. R., & Grotz, R. C. (1970). Progress in development of the Index of ADL. *The Gerontologist, 10,* 20–30.

Kreitler, H., & Kreitler, S. (1970). Movement and aging: A psychological approach. In D. Brunner and E. Jokl, eds., *Medicine and sport: Physical activity and aging,* pp. 302–306. Basel: Karger.

Kuriansky, J., & Gurland, B. (1976). The performance test of activities of daily living. *International Journal of Aging and Human Development, 7,* 343–352.

Larson, R. (1978). Thirty years of research on the subjective well-being of older Americans. *Journal of Gerontology, 33,* 109–125.

Lindsley, O. R. (1964). Geriatric behavioral prosthetics. In R. Kastenbaum, ed., *New thoughts on old age,* pp. 41–60. New York: Springer Publication Company.

Lohr, M. J., Essex, M. J., & Klein, M. H. (1988). The relationships of coping responses to physical health status and life satisfaction among older women. *Journal of Gerontology: Psychological Sciences, 43,* P54–P60.

Martin, A. D., & Brown, E. (1989). The effects of physical activity on the human skeleton. In C. B. Lewis & E. L. Smith, eds., *Bone Changes with Age: Topics in Geriatrics Rehabilitation, 4,* 25–36.

Melin, E., & Steen, E. (1975). *Aldrande och aldringsvard.* Skovde: Esselte Studium.

Milligan, W. L., Powell, D. A., Harley, C., & Furchtgott, E. (1984). A comparison of physical health and psychosocial variables as predictors of reaction time and serial learning performance in elderly men. *Journal of Gerontology, 39,* 704–710.

Molloy, D. W., Richardson, L. D., & Crilly, R. G. (1988). The effects of a three-month exercise programme on neuropsychological function in elderly institutionalized women: A randomized controlled trial. *Age and Ageing, 17,* 303–310.

Morey, M. C., Cowper, P. A., Feussner, J. R., DiPasquale, R. C., Crowley, G. M., Kitzman, D. W., & Sullivan, R. J. (1989). Evaluation of a supervised exercise program in a geriatric population. *Journal of the American Geriatrics Society, 37,* 348–354.

Moritani, T., & deVries, H. A. (1980). Potential for gross muscle hypertrophy in older men. *Journal of Gerontology, 35,* 672–682.

Niinimaa, V., & Shephard, R. J. (1978). Training and oxygen conductance in the elderly. I. the respiratory system. II: The cardiovascular system. *Journal of Gerontology, 33,* 362–367.

Okun, M. A., Stock, W. A., Haring, M. J., & Witter, R. A. (1984). Health and subjective well-being: A meta-analysis. *International Journal of Aging and Human Development, 19,* 111–131.

Orlander, J., & Aniansson, A. (1980). Effects of physical training on skeletal muscle metabolism and ultrastructure in 70 to 75-year-old men. *Acta Physiologica Scandinavica, 109,* 149–154.

Osness, W. (1987). Goals, plans, and work of the Association for Research, Administration, Professional Councils, and Societies fitness task force. American Association for Health, Physical Education, Recreation, and Dance national convention, Las Vegas, Nev.

Ostrow, A. C., & Dzewaltowski, D. A. (1986). Older adults' perceptions of physical activity participation based on age-role and sex-role appropriateness. *Research Quarterly for Exercise and Sport, 57,* 167–169.

Ostrow, A. C., Jones, D. C., & Spiker, D. D. (1981). Age role expectations and sex role expectations for selected sport activities. *Research Quarterly for Exercise and Sport, 52,* 216–227.

Ostrow, A. C., Keener, R. E., & Perry, S. A. (1987). The age grading of physical activity among children. *International Journal of Aging and Human Development, 24,* 101–111.

Paffenbarger, R. S., Hyde, R. T., Wing, A. L., & Hsieh, C. C. (1986). Physical activity, all-cause mortality, and longevity of college alumni. *New England Journal of Medicine, 314,* 605–613.

Panush, R. S. (1989). Exercise and arthritis. *Joint Changes with Age: Topics in Geriatric Rehabilitation, 4,* 23–31.

Paraspiropoutos, S. (1979). Aktiviteter pa en klinik for psykiatrisk aldre vard. *Sosial Medisinsk Tidsskrift, 56,* 309–310.

Perri, S., II, & Templer, D. I. (1985). The effects of an aerobic exercise program on psychological variables in older adults. *International Journal of Aging and Human Development, 20,* 167–172.

Pollock, M. L., Foster, C., Knapp, E., Rod, J. L., & Schmidt, D. H. (1987). Effect of age and training on aerobic capacity and body composition of master athletes. *Journal of Applied Physiology, 62,* 725–731.

Podsiadlo, D., & Richardson, S. (1989). Timed "up and go"—A useful screen of functional mobility. *The Gerontologist, 29,* 257A.

Powell, R. R. (1975). Effects of exercise on mental functioning. *Journal of Sports Medicine, 15,* 125–131.

Powell, R. R., & Pohndorf, R. A. (1971). Comparison of adult exercisers and non-exercisers on fluid intelligence and selected physiological variables. *Research Quarterly for Exercise and Sport, 42,* 70–77.

Prudham, D., & Grimley-Evans, J. (1981). Factors associated with falls in the elderly: A community study. *Age and Ageing, 10,* 141–146.

Ray, R. O., Gissal, M. L., & Smith, E. L. (1982). The effect of exercise on morale of older adults. *Physical and Occupational Therapy in Geriatrics, 2*, 53–62.

Reiter, M. A. (1981). Effects of a physical exercise program on selected mood states in a group of women over age 65. *Dissertation Abstracts International, 42*.

Reuben, D. B., & Siu, A. L. (in press). An objective measure of physical function of elderly outpatients: The physical performance test. *Journal of the American Geriatrics Society*.

Reynolds, B., & Garrett, C. (1989). Effects of exercise on elderly ambulatory functions. *The Gerontologist, 29*, 258A.

Rodin, J. (1986). Aging and health: Effects of the sense of control. *Science, 233*, 1271–1276.

Roe, D. A. (1983). Drugs and nutrients. In E. W. Haller & G. E. Cotton, eds., *Nutrition in the young and the elderly*, pp. 69–80. Lexington, Mass.: Collamore Press.

Rowe, J. W. (1989). *The Charles A. Dana foundation report, 4*, 1–3.

Sager, K. (1984). Exercises to activate seniors. *The Physician and Sportsmedicine, 5*, 144–151.

Seals, D. R., Hagberg, J. M., Allen, W. K., Hurley, B. F., Dalsky, G. P., Ehsani, A. A., & Holloszy, J. O. (1984). Glucose tolerance in young and older athletes and sedentary men. *Journal of Applied Physiology: Respiratory, Environmental, and Exercise Physiology, 56*, 1521–1525.

Seals, D. R., Hagberg, J. M., Hurley, B. F., Ehsani, A. A., & Holloszy, J. O. (1984). Endurance training in older men and women. I. Cardiovascular responses to exercise. *Journal of Applied Physiology: Respiratory, Environmental, and Exercise Physiology, 57*, 1024–1029.

Shapiro, C. M., Bortz, R., Mitchell, D., Bartel, P., & Jooste, P. (1981). Slow-wave sleep: A recovery period after exercise. *Science, 214*, 1253–1254.

Shephard, R. J. (1987). *Physical activity and aging*, 2nd ed. Rockville, Md.: Aspen Publishers.

Sidney, K. H., & Shephard, R. J. (1977). Perception of exertion in the elderly, effects of aging, mode of exercise, and physical training. *Perceptual and Motor Skills, 44*, 999–1010.

Smith, E. (1988). The role of exercise in the prevention of bone involution. In R. Chernoff & D. A. Lipschitz, eds., *Health promotion and disease prevention*. New York: Raven Press, Ltd.

Spirduso, W. W. (1980). Physical fitness, aging and psychomotor speed: A review. *Journal of Gerontology, 35*, 850–965.

Spirduso, W. W. (1986). Physical activity and the prevention of premature aging. In V. Seefeldt, ed., *Physical activity and well-being*, pp. 141–160. Champaign, Ill.: Human Kinetics Publishers.

Spirduso, W. W., & Gilliam-MacRae, P. (1990). Motor performance and aging. In J. E. Birren & K. W. Schaie, eds., *Handbook of the psychology of aging*, 3rd ed. Orlando, Fla.: Academic Press, Inc.

Stamford, B. A., Hambacher, W., & Fallica, A. (1974). Effects of daily physical exercise on the psychiatric state of institutionalized geriatric mental patients. *Research Quarterly, 45*, 35–41.

Stones, M. J., & Kozma, A. (1989). Physical activity, age, and cognitive/motor performance. In M. L. Howe & C. J. Brainerd, eds. *Cognitive development in adulthood: Progress in cognitive development research.* New York: Springer-Verlag.

Stones, M. J., & Kozma, A. (in press). Age, exercise, and coding performance. *Psychology and Aging, 4,* 190–194.

Tinetti, M. E. (1987). Factors associated with serious injury during falls by ambulatory nursing home residents. *Journal of the American Geriatrics Society, 35,* 644–648.

Tinetti, M. E., & Speechley, M. (1989). Prevention of falls among the elderly. *New England Journal of Medicine, 320,* 1055–1059.

Tobis, J. S., Friis, R., & Reinsch, S. (1989). Impaired strength leads to falls in the community. *The Gerontologist, 29,* 256A–257A.

Topp, B., Windsor, L. A., Sands, L. P., Gorman, K. M., Bleiman, M., Cherkas, L., & Posner, J. D. (1989). The effect of exercise on morbidity patterns of healthy older adults. *The Gerontologist, 29,* 192A.

Tredway, V. A. (1978). Mood and exercise in older adults. *Dissertation Abstracts International, 39,* 2531-B.

United States Public Health Service. Physician's Drug Prescribing Patterns in Skilled Nursing Facilities: Washington, D.C., United States Department of Health, Education, and Welfare, June, 1976.

Vitiello, M., Schwartz, R., Abrass, I., Bradbury, V., & Stratton, J. (1989). Increased aerobic fitness is associated with improved sleep quality in healthy aged men. *The Gerontologist, 29,* 258A.

Weiss, S. M., & Kayser-Jones, J. S. (1989). Perceptions of the quality of life of the institutionalized aged. *The Gerontologist, 29,* 311A.

Wells, B. G., Middleton, B., Lawrence, G., Lillard, D., & Safarik, J. (1985). Factors associated with the elderly falling in intermediate care facilities. *Geriatrics and Gerontology, 19,* 142–145.

Willits, F. K., & Crider, D. M. (1988). Health rating and life satisfaction in the later middle years. *Journal of Gerontology: Social Sciences, 5,* 5172–5176.

Windsor, L. A., Lawton, M. P., Gitlin, L. N., Kleban, M., Sands, L. P., Gorman, K. M., & Posner, J. D. (1989). Transitory changes in affect in young and older exercisers. *The Gerontologist, 29,* 192A.

Wiswell, R. A. (1980). Relaxation, exercise, and aging. In J. E. Birren & R. B. Sloane, eds., *Handbook of mental health and aging,* p. 954. Princeton, N.J.: Prentice-Hall.

12

Intellectual Exercise and Quality of Life in the Frail Elderly

TORBJÖRN SVENSSON

Introduction

To function well intellectually is probably one of the most important factors in the ability to lead a full and rewarding life. Intellectual functioning is the foundation of our ability to take in, process, and react to our own inner being and to the outer environment, be it social or physical. From this perspective, it is surprising how little emphasis has been given to intellectual capacity in relation to perceived quality of life. For instance, intellectual functioning is not mentioned as a factor in Larson's (1978) evaluation of 30 years of research on subjective well-being in older Americans. Yet without intelligence, human beings would not even be able to adhere to questions about the nature and evaluation of quality of life. Naturally, intelligence is only one of the aspects that contribute to what is called quality of life; however, it is not recognized to the full extent of its importance.

Just as intellectual functioning appears to be taken for granted in research on quality of life, it is not generally reported as a domain of relevance when people themselves are asked to list such factors in quality of life research (e.g., see Nordbeck, 1989). It also seems that most researchers have overlooked intellectual functioning as a relevant domain when constructing different measurement scales for quality of life, although some do include memory (e.g., Pearlman & Uhlman, 1988) and learning (Flanagan, 1978) as factors influencing quality of life. What is actually needed is for intellectual functioning to be evaluated alongside with health, socioeconomic status, work, and so on. This is not to say that higher intelligence scores should yield a higher quality of life. To most individuals, it is more a matter of using one's abilities in a successful manner than the actual level of abilities that are important when defining their own quality of life. Most likely, with age it is also the degree of change from one's normal level of functioning rather than the level or score per se that decides if a

Copyright © 1991 by Academic Press, Inc.
All rights of reproduction in any form reserved.

person will perceive a lower or higher quality of life. Thus, high intelligence scores do not alone define a good quality of life; however, issues of intellectual performance can contribute considerably to the quality of life of many individuals.

Quality of Life

Quality of life is a global concept that is intuitively understood and to some extent shared by people. In the research literature, however, rather than a single definition there are many and only moderately agreed-upon definitions that have so far been proposed (e.g., Bearon, 1988; George & Bearon, 1980; Lawton, 1983; Maeland, 1989; Nordbeck, 1989; Siegrist & Junge, 1989). When an individual is asked to evaluate his or her quality of life, the response is generally based on an evaluation of the whole life span. It can be assumed to rest upon experiences from former and present periods of life but also on an estimate of the coming period, on future expectations. This would especially be the case if quality of life were measured by one global question.

There seems to be general agreement that quality of life is a global measure or concept. At the same time, it is agreed that quality of life is built upon other concepts, which have been described as domains or attributes. In the present chapter it is proposed that these domains are qualities *in* life. Qualities *in* life are defined as the specific areas a person perceives to be vital to the ability to enjoy life and to feel that it has meaning. It can also be said that these qualities are areas into which an individual puts high meaning and involvement. As such, involvement and meaning are important aspects for measurements that seek to discern what is perceived as a quality in life. Meaning in life particularly must be considered since it involves a global evaluation of the entire life situation, with former, present, future, and perhaps even transcendent aspects of the individual's life content (Kenyon, 1989; Tornstam, 1989).

The concept of *involvement* has been presented by Svensson (1989a) in an attempt to reach a new understanding of the failure of activity theory and disengagement theory to adequately explain the diverging empirical findings that have been made concerning well-being and successful aging. Different forms of involvement or engagement should be addressed in measurements (i.e., both outer and inner involvement). Outer involvement is most often in the form of observable, performed activities that lend themselves to quantification. Inner involvement is understood to accompany a devotion to different forms of ethical, philosophical, and/or "cognitive" values. This could include, for example, religious belief, a strong conviction in a political system, a belief in the possibility of uniting generations, races, and so on, or a conviction that the earth is moving toward an ecological disaster. The last example was chosen to demonstrate that the involvement a person has does not necessarily have to be of a positive kind in order to work as an organizing principle to motivate the individual. What is proposed here is that all human beings are more or less strongly expressing involvement of some kind, outer or inner. Individuals show both types of involvement at the same time in their personal histories but not necessarily at the same moment; at any given time, one or the other might be stronger. It can also be claimed that, as a rule, outer engagement is more prominent during childhood, adolescence, and early adulthood. However, in certain phases of these periods, inner involvement may be the dominating form. As people move into middle age, inner involvement becomes more and more obvious; and at higher ages this type of involvement becomes the dominating pattern. This does not exclude elderly persons from showing high degrees of outer involvement nor suggest that fluctuations over time do not occur. Every phase has its distribution of inner and outer involvements (i.e., areas of high meaning in which the individual has invested a large amount of his or her energy). There is probably continuity in the ways an individual uses and demonstrates involvement over the life course even if there are shifts over periods in life.

In evaluating his or her quality of life, an individual must engage in some form of autobiographical process with the intention of evaluating and synthesizing the meanings and involvements that have been experienced so far. The person who successfully synthesizes his or her life and shows the highest degree of involvement, be it inner or outer, will also be the person who has the best potential for perceiving a good quality of life and for being satisfied with life. Furthermore, such a person would best be able to cope with stressful situations of different kinds and supposedly would be able to choose the most mature forms of coping strategies (Svensson, 1989a).

As noted earlier, several definitions of quality of life have been formulated and used. A new definition is proposed on which the contents of life are concentrated. In the present chapter, overall quality of life is defined as:

> the global evaluation of the fulfillment of what is considered by the individual to be meaningful contents in life in light of former, present, and future experiences and expectations of life.

This proposed definition stresses the importance of the individual's own evaluations and perceptions. This is not to neglect the socionormative aspects of quality of life (see Lawton, Chapter 1), but rather to point to the fact that these are always filtered and interpreted through the individual. Naturally, the norms of what is considered good or bad in life have a great impact on the individual's perception of his or her personal quality of life. What is important to remember, however, is that these norms only have relevance to the extent that they hold meaning to a particular individual.

As with life satisfaction, well-being, and morale, quality of life can be looked upon as a global construct built up of other more domain-specific concepts or constructs. To date, a number of such domains have been recognized in research on quality of life. According to Pearlman and Uhlman (1988), intellectual functioning is one of the qualities *in* life that makes up quality *of* life. Other such qualities noted by these authors are social roles, physical health, life satisfaction, well-being, and emotional state; in addition, one might add socioeconomic status, living conditions, social integration, and mental health.

It is important to note that not only is it important to distinguish what the different qualities *in* life are, but the relative importance of one quality in life as compared with other qualities must also be considered. Stability over time may exist at the global level of quality of life, while at the same time different domains may change in value, function, or importance. Reevaluations of domains can be made by individuals such that no change is seen at the overall level, even though there may be major changes in and between the different qualities *in* life.

Health is often considered important to maintaining a high quality of life (Clark, 1988; Nordbeck, 1989). At the same time, however, cognitive functioning and intellectual capacity is not considered as vital or many times is not even mentioned in the literature. This trend may result because it actually is of low importance or because people, in general, count cognitive capacity or mental health as included in the general health concept. It is necessary then to establish whether there is a difference in ascribed importance between physical and mental health and whether normal cognitive functioning is actually included in the concept of mental health.

Nordbeck's (1989) research demonstrates that there is very little difference in quality of life between those with and without chronic pain, while there is a great difference between those with and without *severe* chronic pain. This may point to the fact that a decline in one quality *in* life does not affect the global concept as long as certain limits are not exceeded. It would indicate the effectiveness of coping and compensation to overcome threats in an aspect of quality. As areas of life with a high ascribed meaning and a high amount of involvement are dealt with, it may also be that the meaning of or the involvement in one area is devalued and others are upgraded to maintain the same overall quality of life.

Intelligence in the Frail Elderly

When intelligence and intelligent behavior in the elderly are discussed in research on quality of life, these concepts should not only be restricted to the form of intelligence that is understood by what is measured with traditional intelligence tests, but also must include everyday competence and wisdom.

Some theories on intelligence (i.e., the cultural norms or notions about what is to be considered intelligent behavior or an intelligent person) are implicit (Sternberg & Berg, 1987). These theories are important in that they tell us what is and is not to be considered appropriate thinking at different stages of the life span. They also have implications for how more formal theories are formulated and how different measures of intelligence are constructed. A parallel to quality of life can be drawn here, as it too includes implicit models or theories of what is to be considered a good or bad quality of life. The problem is that too little interest has been put into understanding these societal theories or norms of quality of life.

Salthouse (1987) stresses the discrepancy that can be noticed between laboratory results and everyday accomplishments by older adults. He points to different interpretations as to why this is the case, one being the idea that what is observed in daily life is an effect of the selection of situations and tasks by the individual him- or herself and that these do not represent the full range of situations and tasks. Another interpretation is that laboratory tasks cover process, while everyday tasks are more directed toward task fulfillment and product. This interpretation is in line with what is proposed by Baltes, Dittmann-Kohli, and Dixon (1984). They discuss the lowered orientation toward cognitive efficacy in the elderly related to the growing importance of other domains, such as social intelligence and everyday functioning. Salthouse (1987) also points out that everyday activities are often used and thereby practiced, pointing to the benefits of not only familiarity but also of training and exercise.

It has been suggested that, as we grow older, intelligence becomes more and more directed to the adaptation to everyday life, which means that the need for more ecologically valid tests is great (Baltes et al., 1984; Sternberg & Berg, 1987). The tests must reflect the different intellectual aspects of the situations that are important to solve the task at hand in a successful manner. It also must be recognized that there are differences over the life span as to the importance and use of different aspects of intelligence. With advancing age there is a shift in importance away from intelligence and other cognitive abilities toward social competence and inner meaning (Baltes et al., 1984; Kenyon, 1989; Svensson, 1989a; Tornstam, 1989). Context, value, and the evaluation of consequences might become more important than managing the task itself. It has been suggested that after reaching the stage of formal operations there are other structural changes taking place during adult cognitive development (see, e.g., Cavanaugh, Kramer, Sinnott, Camp, & Markley, 1985; Riegel, 1973).

As mentioned earlier, tests of a more everyday nature can prove to better tap the important aspects of intelligence and cognition in elderly persons' daily lives. For example, when memory is measured with the technique that Cohen (1981) called Subject Performed Task (SPT; i.e., enacted to-be-remembered material), there are less differences between young and old subjects than can be seen in other tests (Bäckman, 1985; Bäckman & Nilsson, 1985). The SPT test also shows some atypical patterns in the relation between scores on recognition and recall compared with what is found on verbal tasks (Svensson & Nilsson, 1989).

Wisdom must also be discussed in this context, as it might be one of the important aspects of cognitive ability developed later in life. It is not the number of years lived but rather the number and quality of experiences and the person's degree of success in synthesizing his or her life that constitute wisdom (Svensson, 1989a). In a study performed by Clayton and Birren (1980), elderly subjects did not rate themselves as possessing more or less wisdom than middle-aged or younger subjects. On the other hand, both the young and the middle-aged rated the concept of "aged" to be closer to the concept of "wise" than did the elderly themselves. Wisdom probably also embraces a grasp of culture and societal norms. Furthermore, it is important to note that affect and motivation may influence the directions of actions. For these reasons, it is important to deal with wisdom not only as an intellectual capacity but also as reflective of an individual's personality. Here, it is posited that more and more of the personality is integrated into the repertoire of the wise individual so as to also involve the capacity for operating and acting on values, norms, and expectations about reactions to intellectual solutions. Thus, the evaluation of reactions might become more important than whether the actions are correct. In this way, the individual's thinking and acting become more and more the "self" (i.e., the individual becomes more and more integrated and individualized with advancing age). On the other hand, wisdom can be said to be the ability to use generalized knowledge on a specific task or situation. It seems that, one way or the other, wisdom has a relation to problem solving in everyday situations. To be able to act, think, and use feelings wisely and to be looked upon as being wise will add to a person's perception of being successful and thereby add to the perception of quality of life.

When dealing with intelligence and everyday competence, the importance of the environment has to be recognized. Schooler (1987) points to the importance of a complex environment for intellectual development and, especially, for flexibility. A simple, predictable, and monotonous environment can cause decline in intellectual functioning and competence (see also Lawton, 1975; Svensson, 1984), while a complex, stimulating, and rewarding environment promotes development. However, it is not only the degree of complexity and stimulation that is important, but also the congruence, fit, or match of the level of stimulus with the individual's capacity or competence (Kahana, 1975; Lawton, 1975; Svensson, 1984).

Stability and Change

The majority of studies on intellectual capacity during old age have been carried out with the WAIS battery or with national revisions and adoptions of tests in this battery. Most studies in the area have also been cross-sectional and, thereby, have led to an overestimation of the reduction in intellectual functioning with increasing age. Based on these studies (e.g., Doppelt & Wallace, 1955; Eisdorfer, 1963), it was concluded, among other things, that both performance (i.e., the processing of new information and perceptual integrating capacities) and verbal abilities decrease profoundly even if the decrease in verbal functioning is somewhat less prominent. However, these results have not been corroborated in longitudinal research.

From longitudinal studies and studies permitting cohort comparisons (Berg, 1980; Schaie, 1983), the conclusion has been drawn that a high degree of intraindividual stability signifies intellectual development during aging and that a marked cohort difference is at hand, such that younger cohorts exhibit a better intellectual capacity than preceding cohorts. It also has been shown that illnesses and impending death lead to decreases in intellectual functioning, while individuals in good health show good stability. There are suggestions that more prominent changes do occur around the age of 80. However, this has not been subjected to study, although it would be of great value to study aging effects and cohort effects on intellectual functioning after the age of 80. Another reason to study intellectual development in advanced age is the close relation between illness and intellectual functioning and the perspective of an apparent connection between intellectual functioning and adaptation to aging and illness.

Longitudinal studies demonstrate a high degree of stability in intellectual performance into the late 60s and early 70s (Berg, 1980; Schaie & Hertzog, 1983). When decline is observed, it is usually seen in specific abilities and especially in the domain of fluid intelligence (Berg, 1980; Botwinick, 1977; Horn, 1982; Schaie, 1979). At the same time, it has been noted that there are large interindividual differences in the onset of the decline such that some individuals show no signs of decline even in their late 70s and early 80s, while others show a general decline as early as age 60. Even if the general pattern is stability, intellectual growth is possible into advanced age, especially in those functions that depend on experience (i.e., crystallized intelligence) (Cattell, 1971; Horn, 1980). There is evidence that well-practiced abilities show less decline. There is also a profound intraindividual variation in the pattern of decline in different abilities. Individuals can show decline in certain abilities, most possibly fluid, while at the same time they can be stable in other functions and even show a gain in yet others. There is also more and more evidence that training and behavioral intervention can help a person maintain or regain intellectual abilities (Baltes, Dittmann-Kohli, & Kliegl, 1986; Denney, 1979; Labouvie-Vief & Gonda, 1976; Schaie, Willis, Hertzog, & Schulenberg, 1987; Willis & Schaie, 1986).

Intelligence and the use of intellectual abilities are dependent on the context; there is no one answer to whether there is a decline in the ability to deal with everyday situations with advancing age. Intelligence, among other things, is used for adjusting to a changing environment. According to Sternberg and Berg (1987), this can be accomplished by utilizing one of three processes: adjusting to the environment; changing the environment; or moving to a new environment (see also Kahana, 1975). It might be that all three strategies are in operation at the same time, even if it is sufficient to use only one successfully. It could then be assumed that in very advanced age or in elderly persons suffering from some kind of illness there is a growing difficulty in using at least the first two processes mentioned. In such cases, the only strategy left is to leave the present environment. Maybe it is at this point that a threat to the experience of a good quality of life can be seen. To take it one step further, it could be that the last blow occurs when the person is no longer able to even leave the environment of his or her own free will.

Sternberg and Berg (1987) suggest that one way to avoid a decline in performance in the elderly is to train them how to choose and change their environments. This form of training might also be a way to maintain the same level of quality of life.

Primarily, there is a decline in maximum performance and the ability to perform difficult tasks, although it has not been shown that this impedes everyday intellectual functioning (Baltes *et al.,* 1984). That no decline is shown in everyday performance could account for the absence of negative effects in quality of life even though a decline can be seen in different forms of tests for intelligence.

Terminal Decline

One aspect of change in cognitive abilities during aging is the terminal decline phenomenon. Terminal decline, first described by Kleemeier (1962), is strongly related to loss of health and distance from death. Riegel and Riegel (1972) stated that approximately five years prior to death there can be seen an overall decrease in cognitive functioning. It seems that the decline in intellectual functioning observed near the very end of life is more related to proximity to death than to old age per se. Palmore and Cleveland (1976) and Siegler (1975) have also discussed the difference between the linear, more lasting period of decline, "terminal decline," and the curvilinear, accelerated decline in intellectual functioning just before death, "terminal drop." Research by Schaie and Hertzog (1983) demonstrates that there is a general decline in intellectual functioning in later years, especially from the 70s and 80s. The terminal decline phenomenon has also been shown to apply to verbal ability, reasoning (Berg, 1987), and long-term memory (Johansson, 1985). However, it has been questioned whether the decline in cognitive abilities is pervasive or only restricted to certain abilities (White & Cunningham, 1988). Recent results from the Gothenburg longitudinal study speak in favor of a terminal decline in all cognitive functions (Johansson & Berg, 1989). Whether terminal decline leads to a drop in the perceived quality of life still needs to be verified, even if it can be assumed. It is possible that there are effects on quality of life only late in the terminal drop period. This can depend either on the individual's ability to cope or compensate for the loss or on whether the individual shifts his or her investment of meaning and energy to another domain, thereby maintaining the same level of quality of life.

Intellectual Exercise and Training

There has been a growing interest in the training and exercise of intellectual functions in old age. The primary interest of researchers has been in demonstrating whether or not a growth in the latent construct could be established that would then show in the performance on a test of that ability. These experiments have been criticized for only training performance on a particular test rather than showing a growth in the construct itself or that the educational techniques applied might change the character of the tests from measuring fluid intelligence to measuring crystallized intelligence (see, e.g., Donaldson, 1981). Denney (1979) also warned of possible negative effects of interventions to train elderly on intellectual abilities. She pointed out that elderly people usually use problem-solving techniques that are adapted to their particular life situations. If trained on other strategies, they might lose some of their everyday competence and thereby also reduce their overall functioning.

Labouvie-Vief and Gonda (1976) studied effects of training on inductive reasoning problems. They showed a significant increase in performance, especially for the group who received unspecific training in which they themselves had to generate strategies. The results pointed to a generalizability over tasks and that the effects could be registered at a post-test two weeks later.

In a short-term longitudinal study on training of fluid intelligence (Baltes *et al.*, 1986) it was established that elderly persons have a reserve capacity for gaining in performance. The transfer of training is low, but it could be shown that the ability to solve more difficult items increases with training. There was also a heightened accuracy of performance found on the tests.

In the Seattle longitudinal study, Willis and Schaie (1986) trained elderly participants who had declined or had been stable over a 14-year period in either or both spatial orientation and inductive reasoning. Persons who had declined in one of the abilities received training on that particular ability. Those who had declined or had been stable in both were randomly assigned to one of the training programs. Significant improvements resulted from both training programs, but only for the particular ability that had been trained. The interventions were effective in both restoring cognitive decline and improving the performance of stable persons. According to the authors, it should be possible to train a specific declining ability, especially if the person has a known history of intellectual performance such that the training could be individualized. This conclusion could relieve some of the fears raised earlier by Denney (1979).

Possible change of character of the measures, along with the criticism that these kinds of programs only train test efficiency, were issues addressed in another study (Schaie *et al.*, 1987). Studying 401 subjects on a five-hour test battery given as pre- and post-test and where 229 subjects received a five-hour individualized training program, Schaie and his collegues demonstrated that training of the latent constructs produces effects.

Measurements of intelligence are evaluations of the observed or manifest level of functioning. At the same time, the latent, or reserve, capacity that the individual possesses has to be taken into account (Baltes *et al.*, 1984; Sternberg & Berg, 1987); that is, the difference between overt and covert competence must be considered (Svensson, 1984). It is also important to note that the same latent constructs are not valid for young and old adults (i.e., constructs may vary over the life span). Also, even if constructs remain the same, they might not be of the same importance or hold the same meaning at different periods of life. More must be learned about what is really considered meaningful by the elderly in general and by particular individuals before research can progress further into the training of different intellectual functions. Understanding everyday competence may be the route to better understanding the intellectual powers of the elderly.

Quality of Life and Intelligence

Intellectual functioning is probably one of the most neglected qualities *in* life in relation to research on quality *of* life. It is generally taken for granted until the moment when decline sets in. Decline does not necessarily have to be in the form of psychiatric disturbances or dementias of various kinds. It can probably pose a threat to the quality of life in the normal aging process if and when the decline exceeds limits such that the individual can no longer accept or cope with requirements of everyday living.

Intelligence in relation to quality of life is not to be thought of as a score or as a level of functioning, but rather as a quality *in* life as valued by the individual as to its meaning and the perceived level of fulfillment. Intellectual capacity or activity does not necessarily have high meaning for all individuals but can be claimed to do so for some. Such persons would feel a threat to their quality of life if their perceived capacity went down from their former state of functioning, unless they were able to accept the decline and still perceive a high level of meaning in this quality *in* life. In general, intellectual capacity or activity is not reported to have such a high meaning in life. To be considered fatal to the experience of quality of life, the intellect probably must suffer severe damage or decline, for instance, from dementia or other states that influence intellectual functioning.

As noted earlier, for most individuals it is not a high intellectual ability that holds high meaning and thereby adds positively to the perception of quality of life. Rather, it is the possibility of successfully using the abilities that the individual possesses. For this reason, the question of stability and change in intellectual functioning over the life course is important to address. The loss of ability, or a negative change, exceeding the limits where different forms of compensation and coping are effective would have a negative effect on a person's perceived quality of life. This negative effect occurs provided that this quality *in* life is not ascribed less meaning or no meaning at all by the individual, who could eventually relieve the threat by upgrading the meaning of other areas in life. Training and exercise that result in growth in intellectual functioning—positive change—for many individuals would have a positive effect on the intellectual quality *in* life and eventually on the overall quality *of* life. Note that the direct link between quality of life and intelligence is based on the fulfillment of that quality *in* life as valued by the individual, and not based on the intelligence scores. When dealing with aging, and especially with frail elderly, it is often inevitable negative change and the eventual possibility for positive change that must be dealt with. Negative changes of a mild or moderate nature can be handled by using compensation or different coping strategies, but more profound changes pose a threat to the person's perception of fulfillment and success. On the other hand, lasting periods, or even moments, of stability could produce positive feelings of accomplishment. As for people suffering from mental retardation or dementia at a stage where they do not have any experience of or any memory of experiencing any higher level of functioning, this state of stability can also give the perception of fulfillment or at least of positive accomplishments. This means that demented or mentally retarded individuals are not excluded from experiencing a good quality in this area of life. Whether it then also affects their overall feeling of quality of life depends on the meaning this aspect of life holds to the individual. In these cases, however, there is also the possibility that very small negative changes in functioning can have devastating effects on the experience of fulfillment, since the critical point may be reached quickly.

Marcel (1951) argues for the importance of wisdom and alternative models of thought when dealing with the more spiritual aspects of life such as quality of life and well-being. As intellectual abilities build up part of what we call wisdom, it can also be claimed that they play a role in the formation of the global experiencing of quality of life. As Holliday and Chandler (1986) point out, there is no need to compare wisdom to intelligence or to treat them as accounting for the same phenomenon. On the other hand, we still have to be aware of the strong contribution of intellectual ability to the concept of wisdom. The significance of wisdom for the experience of a good quality of life is probably arguable. Nevertheless, it is claimed here that it is of at least some importance and that there is some evidence of the influence of intellectual abilities on the perception of quality of life.

Compensation, coping, and training can take care of the low or moderate decline in intelligence with age. When severe decline or a mental health problem sets in, these strategies are no longer sufficient, and reduction in the perceived quality of life is produced. An example of the former statement can be taken from the Lund 80+ study (Svensson, 1989b), in which 80-year-old subjects rating different aspects of subjective memory stated that they still thought their memory was better or a lot better than other people their own age, even if they thought that their memory had declined with age and that their level of functioning was about the same as the previous year.

According to George (1979), life satisfaction, as one of the important qualities of life, is essentially a cognitive assessment of one's progress toward desired goals. This statement of the cognitive loading of the concept will here serve as a basis for analyzing the relationship between intellectual capacities and life satisfaction. If it is possible to establish a positive correlation, there will also be, thereby, some indication of the importance or validity of intellectual functioning for experiencing a good quality of life. This is not to say that this is the only indirect way intellectual ability relates to quality of life. As already mentioned, intellectual functioning is probably also a component in the perception of good health, as evaluated globally by the individual.

Life satisfaction is mostly characterized as a cognitive component and is often claimed to rest upon the comparison of a person's own situation with that of others' (Staats & Stassen, 1987). On these grounds, it may be claimed that life satisfaction, being cognitively loaded, would correlate with other cognitive measures. In viewing the Neugarten Life Satisfaction Index A (LSIA) with measures of intelligence from the Lund 80+ study, Svensson and colleagues (1990) found a significant correlation between two measures of fluid intelligence: reasoning and spatial ability. Similar findings have been made in a study of cognitive functioning in elderly males (Steen, Hagberg, Johnson, & Steen, 1987).

Adams (1969) found four factors constituting the LSIA: mood tone, zest for life, congruence between desired and achieved goals, and one unnamed residual factor. As stated by George (1979), only the congruence factor should be considered to measure life satisfaction. In the Lund 80+ study, both an analysis of the full LSIA scale and the congruence factor were performed. Both congruence factors as suggested by Adams (1969) and by Liang (1985) were tested. No significant correlations were found between any of the intelligence measures and the congruence factor, while there was a significant correlation between reasoning and spatial ability and the full LSIA scale.

In discussing expertise, Kliegl and Baltes (1987) point to the possibility of using a person's reserve capacity for training of abilities even up to the expert level. This is possible in advanced age provided that the person is motivated and the physical and mental resources lie within normal range. Even if an expert level is not reached or not even set as a goal, an increase in one or more intellectual or cognitive abilities will add to the person's functioning in daily life and thereby to his or her quality of life. On the other hand, from a study by Lawton, Moss, and

Kleban (1984) of marital status, living conditions, and well-being in the elderly, it can be concluded that a good cognitive capacity does not contribute to a good quality of life in situations where other overriding, unfavorable conditions are operating.

Terminal Decline and Quality of Life

It is difficult to assume the possibility of training or exercise having an effect on terminal decline in intelligence factors, as the decline probably depends to a large extent on certain critical limits having been exceeded in different physiological factors. On the other hand, this possibility has not been studied. First, it might be that the onset of terminal decline can be postponed for a shorter or longer period of time through training. This statement is made with recognition that there cannot be any expected influence on the time of death. Second, there is also the slight possibility that the slope of the decline may be less steep or less rapid as an effect of exercise. If the first statement were true, there would be a shorter time before death during which the individual would feel negative effects of intellectual decline to the extent of affecting the perception of quality of life. If the second statement were true, then it would take a longer time from the onset of terminal decline to the point where the individual would feel his or her quality of life being negatively influenced. This would follow from the proposition that as long as the intellectual decline is of a mild or moderate level, the individual can compensate or cope with the effects of the decline and thereby handle the situation such that he or she does not experience a feeling of lowered quality of life. If both situations were true, the investment in different forms of exercises or facilities for intellectual training for older persons would have real payoffs in maintaining a high quality of life despite or regardless of the distance from death.

If it only were true that training had an effect on postponing terminal decline, that is, that there is a compression of the curve of terminal decline, the effect might also be that the slope of the curve gets more steep. This would then result in a situation where there would be a dramatic shrinkage in the amount of time during which the individual could cope with or compensate for the decline. It follows that the period from the onset of terminal decline to the point in time where the individual would experience a loss in quality of life would get considerably shorter. Such effects of training on terminal decline would be of high value as a focus in future research.

Training and Quality of Life

As no close links are as yet established between cognitive functioning (or intelligence) and quality of life, evidence of training effects of mental abilities on the perception of quality of life can only be circumstantial. At the very best, it can be said that intact cognitive functioning is important for experiencing a good quality of life. On the other hand, as intellectual functioning is seldom mentioned as a quality *in* life, we might have to regard as a fair assumption that intellectual ability has an impact on quality of life only when it is declining. In that case, it might also be claimed that training to restore the loss or diminish the decline can have a positive effect on the perception of quality of life.

Earlier in this chapter it was stated that a correlation was found between life satisfaction and fluid intelligence. As life satisfaction is also considered to be one of the domains contributing to quality of life, there is at least some evidence of a link between intelligence and quality of life. With the growing evidence of the possibility of the training of fluid intelligence there is at least the chance of influencing the perception of life satisfaction through training. It remains to be shown if it also influences the quality of life.

The kinds of training experiments that have been mentioned earlier in the chapter are naturally not the only ways to improve cognitive functioning. As discussed, everyday competence is also considered to grow in importance as we get older. The different components of this competence may also be susceptible to change and growth from training. Helping the elderly to regain competence through training in everyday tasks could have an impact on the perception of quality of life. Since the training would involve an aspect of life that is of high meaning to the individual, a heightened level of experienced fulfillment in that particular quality in life could be expected. It is of importance that different kinds of training programs and training facilities be offered for everyday tasks where people experience loss either from aging or illness. Training thus can have a positive effect on the individual's perception of his or her quality of life without any actual change in ability or status. The training in and of itself, along with the social aspects of the situation, can hold meaning to the individual and thereby add positively to his or her perception of quality of life. However, there is also the danger of the reverse effect, in which the person feels the environmental demands are too high and might then experience frustration and failure.

A Tentative Model of Intelligence and Quality of Life

From what has been discussed so far in this chapter, there is a basis for formulating a tentative model of the relation between intellectual functioning and quality of life. The proposed definition of quality of life can serve as the first step of the model. An individual's perception of his or her global overall quality of life is based on the person's evaluation of the fulfillment of meaning in life. To reach this evaluation the individual has to value the extent to which he or she has experienced fulfillment in the areas of life that have been ascribed high personal meaning. The areas of life that a person perceives as holding high meaning can then be called qualities *in* life, areas in which the individual has invested much energy (i.e., highly cathected areas). They are also those parts of life in which the person shows involvement and personal commitment. Thus, these are the areas in life about which we can feel most good; but, at the same time, these areas can hurt the most. Where we are most involved, where we have invested most, and where we experience personal meaning are the domains of life that qualify as qualities *in* life. The level of fulfillment that a person experiences in a quality in life is related to how good or bad he or she feels about that part of life. The individual also has to take into account what he or she has formerly experienced in that aspect of life. The present situation is interpreted in relation to all former experiences. At the same time, the individual will probably also make an estimate of what might eventually happen in that area of life in the future. This means that the individual will make a prediction of his or her chances of experiencing a better or worse situation. This will then be put in relation to both the present and former periods of life to reach an evaluation of that particular quality in life. Then, to arrive at a perception of the global quality of life, the person weighs together all those areas that he or she considers to be qualities in life.

Some of these qualities in life are probably shared by most people and thereby are easy to identify and define. Others are shared by few persons. Still others may be highly personal. There is still the further prospect of making evaluations and measurements of quality of life embracing those qualities in life that are shared by most people and those that are usually mentioned by more than a few. In this way, a better understanding of what is hidden in the global measure could be reached. It would naturally mean that measuring overall quality of life in one single question would be of little value.

It can be expected that the number of qualities in life change throughout the life span. Also, there will probably be alterations in the relative importance or significance of them from one point in life to another. It can be expected that a quality in life can be upgraded in importance (i.e., gain in meaning to the person). Likewise, there can be seen qualities in life that are downgraded over time. If quality of life is measured in a single question at two different times, it might be found that a person scores him- or herself as having the same global quality of life although from other measures he or she is known to have declined in what can be considered important areas of life. This finding could result if the person has devalued one or several qualities in life in which he or she has lost ability or fulfillment, while at the same time investing more meaning in other areas of life. Along the same lines, the individual would be expected to adopt new qualities in life in his or her personal appraisal, areas that would gain meaning and in which the individual could feel involvement. It is possible in this context that, with maturity and/or aging, earlier meaningful qualities might even be totally disqualified by the individual.

What we have, then, is a global overall quality of life concept built upon a number of qualities in life that are defined by their meaning to the individual. As mentioned, some of these qualities in life are easy to identify (e.g., health, work, family relations, dwelling). Others could be in the form of more global measures like life satisfaction and morale.

It is proposed here that intelligence is one quality in life. Intelligence not only has a direct relation to the global quality of life but also relates to one or several of the other qualities in life and, in this way, influences the overall evaluation. Even if it is true that there is a direct relation between intellectual functioning and quality of life, it does not mean that a decrease in intellectual capacity must have a negative effect on the overall quality of life. This follows from the aforementioned possibility of upgrading or downgrading the meaning that an individual ascribes to a certain quality *in* life and its relative importance to the other qualities. We are dealing with a dynamic and highly complex concept, which has to be subject to much thought, theorizing, and research in the future.

Suggestions for Future Research

To get a broader, and possibly better-defined, array of domains, techniques similar to those used by Clayton and Birren (1980) and Holliday and Chandler (1986) in defining wisdom ought to be applied to research on quality of life. These techniques, in brief, had groups of people define what they understood by the concept of wisdom and tell what they thought constituted a wise person.

First, we need to identify the aspects of life to which people attach high meaning. This would define the domains or areas that can be considered as qualities in life. To reach this knowledge, groups of people have to be asked what they think gives them meaning in life and the areas in which they feel most involved. When this has been done and a fair number of qualities have been defined, the next step will be to have people score the relative importance of the different qualities in life. At this stage of research, subjects would be asked to evaluate to what degree they rated themselves as having reached fulfillment in the different areas of life. To test for the influence of intelligence, each individual would be asked to state the relative importance of intelligence to all other qualities in life. Then they would also rate their fulfillment in that domain. Through this process it would then be possible to understand the extent to which people share their experiences of quality of life. It might be of interest to measure the global quality of life in just one question and determine which qualities in life contributed to the global measure and to what degree.

To be able to prove that training of intelligence and everyday competence have an impact on quality of life, experiments must be conducted in which groups of people receive different forms of training. This has to be done as a before-and-after test of quality of life with a control of changes in the different qualities in life that the individuals have. These have to be registered not only if there are changes in magnitude within one quality in life (in this case intelligence), but also if there are changes in their relative meaning. This is to determine if there are merely adjustments within one quality of life or also changes between qualities. Then it has to be established whether the changes take place with or without affecting the overall measure of quality of life.

References

Adams, D. L. (1969). Analysis of a life satisfaction index. *Journal of Gerontology, 24,* 470–474.

Baltes, P. B., Dittmann-Kohli, F., & Dixon R. A. (1984). New perspectives on the development of intelligence in adulthood: Toward a dual-process conception and a model of selective optimization with compensation. In P. B. Baltes & O. G. Brim, Jr., eds., *Life-span development and behavior,* vol. 6, pp. 33–76. New York: Academic Press.

Baltes, P. B., Dittmann-Kohli, F., & Kliegl, R. (1986). Reserve capacity of the elderly in aging-sensitive tests of fluid intelligence: Replication and extension. *Psychology and Aging, 1,* 172–177.

Bearon, L. B. (1988). Conceptualizing quality of life: Finding the common ground. *Journal of Applied Gerontology, 7,* 275–278.

Berg, S. (1980). Psychological functioning in 70- and 75-year old people. *Acta Psychologica Scandinavica, 62* (Suppl. 288).

Berg, S. (1987). Intelligence and terminal decline. In G. L. Maddox & E. W. Busse, eds., *Aging: The universal human experience,* pp. 411–416. New York: Springer.

Botwinick, J. (1977). Aging and intelligence. In J. E. Birren & K. W. Schaie, eds., *Handbook of the psychology of aging,* pp. 580–605. Princeton, N.J.: Van Nostrand Reinhold.

Bäckman, L. (1985). Further evidence for the lack of adult age differences on free recall of subject performed tasks: The importance of motor action. *Human Learning, 4,* 79–87.

Bäckman, L., & Nilsson, L.-G. (1985). Prerequisites for the lack of age differences in memory performance. *Experimental Aging Research, 11,* 67–73.

Cattell, R. B. (1971). *Abilities: Their structure, growth, and action.* Boston: Houghton Mifflin.

Cavanaugh, J., Kramer, D. A., Sinnott, J. D., Camp, C. J., & Markley, R. P. (1985). On missing links and such: Interfaces between cognitive research and everyday problem solving. *Human Development, 28,* 146–168.

Clark, P. G. (1988). Autonomy, personal empowerment, and quality of life in long-term care. *Journal of Applied Gerontology, 7,* 279–297.

Clayton, V. P., & Birren, J. E. (1980). The development of wisdom across the life span: A reexamination of an ancient topic. In P. B. Baltes & O. G. Brim, Jr., eds., *Life-span development and behavior,* vol. 3, pp. 103–135. New York: Academic Press.

Cohen, R. L. (1981). On the generality of some memory laws. *Scandinavian Journal of Psychology, 22,* 267–281.

Denney, N. W. (1979). Problem solving in later adulthood: Intervention research. In P. B.

Baltes & O. G. Brim, Jr., eds., *Life-span development and behavior,* vol. 2, pp. 37–66. New York: Academic Press.

Donaldson, G. (1981). Letter to the editor. *Journal of Gerontology, 36,* 634–636.

Doppelt, J. E., & Wallace, W. L. (1955). Standardization of the Wechsler Adult Intelligence Scale for older persons. *Journal of Abnormal and Social Psychology, 51,* 312–330.

Eisdorfer, C. (1963). The WAIS performance of the aged: A retest evaluation. *Journal of Gerontology, 18,* 169–172.

Flanagan, J. C. (1978). A research approach to improving our quality of life. *American Psychologist, 33,* 138–147.

George, L. K. (1979). The happiness syndrome: Methodological and substantive issues in the study of social-psychological well-being in adulthood. *The Gerontologist, 19,* 210–216.

George, L. K., & Bearon, L. B. (1980). *Quality of life in older persons: Meaning and measurement.* New York: Human Sciences Press.

Holliday, S. G., & Chandler, M. J. (1986). Wisdom: Explorations in adult competence. In J. A. Meacham, ed., *Contributions to human development,* vol. 17. Basel: Karger.

Horn, J. L. (1980). Concepts of intellect in relation to learning and adult development. *Intelligence, 4,* 285–317.

Horn, J. L. (1982). The aging of human abilities. In B. B. Wohlman, ed., *Handbook of developmental psychology,* pp. 847–870. Englewood Cliffs, N.J.: Prentice-Hall.

Johansson, B. (1985). *Memory and memory measurement in old age: Memory structure, context and metamemory.* Jönköping, Sweden: Institute of Gerontology.

Johansson, B., & Berg, S. (1989). The robustness of the terminal decline phenomenon: Longitudinal data from the digit-span memory test. *Journal of Gerontology: Psychological Sciences, 44,* P184–P186.

Kahana, E. (1975). A congruence model of person–environment interaction. In P. G. Windley, T. O. Byerts, & F. G. Ernst, eds., *Theory development in environment and aging,* pp. 181–214. Washington, D.C.: Gerontological Society.

Kenyon, G. M. (1989). Enhancing personal meanings of aging: The importance of biography. Paper presented at the Fourteenth International Congress of Gerontology, Acapulco.

Kleemeier, R. (1962). Intellectual changes in the senium. Proceedings of the Social Statistics Section of the American Statistical Association, 290–295.

Kliegl, R., & Baltes, P. B. (1987). Theory-guided analysis of mechanisms of development and aging through testing-the-limits and research on expertise. In C. Schooler & K. W. Schaie, eds., *Cognitive functioning and social structure over the life course,* pp. 95–119. Norwood, N.J.: Ablex Publishing Corporation.

Labouvie-Vief, G., & Gonda, J. N. (1976). Cognitive strategy training and intellectual performance in the elderly. *Journal of Gerontology, 31,* 327–332.

Larson, R. (1978). Thirty years of research on the subjective well-being of older Americans. *Journal of Gerontology, 33,* 109–125.

Lawton, M. P. (1975). Competence, environmental press and the adaptation of older people. In P. G. Windley, T. O. Byerts, & F. G. Ernst, eds., *Theory development in environment and aging,* pp. 13–83. Washington, D.C.: Gerontological Society.

Lawton, M. P. (1983). Environment and other determinants of well-being in older people. *The Gerontologist, 23,* 349–357.

Lawton, M. P., Moss, M., & Kleban, M. H. (1984). Marital status, living arrangements, and the well-being of older people. *Research on Aging, 6,* 323–345.

Liang, J. (1985). A structural integration of the Affect Balance Scale and the Life Satisfaction index A. *Journal of Gerontology, 40,* 552–561.

Maeland, J. G. (1989). Helse og livskvalitet. Begrepper og definisjoner. *Tidsskrift for den Norske Laegeforening, 109,* 1311–1315.

Marcel, G. (1951). *The decline of wisdom.* London: Harvill Press.

Nordbeck, B. (1989). Quality of life, health and aging. Paper presented at the Fourteenth International Congress of Gerontology, Acapulco.

Palmore, E., & Cleveland, W. (1976). Aging, terminal decline, and terminal drop. *Journal of Gerontology, 31,* 76–81.

Pearlman, R. A., & Uhlman, R. F. (1988). Quality of life in the elderly: Comparisons between nursing home and community residents. *Journal of Applied Gerontology, 7,* 316–330.

Riegel, K. F. (1973). Dialectic operations: The final period of cognitive development. *Human Development, 16,* 346–370.

Riegel, K. F., & Riegel, R. M. (1972). Development, drop, and death. *Developmental Psychology, 6,* 306–319.

Salthouse, T. A. (1987). Age, experience, and compensation. In C. Schooler & K. W. Schaie, eds., *Cognitive functioning and social structure over the life course,* pp. 142–157. Norwood, N.J.: Ablex Publishing Corporation.

Schaie, K. W. (1979). The primary mental abilities in adulthood: An exploration in the development of psychometric intelligence. In P. B. Baltes & O. G. Brim, Jr., eds., *Life-span development and behavior,* vol. 2, pp. 67–115. New York: Academic Press.

Schaie, K. W. (1983). The Seattle Longitudinal Study: A twenty-one year exploration of psychometric intelligence. In K. W. Schaie, ed., *Longitudinal studies of adult psychological development,* pp. 64–135. New York: Guilford Press.

Schaie, K. W., & Hertzog, C. (1983). Fourteen-year cohort sequential analyses of adult intellectual development. *Developmental Psychology, 19,* 531–543.

Schaie, K. W., Willis, S. L., Hertzog, C., & Schulenberg, J. E. (1987). Effects of cognitive training on primary mental ability structure. *Psychology and Aging, 2,* 233–242.

Schooler, C. (1987). Psychological effects of complex environments during the life span: A review and theory. In C. Schooler & K. W. Schaie, eds., *Cognitive functioning and social structure over the life course,* pp. 24–49. Norwood, N.J.: Ablex Publishing Corporation.

Siegler, I. C. (1975). The terminal drop hypothesis: Fact or artifact. *Experimental Aging Research, 1,* 169–185.

Siegrist, J., & Junge, A. (1989). Conceptual and methodological problems in research on the quality of life in clinical medicine. *Social Science and Medicine, 29,* 463–468.

Staats, S. R., & Stassen, M. A. (1987). Age and present and future perceived quality of life. *International Journal of Aging and Human Development, 25,* 167–176.

Steen, G., Hagberg, B., Johnson, G., & Steen, B. (1987). Cognitive function, cognitive style and life satisfaction in a 68-year-old male population. *Comprehensive Gerontology B, 1,* 54–61.

Sternberg, R. J., & Berg, C. A. (1987). What are theories of adult intellectual development theories of? In C. Schooler & K. W. Schaie, eds., *Cognitive functioning and social structure over the life course,* pp. 3–23. Norwood, N.J.: Ablex Publishing Corporation.

Svensson, T. (1984). *Aging and environment: Institutional aspects.* Linköping, Sweden: Department of Education and Psychology, Linköping University.

Svensson, T. (1989a). Involvement theory and biography. Paper presented at the symposium on aging and biography, St. Märgen, West Germany.

Svensson, T. (1989b). Los mas ancianos: Datos demograficos y caracteristicas psicosociales. In *La tercera edad en Europa: Necesidades y demandas,* pp. 293–314. Madrid: Ministerio de Asuntos Sociales.

Svensson, T., & Nilsson, L.-G. (1989). The relationship between recognition and cued recall in memory of enacted and nonenacted information. *Psychological Research, 51,* 194–200.

Svensson, T., Dehlin, O., Hagberg, B., & Samuelson, G. (unpublished). Lund 80+ Study. Lund, Sweden: Gerontology Research Center.

Tornstam, L. (1989). Gero-transcendence: A reformulation of the disengagement theory. *Aging: Clinical and Experimental Research, 1,* 55–63.

White, N., & Cunningham, W. R. (1988). Is terminal drop pervasive or specific? *Journal of Gerontology: Psychological Sciences, 43,* P141–P144.

Willis, S. L., & Schaie, K. W. (1986). Training the elderly on the ability factors of spatial orientation and inductive reasoning. *Psychology and Aging, 1,* 239–247.

V

Autonomy as a Factor in Quality of Life in the Frail Elderly

13

Resident Decision Making and Quality of Life in the Frail Elderly

TERRIE WETLE

Introduction

It is generally presumed that the opportunities for making autonomous choices are diminished for frail elderly, particularly elderly residents in nursing homes (Avorn & Langer, 1982; Baltes & Reisen, 1986; Besdine, 1983; Cohen, 1988; White & Janson, 1986). Moreover, advocates for the aged argue that efforts should be made to enhance autonomy by identifying new opportunities for decision making and encouraging older persons to make decisions and "take control of their lives" (Dubler, 1988; Hegeman & Tobin, 1988; Teitelman & Priddy, 1988). It is recognized, however, that several factors may influence the willingness and capacity of frail elderly, particularly nursing home residents, to fully participate in decision making.

The present chapter examines the exercise of autonomy, as expressed via decision making by nursing home residents, beginning with a discussion of the growing emphasis on autonomy among competing values. This is followed by a brief look at the expressed preferences of frail elderly in nursing homes, distinguishing among "micro" and "macro" decisions, cohort differences, and the influence of institutional settings on preferences and participation. The potential influence of the "sick role" on decision-making preferences is also considered, as are competing values or "contributors" to quality of life. The chapter ends with a discussion of "delegated" and "forced" autonomy.

Autonomy

Whose Value Is It Anyway?

The subject of autonomy is the focus of much attention in the applied ethics literature, but there is limited agreement about what should be done to enhance

Copyright © 1991 by Academic Press, Inc.
All rights of reproduction in any form reserved.

the autonomy of frail older persons. This grows in part out of the fuzzy and rather loose definitions for a word etymologically related to the Greek *autos* (self) and *nomos* (rule). The concept—autonomy—has been used to refer to individual liberty, freedom of choice, independence, will, self-governance, and privacy (Beauchamp & Childress, 1983; Collopy, 1988) and has been further delineated into a variety of subcategories of meanings (Dworkin, 1978; Gadow, 1980; Thomasma, 1984). Collopy (1988), in a landmark piece on autonomy in long-term care, provides six "polarities" within the concept of autonomy: decisional versus executional, direct versus delegated, competent versus incapacitated, authentic versus inauthentic, immediate versus long-range, and negative versus positive. Most discussions of autonomy emphasize that this value is balanced against competing values such as beneficence, concern for the common good, or justice, in virtually any decision (Callahan, 1984; Childress, 1982; Komrad, 1983; McCullough & Wear, 1985; VanDeVeer, 1986; Veatch, 1981).

It should be noted that a focus on autonomy of the individual in practical and legal terms is both time and culture bound. It may be a luxury of modern Western economies that considerations of autonomy are balanced so strongly against perceptions of the common good. It is one matter to discuss "moral autonomy" or the responsibility of individuals to make decisions for themselves, but it is quite another to ensure the rights and opportunities of individuals to make decisions for themselves, particularly frail elderly. The growing importance placed upon informed consent for health care is just one example of the increasing emphasis on autonomy in practical translation. Problems are encountered, however, as autonomy and right to personal decision making are infused into everyday practice, particularly among individuals who, because of physical frailty and/or cognitive deficits, are dependent upon others for some or all of their care.

Moreover, because the emphasis on autonomy has undergone significant change over the last several decades, individuals from separate cultures and different age-cohorts may not share common values regarding the importance of autonomy or the role of the individual in personal and health care decisions. By way of example, the present author's research in Southeast Asia and among Puerto Rican elderly in the continental United States demonstrates important culturally and age-cohort-based differences regarding health beliefs and the appropriate role of elderly persons in decisions regarding their health care (Wetle, Schensul, Torres, & Mayen, 1990). Thus, our understanding of the importance of autonomy for the elderly, among other values, may involve focus on a "moving target." Moreover, issues of central importance to advocates for the aging may not take primacy for specific individuals or groups of elderly.

The Impact of Decision Making

Control and the Illusion of Control

Control over one's environment has long been viewed as a basic human motivation (Rodin, Timko, & Harris, 1985; Baltes & Baltes, 1986; Bandura, 1982), and, more recently, several studies indicate that presence or absence of control exert important influences on emotional and physical well-being (Langer & Rodin, 1976; Perlmutter, Monty, & Chan, 1986; Seligman, 1975). The concept of control has been defined variously as the use of independent judgment, the degree of contingency between a response and an outcome, and expectations regarding internal and external control of reinforcements and perceptions of self-efficacy (Rodin *et al.*, 1985). Several studies have examined the relationship of perceived locus of control and a variety of correlates, including life satisfaction (Reid & Ziegler, 1980; Wolk & Kurtz, 1975); morale and self-esteem (Brown & Granick, 1983; Hunter, Linn, & Harris, 1981); coping (Kuypers, 1972); health (Mancini, 1980; Rodin, 1986); and health behaviors (Bohm, 1983).

Studies examining the causal relationship between feelings of control and a variety of outcomes indicate that changes in perceived control may indeed influence behavior. Piper and Langer (1986) summarize this literature as follows:

> Several researchers have reported the positive effects of this belief in control on various types of behavior, including increases in task performance (Monty & Perlmuter, 1975); reductions in test anxiety (Stotland & Blumentahal, 1964); decreases in preoperative stress (Langer, Janis, & Wolfer, 1975); enhancement in adaptation to aversive stimuli and tolerance for poststimuli frustration (Glass & Singer, 1972; Sherod, Hage, Halpern, & Moore, 1977) and reductions in causal attributions to task difficulty (Overmier & Seligman, 1967). (p. 78)

Nursing-home-based studies provide similar findings. Schulz and Hanusa (1978) demonstrate that perceived control over visits by college students improved measures of activity, satisfaction, and health of nursing home residents as compared to controls. Langer and Rodin (1976) report that an intervention with nursing home residents consisting of a lecture "designed to increase feelings of choice and personal responsibility," combined with being given a plant to care for, significantly increased nurses' ratings of resident happiness, level of activity, and alertness for subjects compared to controls. Banziger and Roush (1983) report similar findings with an intervention consisting of residents taking responsibility for maintaining bird feeders. The longer-term effects of such interventions are less clear. Rodin and Langer (1977) report that over 18 months their intervention group continued to be rated by nurses as more happy, active, sociable, and vigorous than the control groups and also reported differential mortality rates of 15% (intervention group) and 30% (controls). Schulz and Hanusa (1978), on the other hand, did not observe lasting effects of their intervention, perhaps because the visits terminated at the end of the intervention period.

These widely reported studies have refueled interest in the concept of "learned helplessness" (Abramson, Seligman, & Teasdale, 1978), a term used to describe the frequently replicated finding that humans (or animals) exposed to a series of uncontrollable aversive events develop generalized performance deficits (Hiroto & Seligman, 1975; Juhl, 1986; Overmier & Seligman, 1967).

Juhl (1986) models how this might occur:

> A perception of lost control might produce physiological overactivation, a reduction of attentional capacity, or short-term memory overload resulting from intrusive thoughts about the loss. It may activate unconscious conflicts and alter the mode of processing these conflicts; it might change the functional significance of conscious experience or the format of information retrieved from long-term memory; it may result in strenuous attempts to selectively disregard certain information. (p. 4)

Piper and Langer (1986) contrast learned helplessness with "mindful control."

> The physical and social environments of the elderly tend to encourage mindlessness. The mindless individual is caught in a cycle that is quite vicious, even deadly: When s/he is in various ways told that s/he is no longer competent (that his/her responses no longer influence desired outcomes), the individual mindlessly accepts this negative image, loses feelings of self-worth, and, consequently, makes little or no attempt to disprove the label. Instead s/he supports the notion of incompetence by becoming unduly helpless and ill, often terminally so. (p. 71)

Avorn and Langer (1982) demonstrate the inducement of learned helplessness, through a study in which nursing home residents were either "helped" or "encouraged" in completing a puzzle task. Those who were "helped" performed significantly worse than controls, and those who were "encouraged" performed significantly better than controls. Most surprising, perhaps, was the observation that, despite expectations that the "helped" group would improve given practice opportunities, they actually did worse over time. Langer (1975) conducted several studies that support her assertion that it is not the actual level of control which explains these findings, but rather the perception or "illusion" of control. What matters is the individual's *belief* that he or she controls circumstances and outcomes.

Decision-Making Preferences

What Do Frail Elderly Really Want?

Prior studies of patient participation in treatment decisions have focused mainly on acutely ill hospitalized patients (Bedell & Delbanco, 1984; Lo, McLeod, & Saika, 1986) or on outpatients with specific diseases, such as cancer (Cassileth, Zupkis, Sutton-Smith, & March, 1980) or hypertension (Strull, Lo, & Charles, 1984), and have provided somewhat conflicting results. Those patients shown to prefer active involvement in decisions included cancer patients (Cassileth *et al.*, 1980), ulcer patients (Greenfield, Kaplan, & Ware, 1985), seizure patients (Faden, Becker, Lewis, Freeman, & Faden, 1981) and patients using psychotropic drugs (Durel & Munjas, 1982). Other groups of patients preferred to play a more passive role in their medical care and to leave decision making largely to their practitioners. These included patients with hypertension (Strull *et al.*, 1984), diabetics (Ruzicki, 1984), and female surgical patients (Boreham & Gibson, 1978). Chronological literature reviews suggest that patients have reported increasing preference for medical information (DiMatteo & DiNicola, 1982; Lou Harris & Associates, 1982). Many studies have examined communication and information sharing (Hulka, Cassel, Kupper, & Burdette, 1988; Katz, 1984; Smith & Pettegrew, 1986). Few studies have focused specifically on older individuals, but it has been suggested that elderly individuals wish to be involved in medical treatment decisions and actively participate when given the opportunity (Coulton, Dunkle, Goode, & MacKintosh, 1982; Lo, Saika, & Strull, 1985; Lo, McLeod, Saika, 1986).

In an effort to better understand the perceptions and preferences of nursing home residents regarding participation in medical decisions, Wetle, Levkoff,

Table 1 Characteristics of Respondents

	n	%
Age		
60–69	26	13
70–79	40	20
80–89	86	44
Over 90	45	23
Sex		
Male	36	18
Female	162	82
Place of birth		
United States	146	74
Other	51	26

Table 2   Amount and Adequacy of Information Provided

	Amount		Adequacy	
	% Provided by doctors	% Provided by nurses		
Nothing	23	34	Not enough	21.2%
Very little	18	18	Right amount	78.3%
Moderate amount	19	19	Too much	0.5%
Everything there is to know	40	28		

Cwikel, and Rosen (1988) conducted a survey of residents in nine facilities. Of the 232 residents approached to participate, 212 (91%) agreed to be interviewed. Data from 198 completed interviews (85%) constituted the data set. Characteristics of respondents are provided in Table 1.

The interview format used both open-ended and closed questions regarding residents' preferences for involvement in medical decision making and their desire for information about medical care. When asked how much they were told about their medical care (see Table 2), 40% of respondents reported being told "everything there is to know" by their doctors, and 41% reported being told "very little" or "nothing." When asked about the adequacy of this information, most respondents (78%) believed that they had received "the right amount" of information, and 21% reported having received "not enough." Only one respondent (0.5%) reported receiving "too much information."

Residents were also asked about their level of involvement in health care decisions. As shown in Table 3, more than half reported little or no involvement. Despite these low levels of reported involvement, 79% reported that their level of involvement was the "right amount." Those who were completely or moderately involved in care decisions were more likely to report this to be the right amount of involvement (88%) than were those who were not involved (68%). But it

Table 3   Amount and Adequacy of Involvement in Decisions

Amount		Adequacy	
None	40.0%	Not enough	19.5%
Very little	13.7%	Right amount	79.3%
Moderate	25.6%	Too much	1.2%
Complete	20.6%		

should be noted that 71% of those who had little or no involvement in care decisions believed this to be the "right amount" of involvement.

In addition to these more general questions about health care decisions, respondents were asked specifically about "do not resuscitate" orders (DNR), since this is the nontreatment decision most frequently discussed in the literature. After an explanation of what such an order means,[1] 92.6% of respondents reported that they had never been asked about resuscitation or their preferences. Almost two-thirds (61.4%) reported that they would wish to be involved in this decision, with 35.2% wishing to be very involved, and 26.2% wishing to be moderately involved. There were 38.6% who reported that they did not want to be involved in such a decision. Nonetheless, individuals in each of these groups were very willing to express opinions. Among those who wanted to participate in such a decision, the following are samples of comments made:

Of course I would want to be involved, it's my life, who else would decide?

Are you talking about living wills? Where do I sign up?

No tubes, no machines, it's enough already . . . it embarrasses my doctor to talk about it. He's a nice boy, but he gets uncomfortable.

We all talk about that here, we're old, we know the end is coming . . . but it embarrasses the nurses . . . they try so hard . . . they don't want to talk about it.

Among those who did not wish to be involved in the resuscitation decision came the following selected comments:

It's God's will. We shouldn't decide these things. When my time comes, it comes.

That's medical. My doctor will know what to do. I don't want tubes.

Don't talk crazy, of course I want to live.

Once again, a very diverse response pattern was observed. Preferences were not reliably predicted by resident characteristics, but those preferring more

---

[1]The following explanation was provided to study participants.

Resuscitation means mechanically restoring the heart beat and breathing after it has stopped. Sometimes, a decision is made *ahead of time,* when you are well, *not* to attempt resuscitation if you should happen to stop breathing at sometime in the *future.*

After eliciting preferences regarding resuscitation, respondents were then provided the following care vignette, and similar questions were asked as a test of validity and reliability.

A (wo)man named Mr(s). Smith is in fairly good health and lives in a nursing home. One day, Mr(s). Smith's doctor and nurse asked him/her to think about whether he/she would like them to try to resuscitate or revive him/her if his/her heart stops beating.

involvement tended to be younger, to be born in the United States, to have a nurse who knew them well, and to have a doctor who had known them for a relatively longer time but who the respondent believed did not know the resident well. Overall, the study demonstrates a wide diversity among resident experiences and preferences regarding health care decisions.

Micro and Macro Decisions

Who Cares about DNR, I Just Want to Choose My Roommate

Although the literature has focused primarily on the "big ticket" issues such as DNR, discontinuing or withholding life supports, decisions to hospitalize nursing home residents (cf. Besdine, 1983; Lo, McLeod, & Saika, 1986; Lo, Saika, & Strull, 1985; President's Commission for the Study of Ethical Problems in Medicine and Biomedical and Behavioral Research, 1982; Wetle, 1988), it may well be that the decisions that are most important to the sense of control and quality of life of frail elderly are the everyday, mundane decisions that we otherwise tend to take for granted (Caplan, 1990).

Kane and Caplan (1990), in their groundbreaking work on "everyday ethics" in the nursing home, identify a multitude of issues reported to be of significant importance to residents. These include such issues as bedtimes, getting-up times, use of common space and equipment, what and when to eat, smoking, roommates, leaving the facility, phone privileges, and visiting rights. There is general agreement among their project participants that, frequently, resident autonomy is unnecessarily restricted as a matter of staff convenience, resource constraints, insensitivity, or fear of liability. Efforts to expand opportunities for resident choice and enhanced autonomy are under way on several fronts (Hegeman & Tobin, 1988), including regulatory efforts to ease physical restraints in some jurisdictions. It has been argued by Kane and Caplan (1990) and other advocates (Jameton, 1988; Kane, 1990; McCullough, 1990) that such attention to everyday decisions may do more to improve quality of life and perceived control than a focus on the larger issues, such as advanced directives and increased involvement in decision making. At the same time, improved autonomy for the "micro" issues may provide the sense of confidence and mastery necessary to advocate for involvement in the "macro" issues.

Cohort Differences

When You've Seen One Old Person, You've Seen One Old Person

As we suggested earlier in the present chapter, important differences are observed in the decision-making preferences and behaviors in different groups of older persons. The control literature suggests that older persons are more likely to have external loci of control than do younger cohorts. Given that future cohorts of elderly will be better educated, have higher incomes, and will have experienced a health care system that encouraged more participation, they will expect to be involved in decision making even after they become frail and require care (Kane & Caplan, 1990; Wetle, 1988). They may be resistant to learned helplessness and demand active participation in decisions of both the micro and macro variety. Even among current cohorts of elderly, we see important differences in participation and preferences—differences to be considered in any effort to enhance autonomy of nursing home residents.

Influence of Institutional Settings on Decision Making

When a Home Is Not a Home

An important consideration in autonomy is the impact of the setting on willingness and capacity to participate in decision making. The nursing home is a common setting of care for older persons and one in which pertinent issues of decision making are raised (Agree, Lipson, McCullough, & Soldo, 1988; Capran, 1990; Cole, 1987; Freeman, 1990; Moody, 1987; Thomasma, 1985). Nursing homes are, indeed, "total institutions," as defined by Goffman (1961).

> In total institutions there is a basic split between a large managed group, conveniently called inmates, and a small supervisory staff. Inmates typically live in the institution and have restricted contact with the world outside the walls; staff often operate on an eight-hour work day and are socially integrated into the outside world. Each grouping tends to conceive of the other in terms of narrow hostile stereotypes, staff often seeing inmates as bitter, secretive, and untrustworthy, while inmates often see staff as condescending, high-handed, and mean. Staff tends to feel superior and righteous; inmates tend, in some ways at least, to feel inferior, weak, blameworthy, and guilty. (p. 7)

These circumstances result not only in lowered self-esteem but in a diminution of decision-making power as well (Annas, Glantz, & Katz, 1978). On the other hand, Besdine (1983) argues that nursing homes offer distinct opportunities to enhance decision-making participation, particularly by very frail and cognitively impaired elderly. Because residents live in the facility for long periods, they may have the opportunity to get to know the staff well; to make decisions over time; to solicit advice from staff, family, and other advisors; and to change their minds. Unfortunately, such opportunities are often overlooked by harried staff, absent physicians, and bewildered residents. The Retirement Research Foundation initiative on autonomy in long-term care addresses this issue through several projects (Hofland, 1988), which indicate that, although the nursing home as an institution restricts and diminishes autonomy, many residents express preferences for more control in their lives. Moreover, changes in daily routine and administrative process can enhance opportunities for autonomous decision making and improve the quality of life of residents.

Frailty, Chronic Illness, and the Sick Role

When Your Job Is to Comply

The more positive view of the nursing home as a site in which decision making might be enhanced requires consideration of several issues. Parsons (1951), in his compelling description of the "sick role," defined the rights and responsibilities of individuals when they become ill. Rights include being excused from usual work and family responsibility, being provided food and personal care, and having the attention of professionals who prescribe interventions. Responsibilities focus mainly on compliance—following orders and working to get well. This view of the "sick role" assumes a relatively acute period in which the patient either gets better or dies.

Chronic illness confounds our cultural view of the sick role. On the one hand, we believe that patients should be cared for as needed and should be provided interventions to make them better and also that they should comply with the advice of professionals. On the other hand, there is considerable ambivalence regarding exemption from everyday responsibilities. Much of the focus of rehabilitation professionals is on getting the chronically impaired individual back into usual roles and activities, despite disabilities. Nursing homes, as facilities for the chronically ill, are modeled after hospitals, and they encourage, in many direct and subtle ways, acceptance of the sick role by residents. Storlie (1982) provides rich case examples of the many ways in which nursing homes "reshape the old."

> Mrs. S., a 79-year-old retired teacher, sat close to the window in her room, watching the snowflakes fall. Seeing me she laughed, "I'd love to go outside and make a snowball."
>
> "Why don't you?" I asked.
>
> "Are you kidding?" Her face looked incredulous. "The first winter I was here I started to go outside on a day like this. The aide grabbed my arm and said 'Nellie, if you'd slip and fall, I'd never hear the end of it.'"
>
> Then she added quietly, "I've never mentioned it since." (p. 556)

Kane and Caplan (1990) provide numerous case studies in which the erosion of opportunity to make even the simplest decisions reinforces the self-perceptions of patients that they are no longer autonomous adults but rather "childlike" patients in a total institution.

Competing Contributors to Quality of Life

Taking Care of Business and Being Taken Care Of

Beyond the issue of institutional restrictions on autonomy, frail elderly themselves may make decisions to voluntarily restrict autonomy in balance with other desired goals. Nursing home residents may clearly argue that the reason they came to the facility was to be relieved of daily responsibilities for self-care and the burden of decision making (Wetle *et al.*, 1988). Research into the relative importance of autonomy compared with other values indicates substantial heterogeneity of opinion among community-dwelling elder (O'Brien & Whitelaw, 1973), as well as among elders in nursing homes (Wagner, 1984; Wetle *et al.*, 1988). These competing values include safety, security, and relief from anxiety. Obviously, care must be taken to encourage the optimization of all expressed values, before one willingly accepts erosion of autonomy.

Forced Autonomy and Delegated Autonomy

Choosing Not to Choose

Collopy (1988) points out that one form of autonomy is to choose someone else to make decisions, that is, *delegated autonomy*. This type of autonomy is recognized by the courts via instruments such as powers of attorney and by institutions through written designation of decision makers. Many institutions have made arguments that, with entry into the facility, the resident automatically delegates autonomy for many decisions. It would seem that this form of delegated autonomy has rather limited applications. High (1988) and High and Turner (1987) have explored the preference of elderly persons regarding delegated autonomy, and they argue that delegation of decisions to family members "extends" autonomy, particularly around health care decisions. Questions arise, however, regarding the appropriate role of families in decisions and care giving (Areen, 1987; Cicirelli, 1981; Hays, 1984; Seelbach, 1977; Seelbach & Sauer, 1977).

Forced autonomy refers to the insistence that individuals make or participate in decisions against their wills. This has been referred to by some as "terrified consent." We must recognize that some individuals, particularly certain members of current older cohorts, are unused to and uncomfortable with making certain types of decisions. Certainly, efforts should be made to assist them in participating, but their wishes for limited participation are also valid.

Summary

Control over one's life and personal responsibility are a central focus of the American value system, and yet autonomy is severely compromised for frail older persons. Assaults to autonomy may result from several factors, including diminished ability to implement decisions due to physical frailty, dependence upon others for physical and economic support, and impaired ability to participate in decisions because of cognitive impairment. Added to these are institutional rules and regulations, behaviors of staff and families, and experience and assumptions of some frail elderly that nonparticipation is appropriate. Research and special demonstration projects indicate, however, that much can be done to enhance both the willingness and the opportunities for older persons to participate in care decisions and that, for many older persons, such participation preserves and enhances quality of life. Care must be taken, however, to recognize that, for some older persons, withdrawal from the responsibility of some decisions is an expected and welcomed event. The heterogeneity of experience and preferences of individuals should be considered in efforts to enhance autonomy and resident decision making with a goal of improving quality of life.

Directions for Future Research

Several areas of future research are suggested by this review. First, much is yet to be learned from descriptive studies that better define the preferences and experiences of older persons regarding decision making. For example, which resident characteristics predict an interest in participation and under what circumstances? Related research would examine the impact of institutions on resident decision making, including expectations and behaviors of staff, institutional rules or regulatory constraints that diminish autonomy, and physical or environmental characteristics. Demonstration projects that test organizational or physical innovations are certainly needed.

Since the institutional setting is just one environment in which frail elderly live, research that identifies factors influencing quality of life across settings is required. For example, a better understanding of events leading up to institutional placement, including the nature of participation of frail elderly in these decisions, would provide important information regarding subsequent quality of life. Such research should also include an examination of the direct and more subtle forces that influence decision making, including strategies of influence or coercion used by families, health care professionals, case managers, and institutional staff.

The competing needs of residents within facilities provide another fruitful area of research, as the autonomy of one individual is balanced against the common good as reflected by the aggregate needs of other residents and facility staff. This balance includes fiscal constraints imposed by limited reimbursement, as well as the demands of congregate living.

Finally, of utmost importance is the development and testing of innovative approaches that extend the capacity of individuals to function, to participate in decisions, and to control their own lives. This includes a wide array of interventions, such as devices that enhance physical function and/or communication, living environments that provide additional privacy or opportunity for individual life-styles, and community-based services that provide a broader array of choices. Legal processes and documents that encourage individuals to express preferences and to designate surrogate decision makers, as well as regulations and processes that allow individuals and institutions to take "informed risks," may also extend resident autonomy.

Researchers, administrators, and policymakers face unusual opportunities to significantly enrich the quality of life of nursing home residents, as our understanding and skills improve. More must be learned, risks must be taken; and we must be willing to listen to even the frailest voice in the throng. It is worth the effort, though, because quality of life will improve not only for the frail elderly but also for health care professionals, caregivers, and families.

References

Abramson, L. Y., Seligman, M. E. P., & Teasdale, J. D. (1978). Learned helplessness in humans: Critique and reformulation. *Journal of Abnormal Psychology, 87,* 49–74.

Agree, E. A., Lipson, S., McCullough, L. B., & Soldo, B. (1988). Long term care decision making. In W. Reichel, ed., *Clinical aspects of aging,* 3rd ed. Baltimore: Williams and Wildins.

Annas, G., Glantz, L., & Katz, B. (1978). The law of informed consent in human experimentation: Institutionalized mentally infirm. In *Research involving those institutionalized as mentally infirm,* the National Commission for the Protection of Human Subjects of Biomedical and Behavioral Research. DHEW Publication No. (OS) 78-0007, Washington, D.C.: U.S. Government Printing Office.

Areen, J. (1987). The legal status of consent obtained from families of adult patients to withhold or withdraw treatment. *Journal of the American Medical Association, 258,* 229–235.

Avorn, J., & Langer, E. (1982). Induced disability in nursing home patients: A controlled trial. *Journal of the American Geriatrics Society, 30,* 397–400.

Baltes, M. M., & Baltes, P. B., eds. (1986). *The psychology of control and aging.* Hillsdale, N.J.: Lawrence Erlbaum Associates.

Baltes, M. M., & Reisen, R. (1986). The social world in long term care institutions: Psychosocial control toward dependency? In M. M. Baltes & P. B. Baltes, eds., *The psychology of control and aging,* pp. 315–343. Hillsdale, N.J.: Lawrence Erlbaum Associates.

Bandura, A. (1982). Self-efficacy in human agency. *American Psychologist, 37,* 122–147.

Banziger, G., & Roush, S. (1983). Nursing homes for the birds: A control-relevant intervention with bird feeders. *The Gerontologist, 23,* 527–531.

Beauchamp, T., & Childress, J. (1983). *Principles of biomedical ethics.* New York: Oxford University Press.

Bedell, S., & Delbanco, T. (1984). Choices about cardiopulmonary resuscitation in the hospital. *New England Journal of Medicine, 310,* 1089–1093.

Besdine, R. (1983). Decisions to withhold treatment from nursing home residents. *Journal of the American Geriatrics Society, 31,* 602–606.

Bohm, L. C. (1983). *Social support and well-being in older adults: The impact of perceived control.* Doctoral diss., Yale University.

Boreham, P., & Gibson, D. (1978). The informative process in private medical consultations: A preliminary investigation. *Social Science and Medicine, 12,* 409–416.

Brown, B. R., & Granick, S. (1983). Cognitive and psychosocial differences between I and E locus of control aged persons. *Experimental Aging Research, 9,* 107–110.

Callahan, D. (1984). Autonomy: A moral good, not a moral obsession. *Hastings Center Report, 14,* 40–42.

Caplan, A. L. (1990). The morality of the mundane: Ethical issues arising in the daily lives of nursing home residents. In R. A. Kane & A. L. Caplan, eds., *Everyday ethics: Resolving dilemmas in nursing home life.* New York: Springer.

Cassileth, B., Zupkis, R., Sutton-Smith, K., & March, V. (1980). Information and participation preferences among cancer patients. *Annals of Internal Medicine, 92,* 832–836.

Childress, J. F. (1982). *Who should decide? Paternalism in health care.* New York: Oxford University Press.

Cicirelli, V. G. (1981). *Helping elderly parents: The role of adult children.* Boston: Auburn House.

Cohen, E. S. (1988). The elderly mystique: Constraints on the autonomy of the elderly with disabilities. *The Gerontologist, 28,* 24–31.

Cole, T. (1987). Class, culture and coercion: A historical look at long term care. *Generations, 11,* 9–15.

Collopy, B. J. (1988). Autonomy in long term care: Some crucial distinctions. *The Gerontologist, 28,* 10–17.

Coulton, C., Dunkle, R., Goode, R., & MacKintosh, J. (1982). Discharge planning and decision making. *Health and Social Work, 182,* 253–261.

DiMatteo, M. R., & DiNicola, D. D. (1982). Practitioner-patient relationships: The communication of information. In M. R. DiMatteo & D. D. DiNicola, eds., *Achieving patient compliance: The psychology of the medical practitioner's role.* Elmsford, N.Y.: Pergamon Press.

Dubler, N. (1988). Improving the discharge planning process: Distinguishing between coercion and choice. *The Gerontologist, 28,* 76–81.

Durel, S., & Munjas, B. (1982). Client perception of role in psychotropic drug management. *Mental Health Nursing, 4,* 65–74.

Dworkin, G. (1978). Moral autonomy. In H. T. Engelhardt & D. Callahan, eds., *Morals, science and sociality.* Hastings, N.Y.: Hastings Center.

Faden, R., Becker, C., Lewis, C., Freeman, J., & Faden, A. (1981). Disclosure of information to patients in medical care. *Medical Care, 19,* 718–733.

Freeman, I. C. (1990). Developing systems that promote autonomy: Policy considerations. In R. A. Kane & A. Caplan, eds., *Everyday ethics: Resolving dilemmas in nursing home life.* New York: Springer.

Gadow, S. (1980). Medicine, ethics, and the elderly. *The Gerontologist, 20,* 680–685.

Glass, D. C., & Singer, J. E. (1972). *Urban stress.* New York: Academic Press.

Goffman, E. (1961). *Asylums: Essays on the social situation of mental patients and other inmates.* Garden City, N.Y.: Anchor Books.

Greenfield, S., Kaplan, S., & Ware, J. (1985). Expanding patient involvement in care. *Annals of Internal Medicine, 102,* 520–528.

Hays, J. A. (1984). Aging and family resources: Availability and proximity of kin. *The Gerontologist, 24,* 149–153.

Hegeman, C., & Tobin, S. (1988). Enhancing the autonomy of mentally impaired nursing home residents. *The Gerontologist, 28,* 71–75.

High, D. M. (1988). All in the family: Extended autonomy and expectations in surrogate health care decision-making. *The Gerontologist, 28,* 46–51.

High, D. M., & Turner, H. B. (1987). Surrogate decision-making: The elderly's familial expectations. *Theoretical Medicine, 8,* 303–320.

Hiroto, D. W., & Seligman, M. E. P. (1975). Generality of learned helplessness in man. *Journal of Personality and Social Psychology, 32,* 311–327.

Hofland, B. F. (1988). Autonomy in long term care: Background issues and a programmatic response. *The Gerontologist, 28,* 3–9.

Hulka, B., Cassel, J., Kupper, L., & Burdette, J. (1988). Communications, compliance, and concordance between physicians and patients with prescribed medications. *American Journal of Public Health, 66,* 847–853.

Hunter, K. I., Linn, M. W., & Harris, R. (1981). Characteristics of high and low self-esteem in the elderly. *International Journal of Aging and Human Development, 14,* 117–126.

Jameton, A. (1988). In the borderlands of autonomy: Responsibility in long term care facilities. *The Gerontologist, 28,* 18–23.

Juhl, J. (1986). Aging and models of control: The hidden costs of wisdom. In M. M. Baltes & P. B. Baltes, eds., *The psychology of control and aging,* pp. 1–33. Hillsdale, N.J.: Lawrence Erlbaum Associates.

Kane, R. A. (1990). Everyday life in nursing homes: The way things are. In R. A. Kane & A. Caplan, eds., *Everyday ethics: Resolving dilemmas in nursing home life.* New York: Springer.

Kane, R. A., & Caplan, A., eds. (1990). *Everyday ethics: Resolving dilemmas in nursing home life.* New York: Springer.

Katz, J. (1984). *The silent world of doctor and patient.* New York: Free Press.

Komrad, M. S. (1983). A defense of medical paternalism: Maximizing patient autonomy. *Journal of Medical Ethics, 9,* 38–44.

Kuypers, J. A. (1972). Internal-external locus of control, ego functioning, and personality characteristics in old age. *The Gerontologist, 12,* 168–173.

Langer, E. J. (1975). The illusion of control. *Journal of Personality and Social Psychology, 32,* 311–328.

Langer, E. J., & Rodin, J. (1976). The effects of choice and enhanced personal responsibility for the aged: A field experiment in an institutional setting. *Journal of Personality and Social Psychology, 34,* 191–198.

Langer, E. J., Janis, I. L., & Wolfer, J. A. (1975). Reduction of psychological stress in surgical patients. *Journal of Experimental Social Psychology, 11,* 155–165.

Langer, E. J., Beck, P., Janoff-Bulman, R., & Timko, C. (1984). An explanation of the relationships between mindfulness, longevity, and senility. *Academic Psychology Bulletin, 6,* 211–226.

Lawton, M. P. (1980). *Environment of aging.* Belmont, Calif.: Brooks/Cole.

Lo, B., McLeod, G., & Saika, G. (1986). Patient attitudes to discussing of life-sustaining treatment. *Archives of Internal Medicine, 146,* 1613–1615.

Lo, B., Saika, G., & Strull, W. (1985). Do not resuscitate decisions: A prospective study at three teaching hospitals. *Archives of Internal Medicine, 145,* 1115–1117.

Louis Harris & Associates (1982). Views of informed consent and decision making: Parallel surveys of physicians and the public. In *Making health care decisions,* President's Commission for the Study of Ethical Problems in Medicine and Biomedical and Behavioral Research. Washington, D.C.: U.S. Government Printing Office.

Mancini, J. (1980). Effects of health and income on control orientation and life-satisfaction among aged public housing residents. *International Journal of Aging and Human Development, 12,* 215–220.

McCullough, L. B. (1990). Phone privileges. In R. A. Kane & A. Caplan, eds., *Everyday ethics: Resolving dilemmas in nursing home life,* pp. 125–136. New York: Springer.

McCullough, L., & Wear, S. (1985). Respect for autonomy and medical paternalism reconsidered. *Theoretical Medicine, 6,* 295–308.

Monty, R., & Perlmuter, L. (1975). Persistence of the effects of choice on paired-associate learning. *Memory and Cognition, 3,* 183–187.

Moody, H. R. (1987). Ethical dilemmas in nursing home placement. *Generations, 11,* 16–23.

National Institute of Aging (1977). *Protection of elderly research subjects.* Summary of the National Institute on Aging conference. Washington, D.C.: U.S. Department of Health, Education and Welfare.

O'Brien, J., & Whitelaw, N. (1973). *Analysis of community based alternatives to institutional care for the aged.* Portland, Ore.: Institute on Aging.

Office for Protection from Research Risks (1981). *Protection of human subjects.* (Code of Federal Regulations 45CFR46). Washington, D.C.: Dept. of Health and Human Services.

Overmier, J. B., & Seligman, M. E. P. (1967). Effects of inescapable shock upon subsequent escape and avoidance learning. *Journal of Comparative and Physiological Psychology, 63,* 28–33.

Parsons, T. (1951). *The social system.* New York: Free Press.

Perlmuter, L. C., Monty, R. A., & Chan, F. (1986). Choice, control, and cognitive functioning. In M. M. Baltes & P. B. Baltes, eds., *The psychology of control and aging,* pp. 91–118. Hillsdale, N.J.: Lawrence Erlbaum Associates.

Piper, A. I., & Langer, E. J. (1986). Aging and mindful control. In M. M. Baltes & P. B. Baltes, eds., *The psychology of control and aging,* pp. 71–89. Hillsdale, N.J.: Lawrence Erlbaum Associates.

President's Commission for the Study of Ethical Problems in Medicine and Biomedical and Behavioral Research (1981). *Protecting human subjects: The adequacy and uniformity of federal rules and their implementation.* (G.P.O. Stock No. 040-000-0045201). Washington, D.C.: U.S. Government Printing Office.

President's Commission for the Study of Ethical Problems in Medicine and Biomedical and Behavioral Research (1982). *Making health care decisions: A report on the ethical and legal implications of informed consent in the patient-practitioner relationship*, vol. 1. Washington, D.C.: U.S. Government Printing Office.

Reid, D. W., & Ziegler, M. (1980). Validity and stability of a new desired control measure pertaining to psychological adjustment of the elderly. *Journal of Gerontology, 35*, 315–402.

Rodin, J. (1986). Aging and health: Effects of the sense of control. *Science, 233*, 1271–1276.

Rodin, J., & Langer, E. J. (1977). Long term effects of a control relevant intervention among the institutionalized aged. *Journal of Personality and Social Psychology, 3*, 897–902.

Rodin, J., Timko, C., & Harris, S. (1985). The construct of control: Biological and psychosocial correlates. *Annual Review of Gerontology and Geriatrics, 5*, 3–55.

Ruzicki, D. (1984). Relationship of participation preference and health focus of control in diabetes education. *Diabetes Care, 7*, 372–377.

Schulz, R., & Hanusa, B. (1978). Long-term effects of control and predictability-enhancing interventions: Findings and ethical issues. *Journal of Personality and Social Psychology, 36*, 1194–1201.

Schulz, R., & Hanusa, B. (1980). Experimental social gerontology: A social psychological perspective. *Journal of Social Issues, 36*, 30–46.

Seelbach, W. C. (1977). Gender differences in expectations for filial responsibility. *The Gerontologist, 17*, 421–425.

Seelbach, W. C., & Sauer, W. J. (1977). Filial responsibility expectations and morale among aged parents. *The Gerontologist, 17*, 492–499.

Seligman, M. E. P. (1975). *Helplessness: On depression, development, and death.* San Francisco: Freeman.

Sherod, D., Hage, J., Halpern, P., & Moore, B. (1977). Effects of personal causation and perceived control on responses to an aversive environment: The more control, the better. *Journal of Experimental Social Psychology, 1*, 14–27.

Skinner, E. A., & Connell, J. P. (1986). Control understanding: Suggestions for a developmental framework. In M. M. Baltes & P. B. Baltes, eds., *The psychology of control and aging*, pp. 35–69. Hillsdale, N.J.: Lawrence Erlbaum Associates.

Smith, D. H., & Pettegrew, L. S. (1986). Mutual persuasion as a model for doctor-patient communication. *Theoretical Medicine, 7*, 127–146.

Storlie, F. J. (1982). The reshaping of the old. *Journal of Gerontological Nursing, 8*, 555–559.

Stotland, E., & Blumentahal, A. (1964). The reduction of anxiety as a result of the expectation of making a choice. *Canadian Review of Psychology, 18*, 139–145.

Strull, W., Lo, B., & Charles, G. (1984). Do patients want to participate in medical decision-making? *Journal of the American Medical Association, 252*, 2990–2994.

Teitelman, J. L., & Priddy, M. (1988). From psychological theory to practice: Improving frail elders' quality of life through control-enhancing interventions. *Journal of Applied Gerontology, 7*, 288–315.

Thomasma, D. C. (1984). Freedom, dependency, and the care of the very old. *Journal of the American Geriatrics Society, 32*, 906–914.

Thomasma, D. C. (1985). Personal autonomy of the elderly in long-term care settings. *Journal of the American Geriatrics Society, 33*, 225–227.

VanDeVeer, D. (1986). *Paternalistic intervention: The moral bounds of benevolence.* Princeton: Princeton University Press.

Veatch, R. (1981). *A theory of medical ethics.* New York: Basic Books.

Wagner, A. (1984). Cardiopulmonary resuscitation in the aged. *New England Journal of Medicine, 310,* 1129.

Wetle, T. (1988). Ethical issues. In J. Rowe & R. Besdine, eds., *Geriatric medicine.* Boston: Little, Brown.

Wetle, T., Levkoff, S. E., Cwikel, J., & Rosen, A. (1988). Nursing home resident participation in medical decisions: Perceptions and preferences. *The Gerontologist, 28,* 32–38.

Wetle, T., Schensul, J., Torres, M., & Mayen, M. (1990). Alzheimer's disease symptom interpretation and help-seeking among Puerto Rican elderly. *Geriatric Education Center Newsletter, 4,* 1–3.

White, C. B., & Janson, P. (1986). Helplessness in institutional settings: Adaptation or iatrogenic disease. In M. M. Baltes & P. B. Baltes, eds., *The psychology of control and aging,* pp. 297–313. Hillsdale, N.J.: Lawrence Erlbaum Associates.

Wolk, S., & Kurtz, J. (1975). Positive adjustment and involvement during aging and expectancy for internal control. *Journal of Consulting and Clinical Psychology, 43,* 173–178.

14

Sense of Control, Quality of Life, and Frail Older People

RONALD P. ABELES

Introduction

Sense of control and quality of life for older people are intimately interrelated. Sense of control is a pivotal contributor to a wide variety of behaviors (including intellectual performance and coping with stress) and to both mental and physical well-being (Lefcourt, 1976; Phares, 1976), which are essential elements of quality of life. How older people conceive of their control over their own health has a significant impact upon whether and how long they engage in health-promoting or disease-preventing behaviors and how they cope with chronic disability. Moreover, those with little sense of control may be more likely than others to adopt the "sick role," to "prematurely" withdraw from various daily activities, and to exhibit "excess" disability. Conversely, frailty in old age is likely to be a watershed for sense of control. That is, the onset of chronic disability associated with frailty is probably one of life's critical challenges to sense of control.

Yet, little is known about the cultural, social, environmental, behavioral, and biological processes that are involved in shaping sense of control throughout development and aging or that mediate the effects of sense of control on behaviors and well-being in different domains of functioning. This lack of knowledge is especially the case for older people, even though there is strong reason to believe that the role of sense of control in determining well-being may take on added significance with aging (Rodin, 1986a). An improved understanding of the forces that shape sense of control and mediate its impact in old age is essential for the development of environmental, social, and behavioral intervention strategies to help older people achieve an appropriate sense of control and thereby positively influence their quality of life (Elliot & Lachman, 1989; Reich & Zautra, 1989, 1990; Rodin & Timko, 1990).

With the intimacy between sense of control and quality of life in mind, this chapter reviews the conceptual development of sense of control over the past two decades and considers stability and change in sense of control over a person's life course. It goes on to scrutinize the interrelationship between sense of control and quality of life, with special attention to frail older people, and concludes with an agenda for future research on these interrelationships.

Sense of Control

Sense of control is used as an umbrella term to cover several related concepts, such as locus of control over reinforcements (Rotter, 1966), self-efficacy (Bandura, 1977), personal efficacy (Gurin, Gurin, & Morrison, 1978), perceived control (Skinner, Chapman, & Baltes, 1988), and learned helplessness (Seligman, 1975). Sense of control refers to people's interrelated beliefs and expectancies about their abilities to perform behaviors aimed at obtaining desired outcomes and about the responsiveness of the environment, both physical and social, to their behaviors. This concept is deceptively complex, as evidenced by a simple example. Assume that an older woman wants to improve her health through a change in her diet. What role might sense of control play in her decision to engage in the behaviors necessary for changing her diet? First, she needs to know whether she is capable of performing the required steps associated with changing her eating habits (e.g., giving up favorite foods and substituting more healthy alternatives), which involves an assessment of her own abilities. Second, she needs to consider whether her husband will support and join in making these dietary changes, which concerns her evaluations of the social environment. Thus, in order to have a sense of control, she must have simultaneously particular beliefs and expectations about herself and the environment. Note that nothing has been said about her actual skills or the true nature of the environment. The focus is on *subjective* as opposed to *objective* control. The relationship between actual abilities and true environmental contingencies, on the one hand, and a person's perceptions of these abilities and environmental characteristics, on the other, is an empirical issue and beyond the scope of this chapter.

Initial Formulation and Subsequent Elaborations

While not the first, certainly the most widely employed conceptualization of sense of control has been *perceived locus of control for reinforcements* (Rotter, 1966). As originally formulated within the context of social learning theory, locus of control referred to people's expectations about whether rewards and punishments (i.e., valued outcomes) were contingent upon their behaviors (i.e., internal locus of control) or upon powerful other people, fate, or chance (i.e., external locus of control). By employing a single scale of 23 forced-choice items (i.e., respondents must choose among pairs of items reflecting either an internal or an external locus of control orientation), locus of control is operationalized as a bipolar, generalized orientation or a personality trait, which also implies stability over time and across situations (see Figures 1 and 2). The concept of locus

1.	a.	I have often found that what is going to happen will happen. (External)
	b.	Trust to fate has never turned out as well for me as making a decision to take a definite course of action.
2.	a.	No matter how hard you try some people just don't like you. (External)
	b.	People who can't get others to like them don't understand how to get along with others.

Figure 1 Sample items from the Rotter Locus of Control Scale. From Rotter (1966).

of control and the resulting scale have been used to predict a wide variety of behaviors (Lefcourt, 1976; Phares, 1976). In particular, it has been invoked to explain individual differences in behaviors where two people place equal value upon a desired outcome, but only one of them engages in the behaviors directed toward obtaining that outcome. For example, in one early investigation, Seeman (1963, 1967) found that internally oriented reformatory inmates were more likely than their externally oriented compatriots to seek out information about how to obtain parole.

Almost immediately after the publication of the Rotter Locus of Control Scale, various elaborations and disaggregations of the concept and its measuring instrument emerged. For example, during an item-analysis of the original scale, the Gurins and their collaborators (Gurin, Gurin, Lao, & Beattie, 1969; Gurin *et al.*, 1978) noticed that items phrased in the first person (e.g., item 1 in Figure 1: "I", "me") were more highly correlated with outcome measures than items referring to other people (e.g., item 2: "you," "they," "people"). They reasoned that the first-person items reflected beliefs about oneself (personal efficacy),

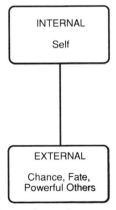

Figure 2 Internal versus external locus of control.

while the other items reflected cultural truisms (control ideology) that were not psychologically meaningful. Similarly, they deduced that a distinction should be made between external explanations invoking fate or chance as opposed to powerful others. Fate and chance connote random processes that cannot be controlled by anyone, reflecting noncontingency between behaviors and outcomes, while powerful others suggest that outcomes are indeed controllable but are contingent upon the behaviors of others rather than oneself. Indeed, a belief in powerful others could be an accurate representation of reality for members of disadvantaged minority groups. Consequently, the Gurins differentiated both the internal and the external poles into two components (Figure 3). Several subsequent studies have confirmed the validity of this approach, especially in regard to the greater predictive value of personal efficacy as opposed to control ideology.

In addition to doubts being raised about the nature of the internal and external poles, the dimensionality of the locus of control concept has been viewed as problematic. Some investigators have questioned the validity of a single locus of control dimension. They have argued for two separate dimensions by pointing out that a person may hold both internal and external beliefs simultaneously (Levenson, 1981). Others have distinguished between control over positively and

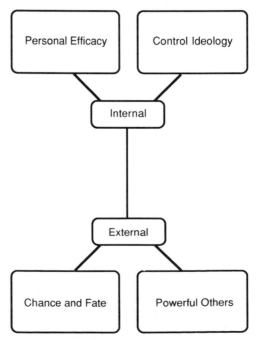

Figure 3 Initial elaborations of locus of control.

negatively valenced outcomes (Gregory, 1981). Still others have opted for the greater conceptual and (presumably greater) predictive value of situation-specific measures of sense of control as opposed to a generalized, global measure (Lachman, 1986a). For example, scales have been developed to measure sense of control in such diverse behavioral domains as health (Wallston, 1989; Wallston & Wallston, 1981), academic achievement (Lachman, 1983; Lachman, Baltes, Nesselroade, & Willis, 1982), and political behaviors (Campbell, Converse, Miller, & Stokes, 1964).

A Model of Sense of Control

These various elaborations have converted a relatively simple construct into a highly differentiated and complex concept. Before considering the relationship between sense of control and quality of life, a model of this elaborated concept first needs to be laid out. Figure 4 synthesizes the major strains in the current literature and provides a model that represents the components of sense of control and schematizes their interrelations. In viewing this model, four points are noteworthy. First, the model refers primarily to internal, cognitive structures and processes. That is, it conceptualizes control in terms of subjective experiences within a person's mind. It is not a model of actual control. (While most elements are internal, a few presumed antecedents and consequences are external to the individual.) Second, sense of control is not a unitary concept but is composed of multiple component beliefs and expectations regarding oneself and the environment. Third, the model postulates processes that are dynamic and also dialectical: These processes include a feedback loop from outcomes back to the hypothesized antecedents of sense of control. This loop implies that accumulating experiences result in both short-term and longer-term changes in sense of control as a person undergoes development and aging. Lastly, the least-elaborated or -specified part of the diagram refers to the hypothesized antecedents of sense of control, which reflects the relative lack of research on antecedents.

As schematized in Figure 4, the model portrays the components of sense of control and their role in influencing whether people will perform a particular behavior and how the results of that behavior feed back to affect the person's sense of control. Sense of control consists of beliefs and expectations about the self and about the environment. According to this model, people's self-beliefs about their own abilities (e.g., skills) and capabilities (e.g., to exert effort) combine with task beliefs about the nature of the task (e.g., how difficult it is, whether it requires skill or luck) to produce their self-efficacy expectations: a sense of whether they could successfully perform the behaviors needed to achieve the particular desired outcome.

People's beliefs about the causal nature of the environment focus upon whether they perceive the environment to be governed by "lawful" or "orderly"

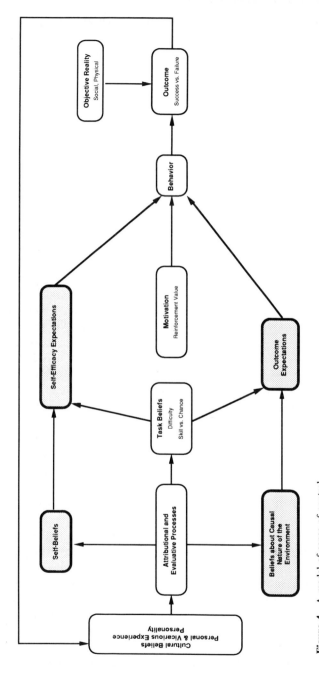

Figure 4 A model of sense of control.

processes such that outcomes (e.g., "success" or "failure") are "contingent" upon people's behaviors as opposed to random forces (i.e., "noncontingent"). Environmental contingency may stem from physical laws (e.g., the laws of nature) or social rules (e.g., norms). Believing that an environment is contingent does not necessarily mean believing that one has control, since one's own outcomes may be (perceived as) more contingent upon the behaviors of others than upon one's own efforts. Beliefs about the causal nature of the environment also combine with task beliefs to produce outcome expectations (i.e., whether performing action α is generally likely to result in outcome β). Thus, a person's sense of control consists of the complex interrelationships among his or her self-beliefs, self-efficacy expectations, beliefs about the causal nature of the environment, and outcome expectations.

Implicit in the model, of course, is the postulate that sense of control is modified by personal experience, as expressed by the feedback loop in Figure 4. After objective reality operates to influence whether people achieve their desired outcomes, people presumably reassess their own performance with reference to the reactions of others and to whether the desired outcome is obtained. Such evaluative and attributional processes may lead to adjustments in their sense of control through changes in beliefs and expectations about the self, the environment, or the task. Similarly, other people's experiences may affect sense of control through social comparison and reference group processes. As social psychologists have long pointed out (Festinger, 1954; Singer, 1980), people compare themselves frequently to others in order to evaluate themselves and their performance, especially under ambiguous circumstances. For example, if other people with perceived similar levels of skills also fail, then one may be more likely to ascribe his or her own failure to external factors, such as the difficulty of the task or interference by powerful others. Conversely, when similar others succeed, then one's own failure is more likely to be interpreted as reflecting something about oneself (e.g., lack of effort or skill).

Furthermore, general cultural beliefs influence the beliefs and expectations constituting sense of control (Abeles, 1990; Atchley, Chapter 10). Cultures provide elaborate belief systems (e.g., science, religion) for explaining how both the social and physical worlds operate, as well as about the appropriate means for achieving desired outcomes, including whether particular outcomes are contingent or noncontingent upon people's behaviors. Furthermore, through stereotypes, cultures provide information about the personal characteristics of culturally defined categories of people. Thus, stereotypes about people of different ages, ageism (Butler, 1975; Crockett & Hummert, 1987), may influence how older people interpret and evaluate their own abilities and those of others, which in turn may affect their sense of control.

Finally, although it is not obvious from Figure 4, people may have more than a single generalized sense of control in that there may be beliefs and expectations specific to many different behavioral domains (e.g., self-care, health, interpersonal, and intellectual behaviors). This possibility can be represented as a Figure 4 specific to each of several behavioral domains, along with a generalized sense of control reflecting some sort of weighted average of the domain-specific senses of control (Paulhus & Christie, 1981).

Sense of Control and Aging

While there is little solid empirical evidence to go by, most analysts postulate that sense of control increases throughout childhood into adulthood and remains fairly stable until old age (Lachman, 1986b; Rodin, 1987; Rodin & Timko, 1991). It is hypothesized that with aging, forces within and without the person lead to a diminishing sense of control. The physical changes accompanying old age (e.g., worsening eyesight and diminishing stamina) and the internalization of negative age stereotypes are believed to attack the older person's self-beliefs and self-efficacy expectations (Lachman, 1983; Lachman & Jelalian, 1984; Lachman & McArthur, in press). Simultaneously, a number of factors appear to undermine the older person's beliefs about the contingent nature of the environment and associated outcome expectations: for example, the loss of significant roles and social status through retirement from work and raising a family; interactions with health care and social service providers who reward dependent over independent behaviors (Baltes & Reisenzein, 1986; Baltes & Wahl, 1991); and treatment by significant others who view one as less capable.

In contrast to this consensual view of diminishing sense of control with aging, the empirical view is far from showing such a clear pattern (Lachman, 1986b; Rodin, 1987; Rodin & Timko, 1991). Contradictory evidence exists for decreasing, stable, and increasing sense of control! Many studies are tainted by the shortcomings that plague much of gerontological research, such as inappropriate cross-sectional and age-comparison designs; small and unrepresentative samples; and the use of nonstandard or inappropriate measures.

In retrospect, the lack of empirical clarity should not come as a surprise. Given that sense of control is now conceived of as having several dimensions and as situation-specific, the reliance on a unidimensional and generalized measure, such as the Rotter Locus of Control Scale, is likely to meet with failure. As the tenets of the life-course perspective remind us (Abeles, 1987; Baltes & Reese, 1984; Riley & Abeles, 1982), it is entirely possible that domain-specific senses of control may have differing age-related trajectories and that the various components of sense of control may similarly show varying patterns of change. Some empirical support for the latter possibility can be found in one longitudinal study in which older people's self-efficacy expectations remained constant while at the same time they came to see the environment as being governed more by chance and powerful others (Lachman, 1986a).

Sense of Control and Frailty

Effects of Frailty upon Sense of Control

People are able to maintain a stable sense of self despite the gradual and slow changes in themselves and their social environment that accompany aging (Atchley, Chapter 10). Assaults against the self, including one's sense of control, are fended off, for example, via common attributional biases (e.g., attributing positive outcomes to stable and internal causes and negative ones to unstable or external causes), shifting standards of comparison (e.g., limiting reference groups to one's age peers), or changing goals (e.g., lowering of aspirations or devaluing activities that can no longer be performed). Since the developmental course of most chronic disabilities is gradual and the overwhelming majority of people remain healthy and active well into their 70s (Abeles & Riley, 1987; Verbrugge, 1989), it might not be until advanced old age that challenges to one's sense of control become sufficiently severe and abrupt to have a negative impact.

What kinds of circumstances might undermine older people's sense of control? The child development and adult cognitive intervention literatures provide some clues about environmental conditions that may link increasing disability with diminishing sense of control. Children and adolescents are likely to develop a positive sense of control when the environment is characterized as offering choice as opposed to constraint and as being contingent, sensitive to one's goals and desires, and supportive (i.e., providing constructive feedback) (Skinner, 1990). Similarly, when older adults are placed in training situations with these same characteristics, they demonstrate improvements in their cognitive performance and their sense of control over those cognitive tasks (Baltes & Willis, 1982; Dittman-Kohli, Lachman, Kliegl, & Baltes, 1990; Schaie & Willis, 1986).

However, with increasing disability, the social and physical world of frail older people may become more and more characterized by the lack of these sense-of-control-promoting properties. Increasing disability may lead to less choice in the activities that frail older people can engage in because of decreased mobility, dexterity, stamina, alertness, or social integration (Harris & Kovar, in press; Rowland, 1989). Obtaining desired goals may become less and less contingent upon one's own behaviors and increasingly contingent upon the behaviors of family, friends, and health care providers. At the same time, the environment may become less sensitive to the disabled older person's desires and more responsive to those of the caretakers who are in the position to organize the physical, temporal, and social environment to their convenience (e.g., the scheduling of meals and baths). Finally, the social environment may be less likely to provide constructive feedback because of diminished social contracts or because of caretakers who reinforce dependent behaviors (Baltes & Reisenzein, 1986; Baltes & Wahl, 1991; Taylor, 1979; Timko & Rodin, 1985; Wills, 1978).

While these speculations imply a steep monotonic decline in sense of control with increasing disability, we should not too readily embrace this hypothesis. One should not forget that "disability is a gap between a person's capability and the environment's demands" (Verbrugge, 1990). As such, functioning can be retained or improved by changes in either the person or the environment (Kiyak, 1991). For example, increasing difficulties in walking may diminish an older person's feelings of self-efficacy. However, being provided with a cane or wheelchair or participating in a strength-building exercise program may restore some lost mobility and simultaneously provide a boost to the older person's sense of control (see Spirduso & Gilliam-MacRae, Chapter 11). In sum, rather than a steady decline in sense of control, a pattern of rises and falls is more likely.

Effects of Sense of Control on Frailty

While the link from sense of control to frailty among older people has not been heavily investigated, both theory and empirical evidence imply such a linkage. An impressive array of correlational, quasi-experimental, and experimental studies indicates a positive relationship between control and both physical and mental health, which may take on added significance as people age. (This literature is too vast to review at this juncture, and extensive reviews are already available: Lachman, 1983, 1986b; Lefcourt, 1976, 1981; Phares, 1976; Rodin, 1986a,b, 1987; Rodin & Timko, 1991). However, it is difficult to say with any definitiveness how sense of control is causally related to health outcomes because often these studies fail to measure sense of control directly. In many intervention studies, *actual* control is manipulated and *sense* of control is treated as an unmeasured intervening construct. The picture is further complicated by the plethora of sense of control measures employed in these studies.

In any event, the consensual view is that sense of control affects mental and physical health, although the exact mechanisms mediating this relationship are as yet to be extensively tested. Sense of control may operate through several physiological, behavioral, and cognitive pathways (Bandura, 1989; Rodin & Timko, 1991). For example, diminished sense of control may directly affect physiological states through the sympathetic adrenal medullary system, the pituitary adrenal cortical axis, or through the immune system. Indeed, Rodin (1986a) argues that physiological declines in these systems make older people particularly vulnerable to negative health consequences stemming from a diminished sense of control. Moreover, sense of control may influence whether actions are taken to prevent or remedy health problems, such as self-care, gathering appropriate information, active interactions with health care providers, or better and longer compliance with medial regimens. For example, among those suffering from hypertension, persons with a greater sense of control are more willing to read information about hypertension than are those with less sense of control (Wallston, Maides, & Wallston, 1976).

By extension, this line of evidence and argument leads to the belief that sense of control, through its effects on actual health, may be a major contributor to disability and frailty in old age.

In addition, sense of control may influence subjective or perceived health through its effects on the salience and labeling of bodily complaints as symptoms (Rodin & Timko, 1991). Several experiments show that when the level of sense of control over environmental events is manipulated, persons who are given little or no control report more physical symptoms that those who feel more in control. This suggests that changes in the social environment and roles (e.g., transition from work to retirement) and perhaps increasing disability may result in a higher salience of symptoms and the assumption of the sick role by older people. Perhaps with aging, older people become more vigilant, perceive more symptoms, attribute these more frequently to aging (an uncontrollable process) than to illness, feel less in control over their health, and thereby become less likely to actively engage in behaviors for promoting health and preventing or treating disease (Lachman, in press). These perceptions and resulting behaviors might then have subsequent consequences for actual health and functioning, leading to a spiral of increasing frailty and decreasing sense of control.

However, this is not universally the case. In fact, older people may be more likely to feel they have control over serious illnesses (e.g., cancer) than do younger people, perhaps because of their greater prior personal or vicarious experience in dealing with serious health crises (Leventhal, Leventhal, & Schaefer, 1991). Moreover, differences among older people in their sense of control may account for differential reactions to disability among older people. For example, those with less sense of control may be likely to suffer from "excess" disability (i.e., to be more disabled than would appear to be warranted by their actual physical condition). That is, perhaps they would be less likely to engage and persist in active attempts to overcome their disability. Such older people may be particularly vulnerable to the downward spiral of increasing frailty and decreasing sense of control, which could ultimately contribute to their institutionalization.

While it is tempting to emphasize the positive effects of sense of control, there are circumstances in which it may have negative health consequences (Folkman, 1984). For example, a sense of control may heighten the threat associated with a stressful event because exercising control in one area may result in costs in others (e.g., attempting to change one's diet may cause conflicts with one's spouse), be antagonistic to a preferred mode of response (i.e., exceed the degree of control usually desired) (Reid & Ziegler, 1981), or imply blame for one's circumstances. Moreover, an orientation toward control may be illusory (Langer, 1975) and fly in the face of reality, thereby dooming attempts at control to failure, which in turn may have negative consequences through heightening one's sense of vulnerability and self-blame.

Sense of Control and Quality of Life

How are sense of control and quality of life related? Are they part and parcel of the same concept, or are they different concepts? Does sense of control have a positive impact upon quality of life? Before turning attention to these questions, a definition of quality of life has to be settled upon. One particularly attractive definition is offered by Lawton (1983; see also Lawton, Chapter 1), who argues for a four-dimensional conceptualization of quality of life: (a) *behavioral compe- tence* is "the social-normative evaluation of the person's functioning in the health, cognitive, time-use, and social dimensions"; (b) *perceived quality of life* refers to "the person's subjective evaluation of function in any of the behavioral competence dimensions"; (c) *environment* affords or hinders particular behaviors and influences perceived quality of life; and (d) *psychological well-being* is "the weighted evaluated level of the person's competence and perceived quality in all domains of contemporary life" and encompasses what is usually thought of as mental health. Now, we can turn to the issue of whether sense of control is related to these dimensions, either conceptually or causally.

The ever-expanding literature on sense of control and aging is most relevant to Lawton's dimensions of behavioral competence and psychological well-being, especially in the domains of physical and mental health and cognitive function- ing. As was just discussed, mounting evidence exists for a relationship between sense of control and health. Similarly, sense of control (as learned helplessness) has been strongly implicated as a determinant of depression (Seligman, 1975) and of cognitive functioning, especially memory, among older people (Elliot & Lachman, 1989; Lachman, 1983; Lachman & Jelalian, 1984). Thus, sense of control is a likely antecedent of these two dimensions of quality of life.

As noted earlier, perceived quality of life refers to "the person's subjective evaluation of function in any of the behavioral competence dimensions." This definition implies some conceptual overlap with self-beliefs and self-efficacy expectations, which are two of the four components constituting sense of control. These are people's own subjective evaluations of their functioning in various behavioral domains. Similarly, environment may be conceptually related to be- liefs about the causal nature of the environment and outcome expectations, the other two components of sense of control (Figure 4), since they refer to whether the social and physical environments are seen as responsive versus nonrespon- sive and facilitating versus inhibiting. Consequently, these aspects of sense of control seem to refer to the subjective evaluation of the environment as a compo- nent in Lawton's concept of quality of life.

Taken together, this brief discussion supports the conclusion that sense of control and quality of life are interconnected. Having a sense of control is likely to have a positive impact on performance or function (e.g., cognition and health) and on the kinds, duration, and extent of coping with adverse events and disabilities

(Folkman, 1984). Furthermore, almost by definition, it is tied to evaluations of the environment and of one's own competencies. Moreover, both the physical and social changes that accompany chronic disability and frailty challenge people's sense of control, with the implication of further deterioration in health and functioning (or quality of life) stemming from a diminished sense of control.

Future Research Directions

While much has been learned about sense of control, much more remains to be learned, especially in regard to changes in sense of control that may accompany aging and frailty. Among possible topics for research are the following.

Antecedents of Sense of Control throughout the Life Course

- What are the antecedents, causes, and origins of sense of control at various ages? How do individuals develop and maintain a sense of control in relation to age-related gains and losses in actual functioning and competence, especially as a result of increasing chronic disability in advanced old age? What is the relationship between perceived and actual efficacy (in specific behavioral domains)?
- What are the roles of biological functioning, health, social comparison processes, personal and vicarious experience, cultural beliefs, and age stereotypes in fostering stability or change in sense of control?
- How do attributional processes, styles, and biases influence sense of control (e.g., reactions to success versus failure)? Do these processes, styles, and biases change with aging?
- Are there different age-related patterns of change in generalized versus situation-specific sense of control? Under what conditions to particular patterns occur? For what domains of function?
- What are the sources of individual and cohort differences in kinds and levels of sense of control?
- How do the characteristics of social situations and roles affect sense of control? Can these characteristics be manipulated, through behavioral and social interventions, to bolster sense of control, and with what consequences?

Consequences of Sense of Control

- How is sense of control related to specific cognitive, behavioral, or health consequences (e.g., memory, morbidity, depression, interpersonal relations, self-esteem, life satisfaction)? Do these relationships change with age, and under what circumstances?

- What processes (e.g., immunological responses, compliance to medical regimens) link sense of control to specific biological, behavioral, and social outcomes (e.g., health, intellectual performance, social relationships)?
- Under what conditions is low versus high sense of control beneficial or detrimental? What are the consequences of discrepancies between the degree of control actually available in the environment and sense of control?
- Are there different consequences stemming from sense of control over the occurrence of an event versus coping with an event after its occurrence?

Conceptual and Methodological Issues

Generalized versus Situation-Specific Sense of Control

- What is the relationship between generalized and situation-specific sense of control? Is generalized sense of control developed from specific situational expectancies? Are some domains more important than others in influencing the development of a generalized sense of control? Are there age-related changes in the relative significance of domains?
- Under what conditions is generalized sense of control a better or worse predictor of behaviors and outcomes than situation-specific sense of control?

Dimensionality of Sense of Control

- How are the various dimensions interrelated? Are there age-related sequences or patterns in the emergence of dimensions or age-related changes in their relationships?

Methodological Issues

- Are existing measuring instruments age-appropriate (i.e., reliable and valid) for generalized and situation-specific sense of control? Are measures sensitive to age-related changes?
- What are the comparative advantages and disadvantages of profiles on several dimensions versus a single, summarizing measure?

Special Populations

- Are there ethnic, racial, or cultural differences in sense of control over the life course? What are their origins and consequences?
- Are there gender differences in levels, origins, and consequences of sense of control? Are they related to the greater life expectancy of women over that of men or to women's comparatively higher levels of morbidity?

Conclusion

The preceding may seem like an extensive list of questions that suggests a lack of knowledge or understanding. However, the contrary is the case. The field has come a long way since the initial conceptualizations of sense of control. In a sense, it is only now that enough is known to pose questions about the nature of sense of control, its origins, and its consequences for people as they age. How older people perceive their control over important domains of their daily life has profound consequences for their health and functioning and, thereby, for their quality of life. Conversely, frailty in old age is likely to be a turning point for sense of control. The sudden commencement of serious disability is most likely a critical threat to one's sense of control.

Acknowledgments

This chapter was prepared as part of the author's duties as an employee of the U.S. Government and is consequently in the public domain. The opinions expressed are those of the author and do not necessarily reflect the position or policy of the National Institute on Aging.

The model of sense of control, represented in Figure 4, has benefited from the insightful and critical comments of several colleagues, but most especially from those of Margret Baltes and Ellen Skinner. The constructive and encouraging comments and advice of the editors of this volume are gratefully acknowledged.

References

Abeles, R. P. (1987). Introduction. In R. P. Abeles, ed., *Life-span perspectives and social psychology*, pp. 1–16. Hillsdale, N.J.: Lawrence Erlbaum Associates.

Abeles, R. P. (1990). Schemas, sense of control, and aging. In C. Schooler, J. Rodin, & K. W. Schaie, eds., *Self-directedness and efficacy: Causes and effects throughout the life course*, pp. 85–94. Hillsdale, N.J.: Lawrence Erlbaum Associates.

Abeles, R. P., & Riley, M. W. (1987). Longevity, social structure, and cognitive aging. In C. Schooler & K. W. Schaie, eds., *Cognitive functioning and social structure over the life course*, pp. 161–175. Norwood, N.J.: Ablex Publishing Corp.

Baltes, M. M., & Reisenzein, R. (1986). The social world in long-term care institutions: Psychosocial control toward dependence? In M. M. Baltes & P. B. Baltes, eds., *The psychology of control and aging*, pp. 315–344. Hillsdale, N.J.: Lawrence Erlbaum Associates.

Baltes, M. M., & Wahl, H. W. (1991). The behavior system of dependency in the elderly: Interaction with the social environment. In M. G. Ory, R. P. Abeles, & P. D. Lipman, eds., *Aging, health, and behavior*. Newbury Park, Calif.: Sage Publications.

Baltes, P. B., & Reese, H. W. (1984). The life-span perspective in developmental psychology. In M. H. Bornstein & M. E. Lamb, eds., *Developmental psychology: An advanced textbook,* pp. 493–531. Hillsdale, N.J.: Lawrence Erlbaum Associates.

Baltes, P. B., & Willis, S. L. (1982). Plasticity and enhancement of intellectual functioning in old age: Penn State's Adult Development and Enrichment Project (ADEPT). In F. I. M. Craik & S. E. Trehub, eds., *Aging and cognitive processes.* N.Y.: Plenum.

Bandura, A. (1977). Self-efficacy: Toward a unifying theory of behavioral change. *Psychological Review, 84,* 191–215.

Bandura, A. (1989). Self-efficacy mechanism in physiological activation and health-promoting behavior. In J. Madden IV, S. Matthysse, & J. Barchas, eds., *Adaptation, learning and affect.* N.Y.: Raven Press.

Butler, R. N. (1975). *Why survive?: Being old in America.* N.Y.: Harper & Row.

Campbell, A., Converse, P. E., Miller, W. E., & Stokes, D. E. (1964). *The American voter.* N.Y.: John Wiley & Sons.

Crockett, W. H., & Hummert, M. L. (1987). Perceptions of aging and the elderly. In K. W. Schaie, ed., *The annual review of gerontology and geriatrics,* pp. 217–241. N.Y.: Springer Publishing Co.

Dittman-Kohli, F., Lachman, M. E., Kliegl, R., & Baltes, P. B. (1990). *Effects of cognitive training and testing on intellectual efficacy beliefs in elderly adults.* Berlin: Max Planck Institute for Human Development and Education and Brandeis University.

Elliot, E., & Lachman, M. E. (1989). Enhancing memory by modifying control beliefs, attributions, and performance goals in the elderly. In P. S. Fry, ed., *Psychological perspectives of helplessness and control in the elderly,* pp. 339–368. Amsterdam: North-Holland.

Festinger, L. (1954). A theory of social comparison processes. *Human Relations, 7,* 117–140.

Folkman, S. (1984). Personal control and stress and coping processes: A theoretical analysis. *Journal of Personality and Social Psychology, 46,* 839–852.

Gregory, W. L. (1981). Expectancies for controllability, performance attributions, and behavior. In H. M. Lefcourt, ed., *Research with the locus of control construct. 1. Assessment methods,* pp. 67–126. N.Y.: Academic Press.

Gurin, P., Gurin, G., & Morrison, B. M. (1978). Personal and ideological aspects of internal and external control. *Social Psychology Quarterly, 41,* 275–296.

Gurin, P., Gurin, G., Lao, R. C., & Beattie, M. (1969). Internal-external control in the motivational dynamics of Negro youth. *Journal of Social Issues, 25,* 29–53.

Harris, T., & Kovar, M. G. (in press). *National statistics on the functional status of older persons.* Hyattsville, Md.: National Center for Health Statistics.

Kiyak, H. A. (1991). Coping with chronic illness and disability. In M. G. Ory, R. P. Abeles, & P. D. Lipman, eds., *Aging, health, and behavior.* Newbury Park, Calif.: Sage Publications.

Lachman, M. E. (1983). Perceptions of intellectual aging: Antecedent or consequence of intellectual functioning? *Developmental Psychology, 19,* 482–498.

Lachman, M. E. (1986a). Locus of control in aging research: A case of multidimensional and domain-specific assessment. *Journal of Psychology and Aging, 1,* 34–40.

Lachman, M. E. (1986b). Personal control in later life: Stability, change, and cognitive correlates. In M. M. Baltes & P. B. Baltes, eds., *The psychology of control and aging,* pp. 207–236. Hillsdale, N.J.: Lawrence Erlbaum Associates.

Lachman, M. E. (in press). When bad things happen to old people: Age differences in attributional style. *Journal of Psychology and Aging.*

Lachman, M. E., & Jelalian, E. (1984). Self-efficacy and attributions for intellectual performance in young and elderly adults. *Journal of Gerontology, 39,* 577–582.

Lachman, M. E., & McArthur, L. Z. (in press). Adulthood age differences in causal attributions for cognitive, physical, and social performance. *Journal of Psychology and Aging.*

Lachman, M. E., Baltes, P. B., Nesselroade, J. R., & Willis, S. L. (1982). Examination of personality-ability relationships in the elderly: The role of contextual (interface) assessment mode. *Journal of Research in Personality, 16,* 485–501.

Langer, E. (1975). The illusion of control. *Journal of Personality and Social Psychology, 32,* 311–328.

Lawton, M. P. (1983). Environment and other determinants of well-being in older people. *The Gerontologist, 23,* 349–357.

Lefcourt, H. M. (1976). *Locus of control: Current trends in theory and research.* Hillsdale, N.J.: Lawrence Erlbaum Associates.

Lefcourt, H. M. (1981). *Research with the locus of control construct. 1. Assessment methods.* N.Y.: Academic Press.

Levenson, H. (1981). Differentiating among internality, powerful others, and change. In H. M. Lefcourt, ed., *Research with the locus of control construct. 1. Assessment methods,* pp. 15–66. N.Y.: Academic Press.

Leventhal, H., Leventhal, E. A., & Schaefer, P. (1991). Vigilant coping and health behavior: A life-span problem. In M. G. Ory, R. P. Abeles, & P. D. Lipman, eds., *Aging, health, and behavior.* Newbury Park, Calif.: Sage Publications.

Paulhus, D., & Christie, R. (1981). Spheres of control: An interactionist approach to assessment of perceived control. In H. M. Lefcourt, eds., *Research with the locus of control construct. 1. Assessment methods,* pp. 161–188. N.Y.: Academic Press.

Phares, E. J. (1976). *Locus of control in personality.* Morristown, N.J.: General Learning Press.

Reich, J. W., & Zautra, A. J. (1989). A perceived control intervention for at-risk older adults. *Psychology and Aging, 4,* 415–424.

Reich, J. W., & Zautra, A. J. (1990). Dispositional control beliefs and the consequences of a control-enhancing intervention. *Journal of Gerontology: Psychological Sciences, 45,* 46–51.

Reid, D. W., & Ziegler, M. (1981). The desired control measure and adjustment among the elderly. In H. M. Lefcourt, ed., *Research with the locus of control construct. 1. Assessment Methods,* pp. 127–160. N.Y.: Academic Press.

Riley, M. W., & Abeles, R. P. (1982). Life-course perspectives. In M. W. Riley, R. P. Abeles, & M. S. Teitelbaum, eds., *Aging from birth to death. 2. Sociotemporal perspectives,* pp. 1–10. Boulder, Colo.: Westview Press.

Rodin, J. (1986a). Aging and health: Effects of the sense of control. *Science, 233,* 1271–1276.

Rodin, J. (1986b). Health, control, and aging. In M. M. Baltes & P. B. Baltes, eds., *The psychology of control and aging,* pp. 139–165. Hillsdale, N.J.: Lawrence Erlbaum Associates.

Rodin, J. (1987). Personal control through the life course. In R. P. Abeles, ed., *Life-span perspectives and social psychology,* pp. 103–120. Hillsdale, N.J.: Lawrence Erlbaum Associates.

Rodin, J., & Timko, C. (1991). Sense of control, aging, and health. In M. G. Ory, R. P. Abeles, & P. D. Lipman, eds., *Aging, health, and behavior.* Sage Publications, Newbury Park, California.

Rotter, J. B. (1966). Generalized expectancies for internal versus external control of reinforcements. *Psychological Monographs, 80.*

Rowland, D. (1989). *Help at home: Long-term care assistance for impaired elderly people.* Commonwealth Fund Commission on Elderly People Living Alone.

Schaie, K. W., & Willis, S. L. (1986). Can decline in adult intellectual functioning be reversed? *Developmental Psychology, 22,* 223–232.

Seeman, M. (1963). Alienation and social learning in a reformatory. *American Journal of Sociology, 69,* 270–284.

Seeman, M. (1967). Powerlessness and knowledge: A comparative study of alienation and learning. *Sociometry, 30,* 105–123.

Seligman, M. E. P. (1975). *Helplessness: On depression, development, and death.* San Francisco: Freeman.

Singer, J. E. (1980). Social comparison: The process of self-evaluation. In L. Festinger, ed., *Retrospections on social psychology,* pp. 158–179. N.Y.: Oxford University Press.

Skinner, E. A. (1990). Development and perceived control: A dynamic model of action in context. In M. Gunnar & L. A. Sroufe, eds., *Minnesota symposium on child development,* pp. 167–215. Hillsdale, N.J.: Lawrence Erlbaum Associates.

Skinner, E. A. Chapman, M., & Baltes, P. B. (1988). Control, means-ends, and agency beliefs: A new conceptualization and its measurement during childhood. *Journal of Personality and Social Psychology, 54,* 117–133.

Taylor, S. E. (1979). Hospital patient behavior: Reactance, helplessness, or control? *Journal of Social Issues, 35,* 156–184.

Timko, C., & Rodin, J. (1985). Staff-patient relationships in nursing homes: Sources of conflict and rehabilitation potential. *Rehabilitation Psychology, 30,* 93–108.

Verbrugge, L. M. (1989). Recent, present, and future health of American adults. *Annual Review of Public Health, 10,* 333–361.

Verbrugge, L. M. (1990). The iceberg of disability. In S. M. Stahl, ed., *The legacy of longevity,* pp. 55–75. Newbury Park, Calif.: Sage Publications.

Wallston, K. A. (1989). Assessment of control in health-care settings. In A. Steptoe & A. Appels, eds., *Stress, personal control, and health,* pp. 85–105. N.Y.: John Wiley & Sons.

Wallston, K. A., & Wallston, B. S. (1981). Health locus of control scales. In H. M. Lefcourt, ed., *Research with the locus of control construct. 1. Assessment methods,* pp. 189–244. N.Y.: Academic Press.

Wallston, K. A., Maides, S., & Wallston, B. S. (1976). Health-related information seeking as a function of health-related locus of control and health value. *Journal of Research in Personality, 10,* 215–222.

Wills, T. H. (1978). Perception of clients by professional helpers. *Psychological Bulletin, 85,* 968–1000.

15

Personal Autonomy for Residents in Long-Term Care: Concepts and Issues of Measurement

ROSALIE A. KANE

With its inspiring language about "life, liberty, and the pursuit of happiness," the preamble to the Declaration of Independence asserts the primacy of freedom for its citizens as a dominant value in the United States. This commitment is further embodied in the Bill of Rights to the U.S. Constitution and is held up by centuries of case law. Autonomy is also ensconced as one of the most central ethical values among philosophers in the United States (Beauchamp & Childress, 1983; Dworkin, 1976). For some (e.g., Childress, 1984; Englehardt, 1986), autonomy is the highest value, trumping principles of beneficence, justice, and community good.

To many philosophers, the principle of autonomy is derived from respect for persons as an end rather than a means to an end and, therefore, is one espoused for its own sake rather than for any utilitarian implications. However, over the last few decades psychologists have added utilitarian fuel to the autonomy fire, pointing out that people who perceive that they are in control of their lives and that they have choices are likely to be less depressed, to be healthier, and even to live longer (Avorn & Langer, 1982; Langer & Rodin, 1986; Rodin, 1986; Rodin & Langer, 1977; Schulz, 1976).

Whether living at home, in a nursing home, or in another type of residential setting, the long-term care client is often in a poor position to exercise personal autonomy. The typical nursing home in the United States is the nadir for expression of personal autonomy (Kane & Caplan, 1990). Few nursing home residents have control over and choice in the basic conditions of their daily life and care. Many have not had control even over the initial admission and the associated disposition of their household goods.

If social scientists are systematically to study the relationship between the personal autonomy of long-term care recipients and their quality of life, it becomes

Copyright © 1991 by Academic Press, Inc. All rights of reproduction in any form reserved.

imperative to be able to measure the presence or absence of autonomy. But autonomy has many shades of meaning and can be made operational in many different ways. This chapter discusses the concept of autonomy, its various meanings in the long-term care context, and difficulties inherent in making meaningful measures of it.

Autonomy: The Concept

Autonomy as Self-Rule

The simplest meaning of autonomy as discussed by philosophers is self-rule. It refers to taking actions and decisions to direct one's own life. However, as Collopy (1988) points out, self-rule can be further elaborated or paraphrased into "a whole family of value-laden ideas, including individual liberty, privacy, free choice, self-governance, self-regulation, and moral independence." To quote Collopy:

> . . . autonomy is understood as a cluster of notions including self-determination, freedom, independence, liberty of choice, and action. In its most general terms, autonomy signifies control of decision-making and other activity by the individual. It refers to human agency free of outside intervention and interferences. (p. 10)

In a reflective essay on the place of autonomy in bioethics, Childress (1990) stresses that the principle should be formulated as respect for autonomy, not autonomy itself. Thus, the philosophical principle asserts not that one should make autonomous choices and act autonomously but that one is obliged to respect the autonomous choices and actions of others. He further discusses the multiple meanings of the term *respect,* which include: to consider or have regard for; to esteem or value; and to refrain from interfering with the autonomous choices and actions of others. Childress argues that, although the principle is paramount, it is also a limited and limiting principle in several ways.

There are at least two qualifiers to the philosophic principle of respect for autonomy that will also have face validity for nonphilosophers: First, the principle does not give license to one person to limit or interfere with the autonomy or rights of another person. Second, the principle recognizes that some people cannot be autonomous because of impaired decision-making capacity. Both of these conditions, however, are hard to measure.

In the context of health decisions, Drane (1984, 1985) argues that the greater the importance of the decision and the greater the benefits or risks of potential actions, the higher the expectation for competence in the decision maker. Under this rule, a less-stringent test of decision-making ability would be required for the principle of autonomy to apply to refusal of a minor elective health procedure than to refusal of life-saving, low-risk surgery. But, however the thresholds for competence are set, and regardless of whether the thresholds vary for different kinds of decisions, autonomy implies an autonomous agent capable of making a decision. Thus, the concept of personal autonomy, as it refers to self-rule, is virtually irrelevant for people who do not achieve the threshold.

The principle of respect for autonomy is entrenched as a value in the social work profession, where it is usually called "self-determination." But self-determination has been notoriously difficult to define and apply to practice, leading one commentator (Rothman, 1989) to suggest that the value should be abandoned and replaced by a continuum for desirable directiveness on the part of the clinical social worker.

Autonomy as Informed Consent

The most visible manifestation of the pursuit of autonomy in acute care settings is informed consent. The ethics literature has promulgated conditions that must be met before one can say informed consent has been given. These include freedom from coercion, availability of choices, capability of understanding the consequences of each alternative choice, and, in some views, an ability to relate these choices to one's own values and preferences.

Thus, an autonomous decision to consent to treatment is made freely, with choices, information, and understanding. Although such a list of attributes seems sensible, each one is difficult to make operational. For example, coercion comes in blatant and subtle forms, including conscious manipulation of information about risks and benefits. Furthermore, few people make decisions alone, nor should they be forced to do so, and it is sometimes difficult to distinguish coercion from persuasion or even from family and professional advice.

Some might go so far as to argue that, by definition, nursing home residents, like prison inmates, are not free from coercion and, therefore, can never be autonomous. But without making that leap, it is certainly clear that the very dependency of a physically frail nursing home resident or home care client on his or her caretakers may introduce an element of coercion. This element may also be present when extremely disabled persons depend on others for care in their own homes.

Similarly, measuring the ability to comprehend information related to choices and to weigh the consequences of these choices against one's own values is difficult. One strategy is to measure cognitive ability directly through a host of approaches ranging in detail and scope from brief screening tests to more elaborate batteries. For example, Wang & Ennis (1986) developed their cognitive competency test in an effort to measure directly the skills needed in everyday life, including exercises that test problem solving in areas such as household tasks and way finding. Others argue that competence can never be adequately assessed by a standardized test and that assessment of competence is better approached by a multidisciplinary group that has ample opportunity to observe the subject over time and discuss the context in which competence is to be exercised (Silberfeld, Harvey, Dickens, & Pepper-Smith, 1988).

Some researchers have attempted to measure the ability to make decisions and reason adequately in a way that goes well beyond general tests of intellectual capacity. One approach involves interviewing the patient after a medical recommendation has been made to determine what the patient understood about the condition, the recommended treatment, the risks, and the benefits (Kaplan, 1988). Another approach asks the person whose capability is being tested to respond to fixed medical scenarios, also giving their decisions and their reasons (Fitten, 1990; Tymchuk, Ouslander, Rahbar, & Fitten, 1988). It is, presumably, the reasons rather than the decision itself that allow the researcher or health care provider to know whether a decision not to follow medical recommendations is based on understanding of the likely consequences in light of the patient's own values.

As far as could be determined, there has been no effort to measure decision-making capability with regard to the more diffuse and ordinary decisions that are made in a social context—for example, to spend money on a particular item, to move to a long-term care facility, to risk a fall by rejecting physical restraints, or to accept or refuse home health care. Indeed, it is much harder to pinpoint actual decision points in matters that are drawn out over time or that may involve repeated decisions (e.g., multiple purchases) in contrast with relatively defined decisions about, say, to do surgery or not or to have chemotherapy or not. Moody (1988) argues that the paradigm of informed consent that involves determining whether a person is capable, has choices, and is free from coercion and then involves respecting their choices is faulty in long-term care. He proposes a model of negotiated consent that takes into account varying capacity, competing interests, and appropriate paternalism.

Autonomy as Authenticity

Although not all agree, some philosophers have introduced the element of authenticity to the discussion of autonomy (Dworkin, 1976; Miller, 1981). An authentic action or decision is one that is consistent with previously expressed values and, therefore, seems characteristic of the person. (According to some tests, authenticity is also a part of decision-making capability, discussed above.) To take Caplan's (1990a) example, if an unathletic university professor decides in his middle years to join the circus, family and friends might rightly question whether this was an autonomous decision on the grounds of authenticity. Caplan (1990b) argues elsewhere that older people may be at the best part of the life stage for realization of full autonomy, including the criterion of authenticity. In contrast, an adolescent in the throes of forming a personal identity is less capable of a fully autonomous decision than someone mature in years. By that token, an elderly, cognitively intact person should be the *most* capable of autonomy in the sense of authenticity because he or she has had a lifetime to understand and refine his or her own values.

Like self-direction, freedom from coercion, and decision-making capability, authenticity is also a difficult concept to make operational. It would seem to require advance knowledge of the person's values and priorities with which to compare the person's present decision. Theoretically, the notion of authenticity has another problem: If carried to an extreme, a person who would not be able to make anything other than minor changes in direction or focus would still be considered autonomous.

Autonomy in Everyday Matters

In biomedical ethics, most attention to autonomy has concerned decisions to use or refrain from using various life saving medical technologies or to choose among an array of possible therapies, each with its likely benefits and risks. Here the law seems quite clear that competent adults may make their own health decisions even if they fly in the face of medical advice, as long as the only risk they are taking is to themselves.

But residents of long-term care facilities typically find their autonomy restricted in an all-encompassing way by the rules and routines of the organization, their own physical need for help, and the unfavorable balance of power between themselves and everyone else in the environment. In the most dramatic sense, older persons may be physically restrained (e.g., tied in bed or in a chair, or confined to a geri-chair, which somewhat resembles a high chair for grownups). Or they may be given high doses of sedatives and other mind-altering drugs. The informed consent processes for either of these strategies are often skipped over or assumed to have been incorporated in the general consent to care given by the person when admitted to the facility.

Other restrictions to autonomy are more subtle, but pervasive. The resident is expected to get up at a particular time and, usually, to go to bed by a particular time. He or she is expected to take meals when they are offered, be available for baths and other personal care procedures when the staff schedules them, and not be overly particular about who shares his or her room. For their safety, nursing home residents are usually not permitted to go outside the building unsupervised. They are expected to adhere to their diets and will not have the prerogative enjoyed by so many Americans of all ages to cheat on the diet a bit. Because of federal and state regulations as well as facility routines, they are not free to arrange their furniture (e.g., put the bed against the wall) or to keep equipment in their rooms that might be considered dangerous (perhaps including candles, scissors, and various toiletries that are poisonous if ingested). Whereas disabled people in their own homes can arrange all their necessities to be within their reach, nursing home residents may be forced to store everyday items in a locked drawer that they cannot gain access to themselves. Typically, the nursing home resident has no direct access to his or her own money either, and cannot freely initiate purchase of goods or services. In summary, the small details of nursing home residents' lives are governed by their care plans, which lay out in considerable detail what they will be permitted to do (Kane & Caplan, 1990).

The above, admittedly overgeneralized, portrait does not sound like a prescription for autonomy. Yet, there are few clear-cut decisions around which one can say autonomy has been violated. Activities such as eating, getting up or going to bed, having a bath, or taking a walk down the street are barely matters of conscious decision making for most people. It is only when freedom is lost in those small details that the restriction of autonomy is noticed (Caplan, 1990a).

Long ago, Goffman (1961) described the characteristics of total institutions, in which the inmates are relatively powerless. Although Goffman was referring to prisons and mental hospitals, some commentators (Foldes, 1990; Gubrium, 1975; Shield, 1988) have extended the analogy to nursing homes.

If a nursing home is a total institution as is a prison, personal autonomy as a concept has little relevance. Although surely nursing homes are somewhat less than total institutions, the physical dependency of the clientele, the power of the staff over the lives of the residents, and the unshakable routines of the organization (which are, in part, driven by resource constraints) all militate against the expression of personal autonomy. More excusable—perhaps inevitable—are constraints on the personal autonomy of each resident derived from the nursing home being a collective, residential setting where the interests of an individual may need to give way to those of the group. To the extent that the environment and program is structured to afford privacy, the group is less likely to impinge on the individual.

Note that personal autonomy on small matters can be compromised in ways presumably injurious to quality of life even when older persons receive long-term care in their own homes. There, too, the disabled person depends on the availability and goodwill of others—family members, paid caregivers, or both. The scheduling problems of a home care agency may mean that older people have little control over their daily movements or the timing of care routines, including going to bed and getting up.

Autonomy as Independence

In common parlance, autonomy is often equated with independence. The ability to perform daily activities independently is seen as at least a covariant that is associated with greater autonomy if not a necessary condition or even a synonym for autonomy. Indeed, a French scale for measuring ability to perform activities of daily living (ADLs) is billed as a measure of "autonomy" (Israel, Kozerevic, & Sartorius, 1984).

One of the primary goals of long-term care is to improve, maintain, or prevent a client's deterioration in physical functioning as measured by ADL scales. And because people who can walk themselves, dress themselves, and perform a variety of functions independently are in a better position to exercise autonomy, it is easy to glide into equating personal autonomy with physical independence. This seems to be a conceptual error, however. Some autonomy in the sense of self-rule can be exercised by people with substantial disabilities. Granted, the more disabled a person is, the more likely he or she will be to depend on the goodwill and good offices of others to carry out autonomous designs. At some levels of disability, autonomy is maintained only with the cooperation of helpers and agents of various kinds. But unless the two concepts—physical functioning and personal autonomy—are kept separate, it will be impossible to study the extent to which increasing physical disability is correlated with reduced personal autonomy.

To illustrate how personal autonomy can be maintained in the face of severe functional disability, consider Franz Rosenzweig, an influential Jewish philosopher afflicted with amyotrophic lateral sclerosis (ALS) who for the last eight years of his life had rapidly progressing paralysis of all his limbs and speech organs. In the age before computers, he lived and worked in a Berlin upper-floor apartment, communicating painstakingly by pointing to the keys on a typewriter and, when he could no longer point, affirming the choice of the key made by someone else. Conversation required his wife to run repeatedly through the alphabet, choosing the characters letter by letter according to her husband's facial cues and sometimes speeding things up by guessing his intended word. Under this painful circumstances, Franz Rosenzweig conducted a voluminous correspondence, continued his studies and publications, and, in collaboration with Martin Buber, made a definitive translation of the Old Testament from Hebrew to German.

Rosenzweig's physician and other visitors have left an account of his daily life (Glatzer, 1961). From his doctor, we learn that he was taken out of bed each morning at 8 a.m., and the process of getting him out of bed, dressed, and seated in his chair took about two to two and a half hours. Eating breakfast took another hour. He usually worked for an hour and a half before lunch and again after an afternoon nap until dinner at eight, after which he read until midnight. His nurses were summoned to turn pages by his clearing his throat or turning his head.

Despite extreme physical dependency, Rosenzweig is described as being in charge:

> F.R. took an active part in the creation of this supporting apparatus [a head

support], as well as in the preparation of the typewriter. He was never simply a passive object of medical treatment and feminine nursing, but always the master of the house, whose wish, after the question had been discussed from every side, finally prevailed.

F.R. was the dominant, active center of all domestic affairs—at least to the extent that a man is concerned with such things—as well as of all social contacts. In this regard, too, he planned and organized everything in advance. Visitors were asked to arrive punctually at a specified time. For parties and festivities, everything was prepared down to the smallest detail. When the guests arrived the patient was already sitting in his chair; he liked to drink coffee beforehand to make himself alert for conversation. . . . All conversation was managed through Mrs. Rosenzweig.

. . . just as he never, despite his muteness and extreme difficulty of conversation, would renounce such apparently superfluous interjections as "For heaven's sake!"—with a little experience one could anticipate them from the mildly shocked expression of his face and mouth—in the same way he insisted in maintaining by every possible means a manner of life consistent with his great gifts and numerous human relationships (Glatzer, 1981, pp. 141–142).

As the descriptions show, despite his great functional incapacity, Rosenzweig was in control. But without the cooperation of his wife and nurses, he could not have exercised such decision-making power. Without the willingness of his family, friends, and colleagues to help him study, work, and communicate, he could hardly have "insisted" on anything.

The subtle relationship between personal autonomy and physical independence is at the heart of a paradox in long-term care. Professionals who operate from a rehabilitation paradigm assume that the more patients or clients can do for themselves the more autonomous they are and the better off they will be. Thus, some commentators indict the nursing home for a lack of rehabilitation focus. This may unintentionally lead some of the most sincere advocates for older people into downplaying the importance of a responsive attitude to requests from someone who is physically impaired.

For example, one nursing study (Barton, Baltes, & Orzech, 1980) observed nurses' aides as they offered care and labeled as dependency-generating all responses wherein the aide fulfilled requests in an unquestioning way. Encounters in which the aide encouraged the resident to do the activity him- or herself were called independence-generating. But this construct may ultimately deprive long-term care clients, in nursing homes and the community, of autonomy in precisely the small, daily matters that seem so related to well-being and quality of life. A rehabilitation plan may require a hardheaded attitude to promote recovery to an expected level of functioning, and the resulting increased physical independence will be associated with potential greater autonomy. But many long-term care clients will always have functional limitations. Their ability to exercise choice and control may depend on the willingness of their helpers to accede to their requests on their timetables. It would be ironic if a stance toward rehabilitation, improperly applied, were to effectively further limit the choice and control of persons who are already so limited physically.

Thus, autonomy for the extremely impaired may be limited to decision making. Whether and how decisions are carried out depends on the willingness of others. The subtleties of how quality of life is related to this two-part scenario is unclear. We do not know whether exercising autonomy in making decisions relates positively to quality of life, regardless of the extent to which the decision is carried out.

Autonomy as Advance Directives

Autonomy in the sense of self-rule is impossible for many persons with severe or even moderate senile dementia such as that caused by Alzheimer's disease. Some would argue that, although it is morally imperative to treat such people with dignity and kindness and to respect their authenticity based on their previous identities, autonomy is entirely irrelevant to this group. Persons officially labeled as having Alzheimer's disease will still often retain the ability to express preference (perhaps for food or activities), and one should be mindful that honoring those preferences would cause no harm. In other matters, one should act to promote the cognitively impaired person's well-being to the best of one's understanding.

Oddly enough, however, a great deal of attention has been given to the autonomy of people who can no longer exercise it in any easily understood sense of the word. The generally accepted way of respecting autonomy for the cognitively impaired is by working through their agents or surrogates and by following any previous directives that the impaired person made for how they would wish to be treated in the event they could not make their own decisions. In some instances, the advance directive might indicate whom the cognitively impaired person wishes to have act as an agent.

This sense of autonomy as executed through advance directives is conceptually confusing. It is possible, for instance, that an advance directive would assert a preference incompatible with the person's current preferences as far as they can be discerned. To take a hypothetical example, if a person with an advance directive stating opposition to ever moving to a nursing home seemed most content while living in a nursing home and highly resistant to leaving it, which course is more respectful of autonomy—adhering to the advance directive or to what seems to be the present wish? Or, if the surrogate decision maker named in the advance directive ordered caregivers to use physical restraints, and the older person seemed vehemently opposed to those restraints, which is more respectful of autonomy: to scrupulously let the surrogate decision maker make the judgments or to follow cues given by the patient despite his or her diminished competence and overrule the advance directive? It is unclear whether honoring advance directives always promotes the vestiges of autonomy of which a person may be capable.

Because it is virtually impossible to anticipate one's reaction to an unknown condition such as an altered physical state or to life with a serious disability, preferences expressed about such circumstances must be based on experience and understanding. Sighted people may believe that conditions such as blindness are worst than death but, on becoming blind, may learn that they prefer life in that state to death after all. It is particularly impossible to predict how one would value life in a state of seriously diminished cognitive capacity, because the feedback available from persons in those states is so limited.

So far, advance directives have been applied only to prohibitions against heroic medical treatments or to identifying the surrogate decision maker whom the person making the directive trusts. These advance directives impose few costs or burdens on others. An advance directive requiring a high-cost treatment or insisting on care of a particular sort and from a particular family member or organization would surely have no force unless cemented by a legal contract.

Measurement and Relationship to Quality of Life

The bulk of this chapter has dealt with the concept of autonomy. Given the complexity of the concept and its roots in philosophy, however, it is not surprising that the measurement of autonomy is embryonic and rarely direct.

In the last decade, the Retirement Research Foundation conducted an initiative in personal autonomy in long-term care. This consisted of a series of several dozen interrelated research, development, and demonstration projects, funded in two phases over a four-year period. The overall purpose was to further explore the nature of personal autonomy in long-term care, along with the conditions associated with it and ways to enhance it. The initial set of projects can be grouped into three categories according to the slant each held on autonomy: projects focusing on individual rights and protection of freedom of choice; projects emphasizing the individual's capacities to express and implement a choice; and projects exploring the preferences of the individual and his or her significant others (David, 1986). The second round of projects continued these emphases but also included those designed to measure phenomena related to autonomy, including a project to develop and use a form for measuring values of older long-term care clients (Gibson, 1990) and a project to develop a measure of paternalistic tendencies in family members of the elderly.

The Retirement Research Foundation projects have, collectively, greatly increased the common understanding of personal autonomy as a concept relevant to long-term care. They have also documented the abridgments of freedom and choice that occur in long-term care settings. But they actually skirted the measurement of autonomy per se. None of the projects, including our own (Kane & Caplan, 1990), directly measure this elusive concept, though many measure conditions (e.g., admission contracts for nursing homes, informed consent processes, satisfaction with choices) that should be related to autonomy or to perceived autonomy. Perhaps the nature of this concept—part philosophical and part empirically observable, part a condition that pertains to a person and part a characteristic of an action or a decision—renders it exceedingly difficult to measure.

Several approaches to approximating autonomy are discussed below.

Case Analysis

Autonomy as a moral imperative—that is, as a principle that *should* be followed—cannot be measured in the sense that a social scientist would think of measurement. Rather, on a case-by-case basis, moral philosophers can consider whether the principle of autonomy was properly respected, and any two philosophers may well disagree in a particular case.

Furthermore, even if a consensus could be achieved about whether the principle was upheld or violated in a particular case, hypotheses about resultant quality of life are unclear. Quality of life as it is usually measured in long-term care— that is, by a client's expressed well-being or satisfaction or by various objective indicators of physical, emotional, or social well-being—may not be correlated with whether that person's autonomy was respected in the sense of meeting a philosopher's caveats. People can autonomously make bad choices or can make choices that involve self-sacrifice or that put priority on something other than their own happiness. Sometimes, there are no good choices to be made in terms of their results.

Methods could be devised to examine cases and strive toward an imperfect philosophical consensus on what is appropriate recognition of autonomy. For example, in our own work, we have made a beginning of this (Kane and Caplan, 1990) by accumulating the kind of cases affecting everyday autonomy that actually arise in nursing home life and by asking philosophers to discuss them. Such cases include questions over who has the right to control a television channel, who gets the next single room, and whether staff should isolate or integrate a person with dementia who is disturbing the group. This exercise culminated in a working conference where considerable agreement was reached that personal autonomy is inappropriately abridged in nursing homes. For instance, no ethical justification could be found for insisting on uniform rising times or bedtimes, prohibiting time alone outdoors or trips outside the nursing home without escort, withholding alcohol or over-the-counter medicines from *all* residents, or strictly controlling residents' mail, phone calls, or funds. Implicit was the belief that the quality of life of nursing home residents on average might have been higher had respect for personal autonomy been greater, but our approach could not have begun to test that assumption.

Autonomous Decisions

Autonomy typically is examined in the context of a decision. Most studies of the decisions of older people cluster around two topics: residential decisions—especially decisions to move to a nursing home—and, more recently, decisions about whether to accept life-sustaining medical treatments in various circumstances. Particularly with the former category of decision, efforts have been made to determine whether control and choice over the decision was associated with the older person's quality of life and health outcomes, measured in a variety of ways.

Without reviewing this extensive literature (see Lieberman, Chapter 6), some comments could be made about using such decisions as a proxy for autonomy. First, the information is almost always gathered retrospectively, and it seems that there are no studies that compare people's comments on a decision at the time of the decision with their reconstruction of the same decision later on. Investigators typically must content themselves with the responses to a few questions that tap whether the persons in question felt they were in control of the decision, the extent to which others assisted them in decision making, and, perhaps, whether they wanted to take the action in question. For example, Reinardy (1990) examined the relationship between various outcomes of nursing home life, perceived control over the decision to move there, and perceived desirability of the move, separately and in interaction with each other. But he acknowledges the great difficulty of working with scanty information, collected retrospectively. (Even if one had excellent and full information collected prospectively, it would still be difficult to know how to incorporate the help of others into the determination that a decision was or was not autonomous, but the objective aspects of the decision such as who was involved, the choices considered, the opinions of all concerned, and the reasons cited by all parties for the final decision could indeed be measured).

In their classic work on the psychology of decision making, Janis and Mann (1977) remind us of the human propensity to justify and bolster a decision already made. They theorized that ideal decision making includes an appraisal of the practical implications of all the available alternatives for the decision maker, those he or she cares about, and the implications for self-esteem (How would I feel about myself if I made that choice? How would others I care about feel about me?). Having made a decision that way, they hypothesized less postdecisional regret, even if the decision involved unhappy choices or if later events proved the decision to have been unfortunate. In theory, if one has made the best decision one could have at the time, regret is minimized. The two factors most associated with inadequate decision making in this model are a sense of despair about the alternatives and a sense of panic about the time available. Both these features may be present for elderly long-term care clients.

The Janis and Mann model of decision making, which has had only sporadic empirical testing, is compatible with the concept of an autonomous decision in the informed consent literature—both emphasize uncoerced choice, information seeking, and testing the alternatives against one's values and preferences.

Measuring autonomy around decision making is of somewhat limited utility in studying the relationship between autonomy or perceived autonomy and the quality of life of long-term care users. The following problems arise:

- The samples usually include only those who have made a particular decision, such as relocation, and omit those who considered the option and decided not to take action.
- The decision approach gives too much weight to the characteristics of a particular decision as evidence of autonomy or lack of it rather than examining a pattern of decision.
- Although memorable decisions are of interest, a person's autonomy may also rest on the numerous small decisions that are regularly made. (This is reminiscent of the old joke about the man who made all the big decisions— whether to go to war, how to save the national economy—while permitting his wife to make the small decisions—what to eat and how to spend their money and their time.)

Everyday Autonomy, Choice, and Control

As mentioned above, psychologists have studied the relationship between perceived control and choice and quality of life (some of this material is reviewed by Abeles, Chapter 14). Indeed, there is some overlap between the concept of perceived control and autonomy, although the ideas are distinct.

In recent studies at the University of Minnesota, Kane and colleagues (1990) have attempted to examine personal autonomy in the everyday life of nursing home residents. However, they found it necessary to approximate the subject rather than try to measure that autonomy directly. In the first exploration, they attempted to learn how important choice and control was to nursing home residents concerning selected mundane matters of everyday life. For that study they randomly selected 25 facilities in the Twin Cities and then randomly selected three cognitively intact residents in each facility, stratified to include one resident who had been in the facility less than six months. The process was replicated in five homes in four other cities—Santa Fe, Little Rock, Los Angeles, and New

York. They also were interested in how nurses' aides, the staff members most in contact with residents, perceived these same everyday matters. A sample of nurse's aides was drawn from the same 45 facilities, stratified to select a day shift, evening shift, and night shift employee from each facility.

Table 1 shows the items included and the responses from residents. Given the option of rating a topic as very important, somewhat important, or not important, over half the residents thought it very important to have control over most of the matters listed. Two-thirds thought control and choice over leaving the facility for short times and over access to a telephone very important, and 56% thought control over roommate selection very important (a proportion that would be higher if those with single rooms had been excluded from the denominator). The last column indicates the proportion who were very satisfied with the control and choice available to them on these items.

Table 2 shows how nurses' aides viewed the same items. For the most part, these staff members also thought choice and control on these matters was important to residents. Staff were more likely than residents to rate items as very important (perhaps because nursing home residents tend away from extreme opinions), but the rank order of importance perceived by staff also differed somewhat from that perceived by residents. More telling was the pessimism of aides in their view of how likely it is for nursing home residents to have choice in these matters. For instance, only 19% saw residents as having choice most of the time in the particulars of when they got up in the morning.

This study did not attempt to measure quality of life of nursing home residents

Table 1   Residents' Desire for and Satisfaction with Control over Selected Aspects of Everyday Life

Topical Areas Ranked by % of Residents Saying Area Is Very Important to Them	% of Residents Saying Area Is Very Important	% of Residents Very Satisfied with Amount of Choice in Area
Leaving the facility for short times	67.4	37.8
Phone use or mail receipt	66.7	39.3
Choice of roommates	56.3	26.7
Nursing home activities	56.3	35.6
Food	55.6	21.5
Care routines	54.1	31.1
Money matters	53.3	33.3
Getting up in morning	52.6	40.0
Going to bed	48.9	42.2
Visitors	40.0	36.3

Note: Data obtained from a study of 135 residents, representatively sampled from 45 nursing homes in five states in a project funded by the Retirement Research Foundation (Kane et al., 1990).

Table 2 Views of Nurse's Aides on the Importance and Feasibility of Resident Control over Selected Aspects of Everyday Life

Topical Areas Ranked by % of Aides Saying Area Is Very Important to Residents	% Aides Saying Area Is Very Important to Residents	% Aides Saying Residents Have Choices in Area Most of the Time
Nursing home activities	80	63
Leaving the facility for short times	72	48
Visitors	71	51
Food	69	24
Getting up in morning	65	19
Choice of roommates	64	13
Care routines	63	33
Going to bed	58	33
Money matters	51	44
Phone or mail use	49	52

Note: Data obtained from a study of 134 nurses' aides, representatively sampled from 45 nursing homes in five states in a project funded by the Retirement Research Foundation (Kane et al., 1990).

and equate it with their satisfaction with choice and control over matters that they deemed important. Even the measures of choice and control were far from precise—for example, the researchers did not offer uniform definitions of the items. Despite this, the exercise did convince us that there are vast areas of nursing home routine that compromise personal autonomy in fundamental ways that many residents care about.

Perceived Latitude of Choice

Various investigators have attempted to develop measures to capture how well older people realize choice and control over matters of importance to them. These embryonic measures were reviewed a decade ago in a compendium on assessment of the elderly (Kane & Kane, 1981). Since then, the investigators working in the area have continued with the development and application of their measures.

The Locus of Desired Control Scale (Reid, Haas, & Hawkins, 1977) contains seven items that are rated on a 4-point scale in terms of how desirable and important they are for the person (namely, to receive regular visits from family or friends; to decide on one's own daily activities; to place one's possessions where one wants them; to receive attention and recognition from those around one; to see one's doctor when one asks for him or her; to find privacy from others; and to be with friends at the nursing home when one wants). Respondents then rate the extent to which they can achieve these seven ends on a 4-point scale from "never" to "always." The scores for the desirability column are multiplied by the scores for the control column to get a total score for each item and the scale. Reid and Ziegler (1980) report that the scores are correlated with overall life satisfaction.

The Latitude of Choice measure is a more elaborate approach to examining actual choice in relation to desired choice, and more work has been reported with this scale (Hulicka, Cataldo, Morganti, & Nehrke, 1983; Hulicka, Morganti, & Cataldo, 1975; Morganti, Nehrke, & Hulicka, 1980). It consists of 37 statements that are rated first by their importance and then by the choice the individual actually has. It was designed for use in institutional or residential settings for people of all ages. Context of the statements include: whom to sit with at meals; whom to have for friends; what time to get up; where to spend free time; what type of haircut to have; what to spend money on; whether to associate with other people; what name to be called; what papers or books to read; what personal possession to have; where to work; what type of work to do; and whether to live at the same place or go elsewhere. Importance and choice are each rated on Likert scales and the scores multiplied for each item. Thus, a score of 9 for an item connotes a combination of maximum importance and maximum choice, whereas a score of 1 connotes an item with maximum importance and no choice. The authors suggest that the latter can be equated with low perceived autonomy. They found that on average, the items were rated as more important by women in non-VA nursing homes, as compared with male veterans in a domiciliary home. The authors found that latitude of choice scores correlate with life satisfaction and in some populations with self-esteem, but the associations were stronger in a population of frail institutionalized women than in a population of relatively functionally intact veterans living in a domiciliary home.

These measures that weight the availability of choice and control to emphasize matters that the older person indicates are important have face validity as an approach to examining perceptions of autonomy. Even these are limited by the presentation of a fixed list (the subject may have experienced a loss of autonomy on some very important matter that was not on the list), and the scoring (which gives equal importance to each item) may not accurately reflect the overall perceptions of autonomy. However, this was the most direct approach to measuring autonomy that could be identified. It is important to recognize that what is measured here is perceived latitude of choice and, by extension, perceived autonomy rather than autonomous actions.

Autonomy-Respecting Environments

Elsewhere, Kane (1990) identified four Rs as enemies of personal autonomy—routine, regulation, restricted capacity, and resource constraints. The last item, resource constraints, militates against creating the environment or the staffing ratios that might permit autonomy to flourish. Regulation is peculiarly intensive in the nursing home sphere where the same regulations designed to protect residents also restrict them, often in minute and intimate ways. Routines established for administrative convenience can have a similarly dampening effect on autonomy. All four Rs interact.

Future work might nominate aspects of the environment and programs that promote personal autonomy on everyday matters so that nursing homes and other care settings could be rated according to their presence or absence. Some obvious features include single rooms, quick response time to call buttons from staff members, telephone technology that permits easy use by disabled residents, staggered meal times, choice of menus, and choice of schedule for care routines, including time for getting up and going to bed.

Few of these may seem feasible in the current regulatory and care environments. If so, perhaps thought should be given to how cognitively intact persons could be enabled to receive long-term care without a sacrifice of small daily freedoms. Policy and administrative changes may be necessary, some of which require action from outside the nursing home. For example, to facilitate residents taking short trips away from the facility, the issue of liability for unaccompanied trips needs to be solved (perhaps residents could waive liability), and the issue of transportation may require that nursing home residents be considered eligible for subsidized transportation for the elderly.

Conclusion

Without being able to measure autonomy directly and without a large body of research as yet to link personal autonomy to quality of life, it seems "self-evident" (to again invoke language from the Declaration of Independence) that personal autonomy is an important human desire. Autonomy does not mean getting everything one wants, but it does seem to mean having a chance to exercise some control and choice and to make decisions concerning oneself. It also seems self-evident that such autonomy is sadly and unnecessarily abridged for many people needing long-term care. Resources will probably always be insufficient to permit full autonomy to persons who require the constant help of one or more people to bring it about, but it should surely be feasible to improve on the current situation. The desire to protect through regulation could also be tempered by respect for personal autonomy and, perhaps, for greater priority in enforcing those regulations that demand respect for autonomy over those that emphasize safety. In order to accomplish this, we must learn what areas of personal autonomy are most precious to long-term care clients, and clients must be involved on an individual basis in deciding how they would like to use the personal help available to them in the service of their own autonomy.

References

Avorn, J., & Langer, E. (1982). Induced disability in nursing home patients: A controlled trial. *Journal of the American Geriatrics Society, 30,* 397–400.

Barton, E. M., Baltes, M. M., & Orzech, M. H. (1980). Etiology of dependence in older nursing home residents during morning care: The roles of staff behavior. *Journal of Personality and Social Psychology, 38,* 423–431.

Beauchamp, T., & Childress, J. F. (1983). *Principles of Biomedical Ethics.* New York: Oxford University Press.

Caplan, A. L. (1990a). Morality of the mundane: Ethical issues arising in the daily lives of nursing home residents. In R. A. Kane & A. L. Caplan, eds., *Everyday ethics: Resolving dilemmas in nursing home life,* pp. 37–52. New York: Springer Publishing Company.

Caplan, A. L. (1990b). The values baseline—A solution or an obstacle to enhancing the autonomy of the elderly. Paper prepared for Working Conference on Values Baseline Assessment, University of Minnesota Long-Term Care DECISIONS Resource Center, April 24–25 (mimeo). Minneapolis, Minn.

Childress, J. F. (1984). Ensuring care, respect, and fairness for the elderly. *Hastings Center Report, 14,* 27–31.

Childress, J. F. (1990). The place of autonomy in bioethics. *Hastings Center Report, 20,* 12–17.

Collopy, B. (1988). Autonomy in long-term care: Some crucial distinctions. *The Gerontologist, 28,* (Suppl.), 10–17.

David, D. (1986). An evaluation of initiative projects: Research issues in operationalizing autonomy. Paper presented at Gerontological Society of America, November, Chicago, Ill.

Drane, J. F. (1984). Competency to give an informed consent. *Journal of the American Medical Association, 252,* 925–927.

Drane, J. F. (1985). The many faces of competency. *Hastings Center Report, 15,* 17–21.

Dworkin, G. (1976). Autonomy and behavior control. *Hastings Center Report, 6,* 23–28.

Englehardt, T. (1986). *The foundations of biomedical ethics.* New York: Oxford University Press.

Fitten, L. J. (1990). Assessing treatment decision-making capacity in elderly hospitalized patients and nursing home residents. In deciding whether the client can decide: Assessment of Decision-Making Capability, R. A. Kane & C. D. King, eds., pp. 112–117. University of Minnesota Long-Term Care DECISIONS Resource Center, December 18–19, 1989 (mimeo). Minneapolis, Minn.

Foldes, S. F. (1990). Life in an institution: A sociological and anthropological view. In R. A. Kane & A. L. Caplan, eds., *Everyday ethics: Resolving dilemmas in nursing home life,* pp. 21–36. New York: Springer Publishing Company.

Gibson, J. M. (1990). National values history project. *Generations, XIV* Supplement, 51–64.

Glatzer, N. N., ed. (1961). *Franz Rosenzweig: His life and thought,* 2nd rev. ed. New York: Schocken Books.

Goffman, E. (1961). *Asylums: Essays on the social situation of mental patients and other inmates.* Garden City, N.Y.: Anchor Books.

Gubrium, J. (1975). *Living and dying at Murray Manor*. New York: St. Martin's Press.

Hulicka, I. M., Morganti, J. B., & Cataldo, J. F. (1975). Perceived latitude of choice of institutionalized and noninstitutionalized elderly women. *Experimental Aging Research, 1,* 27–39.

Hulicka, I. M., Cataldo, J. F., Morganti, J. B., & Nehrke, M. F. (1983). Perceptions of choice and importance by the elderly: Implications for intervention. *Interdisciplinary Topics in Gerontology, 17,* 25–39.

Israel, L., Kozerevic, D., & Sartorius, N. (1984). *Source book of geriatric assessment*. New York: S. Karger.

Janis, I. L. & Mann, L. (1977). *Decision-making: A psychological analysis of conflict, choice, and commitment*. New York: Free Press.

Kane, R. A. (1990). Everyday life in nursing houses: The way things are. In Everyday ethics: Resolving dilemmas in nursing home life. R. A. Kane and A. L. Caplan, eds., pp. 3–20. New York: Springer Publishing Company.

Kane, R. A., & Caplan, A. L., eds. (1990). *Everyday ethics: Resolving dilemmas in nursing home life*. New York: Springer Publishing Company.

Kane, R. A., & Kane, R. L. (1981). *Assessing the elderly: A practical guide to measurement*. Lexington, Mass.: D. C. Heath.

Kane, R. A., Freeman, I. C., Caplan, A. L., Aroskar, M. A., & Urv-Wong, E. K. (1990). Everyday autonomy in nursing homes. *Generations, XIV* Supplement, 69–71.

Kaplan, K. H. (1988). Assessing judgment. *General Hospital Psychiatry, 9,* 202–208.

Langer, E., & Rodin, J. (1986). The effects of choice and enhanced personal responsibility for the aged: A field experiment in an institutional setting. *Journal of Personality and Social Psychology, 34,* 191–198.

Miller, B. (1981). Autonomy and the refusal of life-saving treatment. *Hastings Center Report, 11,* 22–28.

Moody, H. R. (1988). From informed consent to negotiated consent. *The Gerontologist, 28* (Suppl.), 64–70.

Morganti, J. B., Nehrke, M. F., & Hulicka, I. M. (1980). Residents and staff perceptions of latitude of choice in elderly institutionalized men. *Experimental Aging Research, 6,* 367–384.

Reid, D. W., & Ziegler, M. (1980). Validity and stability of a new desired control measure pertaining to the psychological adjustment of the elderly. *Journal of Gerontology, 35,* 395–402.

Reid, D. W., Hass, G., & Hawkins, D. (1977). Locus of desired control and positive self-concept of the elderly. *Journal of Gerontology, 32,* 441–450.

Reinardy, J. (1990). *Personal control in the decision to enter a nursing home as a predictor of post admission well-being*. Doctoral diss., University of Minnesota School of Social Work.

Rodin, J. (1986). Aging and health: Effects of the sense of control. *Science, 233,* 1271–1275.

Rodin, J., & Langer, E. (1977). Long-term effects of a control-relevant intervention with the institutionalized aged. *Journal of Personality and Social Psychology, 35,* 897–902.

Rothman, J. (1989). Client self-determination: Untangling the knot. *Social Service Review, 63,* 598–612.

Schulz, R. (1976). The effects of control and predictability on the psychological and physical well-being of the institutionalized aged. *Journal of Personality and Social Psychology, 36,* 1194–1201.

Shield, R. R. (1988). *Uneasy endings: Daily life in an American nursing home.* Ithica, N.Y.: Cornell University Press.

Silberfeld, M., Harvey, W. R. C., Dickens, B. M., & Pepper-Smith, R. R. J. (1988). A competency clinic for the elderly at Baycrest Center. *The Advocate's Quarterly, 10,* 23–27.

Tymchuk, A. J., Ouslander, J. G., Rahbar, B., & Fitten, L. J. (1988). Medical decision-making among elderly people in long-term care. *The Gerontologist, 28,* (Suppl.), 59–63.

Wang, P. L., & Ennis, K. E. (1986). Competency assessment in clinical populations. In B. Uzzell & Y. Gross, *Clinical neuropsychology of intervention.* Boston: Martius Nijhoff Publishing.

16

Science of Quality of Life of Elders: Challenge and Opportunity

SIDNEY KATZ
BARRY J. GURLAND

This chapter discusses a fundamental concept that challenges scientists and practitioners who are interested in the quality of life of elders, namely the concept of holism. Applied to elders, the concept proposes that the quality of their lives is made up of an irreducible combination of the following interdependent parts: elders themselves, the environment in which they live, and their life experiences in space and time. After describing the need for information about quality of life, a review is presented of the relatively recent emergence of efforts to meet that need by contemporary scientific disciplines. The concept of holism is then discussed, a concept critical to the development and use of information about the quality of life of elders.

A Science of Quality of Life: Why Now?

In the developed countries, increases in longevity and significant increases in the numbers of elders have been associated with expanding personal needs and costly demands for health and social resources. With regard to quality of life, prominent concerns center on the following:

1. Onset of dependency and the prospect of helplessness and death
2. Dislocation from home
3. Transitions from parental and other meaningful, decision-making roles
4. Blows to dignity and self-esteem
5. Loss of respect and affection from others
6. Stresses of changes in physical, mental, social, and economic status on self and family

*The Concept and Measurement of
Quality of Life in the Frail Elderly*

Copyright © 1991 by Academic Press, Inc.
All rights of reproduction in any form reserved.

7. Needs for costly services that are in limited supply and that present individuals, families, and society with tragic choices (e.g., high-risk surgery versus permanent disability)
8. Needs for subsistence, safety, and comfort

During the years ahead, the aging trend is expected to accelerate, and related material and moral dilemmas will surely intensify. Somers has called this trend the "geriatric imperative" (Somers, 1981).

Examples of current activities that deal with the geriatric imperative include the following:

• Self-help in a variety of community-based settings
• Informal assistance by family and friends
• Social and medical services
• Treatment or care in institutions
• Public assistance for subsistence and care

In no instance is there solid evidence about the effectiveness of these activities. Reviews by policy analysts make two points clear. First, society is ill prepared to deal with the geriatric imperative (Callahan & Wallack, 1981; Morris & Youket, 1981; Rivlin & Wiener, 1988, 3–37; Scanlon, Difederico, & Stassen, 1979). Second, the available information is inadequate to justify current actions much less controversial alternatives for future actions (Kurowski & Shaughnessy, 1983; Liu, Manton, & Alliston, 1983). Information about what is done, at what cost, and with what result is in woefully short supply, particularly in terms of the relative benefits and risks of alternative ways of dealing with the geriatric imperative.

With respect to benefits and risks, experts who currently assess service technologies emphasize that services must be evaluated comprehensively (Collen, 1985; Committee for Evaluating Medical Technologies in Clinical Use, 1985; Fusfeld, 1979; Lindberg, 1979; Lohr, 1989; Nelkin, 1979). They state that risks and benefits should be assessed in terms of broad health outcomes and long-term social, economic, and ethical consequences, as well as in terms of immediate and traditional disease-related results. They recognize the holistic implications of assessment and point out that "existing research does not provide a firm basis for comprehensive assessment of usefulness" (Committee for Evaluating Medical Technologies in Clinical Use, 1985). In other words, studies of approaches to the geriatric imperative must take into account more than whether an individual survives or whether blood tests show improvement; it is as important to consider the effects on overall well-being and quality of life, that is, on one's ability to adapt and to find life satisfying.

Interest in the quality of life of elders has been demonstrated at high policy-making levels. The topic was discussed, for example, at a hearing of the U.S. Senate, where one of the summary statements asserted: "Reshaping national programs that concern the elderly through priorities that recognize their functional well-being and the quality of their lives is a challenge that we face and can meet" (Katz, 1984).

Widespread concern about the well-being of residents in nursing homes is another illustration of national interest in the quality of life of elders. Since nursing homes serve as "homes" as well as places of care for those who live out their lives there, moral dilemmas with regard to the quality of life and quality of care invariably accompany the responsibility of providing humane and appropriate living conditions and care. Material dilemmas stem from a growing need for nursing home beds and an expected rise in expenditures from $33 billion in 1986–1990 to $98 billion in 2016–2020, assuming a 5.8% inflation rate (Rivlin & Wiener, 1988, 41–42). Furthermore, qualified service personnel are, and will continue to be, in short supply. Lacking clear information on what to decide about care and living conditions, national nursing home policies are now based on poorly informed judgments and demands (Pifer, 1986, 392–393; Scanlon, Difederico, & Stassen, 1979).

Between 1983 and 1986, an expert committee of the Institute of Medicine of the National Academy of Sciences completed a study of the quality of care and life in nursing homes. The committee observed that professional, nursing home standards did not "explicitly recognize the importance of quality of life" (Committee on Nursing Home Regulation, 1986a). The committee recommended adding a new condition of participation concerning quality of life to certification regulations, a condition based on systematic assessment of all residents (Committee on Nursing Home Regulation, 1986b). Although the committee described factors that are important indicators of quality of life, no scientific evidence was found on which to base a requirement for specific indicators and standards. Research to fill the gap was strongly recommended (Committee on Nursing Home Regulation, 1986c).

Long life spans and the large number of elders only partly explain the prominent interest in the quality of life of elders. Other contributing forces include continuing social and technological changes that affect people of all ages. For example, new production processes and products lead to concerns about the harmful effects of polluted water, radiation, acid rain, and pesticides. Concerns also prevail about the ultimate effects of such technical processes as organ transplants, genetic manipulation, and artificial methods of life support. As a result, manufacturers and those who provide services find themselves increasingly accountable, through regulation and litigation, for mishaps associated with their products and services. In the fields of communication and transportation, technical advances simplify the transfer of information. Thereby, consumers are better informed about possible threats to their ways of life; and they advocate, effectively, for social changes that will improve the quality of their lives (e.g., equal opportunity in work, economic security, education, equal access to health care, and ethical behavior in business, government, law, and medicine).

Beginnings of a Science

Researchers are acutely sensitive to the current scarcity of clear, useful information about the quality of life of elders. Although it is within the province of research to fill informational gaps, the fundamental concepts and methods for producing information about quality of life are yet to be established. In this section, the authors trace the history of the emerging science of quality of life; in the next section, a description is presented of a central concept that challenges pioneers in the field.

For centuries, philosophers and theologians have carried out intellectual explorations of the essence of a good life. Many have viewed the search for a better life as a combination of compelling forces that sets humans apart from lower forms of life (Lovejoy, 1936; Pirsig, 1974; Schumacher, 1977). They have emphasized that forces invisible to the five senses help human beings to shape their environment and their future in search of a better life. Among important examples of these invisible forces are "self-awareness" (Schumacher, 1977), which allows humans to analyze information purposefully, and "diversity" (Lovejoy, 1936, 283–333), which presents contrasting, comparative information that contributes both conflict and empowerment to the process of human reasoning.

Despite this long history, contemporary scientific disciplines have not made a commitment to programs of research into quality of life. Relatively recently, fragmentary interest appeared within the health and social sciences. Szalai (1980) related that sociology colleagues participating in symposia on quality of life in 1978 recalled meeting this term for the first time in the late 1950s and early 1960s, "but not in a scholarly context, rather in popular discussions or general-purpose publications (magazines, newspapers, leaflets, etc.) mostly in connection with problems of environmental pollution, the deterioration of urban living conditions, and the like." Szalai then systematically reviewed the 17-volume *International Encyclopedia of the Social Sciences,* published in 1968, and found no trace of the phrase in its comprehensive index or in its articles and bibliographies on related issues. In another search through 20 encyclopedias and dictionaries published in five world languages between 1968 and 1978, he "could not find a single entry having quality of life as its subject or making a direct reference to it." One indirect reference, "buried in an article about pollution on pages 9638–9 of the great Larousse," stated that the French Ministry of Environment had been renamed "Ministère de la Qualité de Vie" in 1974. Szalai's reviews indicated that up-to-date monitoring in social science literature began only in the 1970s.

In a related effort, the present authors found no record of the phrase in a review of the original *Oxford English Dictionary,* the largest single source of English quotations, indicating that the phrase was rarely used before the present century. Nor did the authors find the phrase in the 1961 unabridged edition of *Webster's International Dictionary* or the 1980 edition of *Bartlett's Quotations.* In a supplemental volume of the *Oxford English Dictionary,* the phrase *quality of life* first appeared in the late 1970s, where eight nonacademic references were cited, one in an environmental context and seven in social, political, or economic contexts. The seven references were to writings or speeches of Adlai Stevenson, Eric Sevareid, and Arthur Schlesinger. No citation was in a health-related context. The first health-related citations were 10 references in *MEDLINE* between 1966 and 1971. In 1978, the phrase *quality of life* was recognized by both the Ninth World Congress of Sociology (Uppsala) and the National Library of Medicine. Since then, academic references to the subject have multiplied manyfold.

As an example of recent, scientific interest in quality of life, behavioral, medical, and social scientists met at the Portugal international conference on the science of quality of life (Katz, 1987). The participants "strongly endorsed the importance of quality of life for a broad range of decisions, extending from clinical decisions for recipients of services to social decisions for program planning and policy making." They emphasized the need "to fulfill the potential usefulness of measures of quality of life" and expressed a need for

> new measures based on alternate constructs of quality of life, studies of the interrelationships among constructs and measures, and validations of usefulness. (Katz, 1987, p. 462)

Challenge to Science

Originating from the ideas of past and present scholars in the humanities, the concept that quality of life is a holistic phenomenon presents major challenges to those who would develop a science of quality of life. Applied to elders, this central concept proposes that the quality of life of elders is made up of an irreducible combination of the following:

1. Elders themselves (i.e., their makeup in terms of body, mind, and spirit)
2. Elders' living and nonliving environments
3. Elders' experiences in space and time

It is clear that, in order to understand the quality of life of elders, one must understand the network of combined parts, since the process of living is not explained by one of the parts alone; nor are life's important decisions made by considering single parts in isolation from others. For example, a daughter who chooses a nursing home for her mother takes into account a combination of many factors, such as service needs, finances, values, beliefs, and the environment.

Bennett (1970) illustrated the interdependence of features in the preceding model as they affect health-related quality of life. Referring to four elements that Cath (1963, 98–99) had termed "anchorages" (i.e., an intact body and mind image, an acceptable home, a socioeconomic anchorage, and a meaningful purpose to life) Bennett pointed out, "These four anchorages provide the structure within which the individual performs the required developmental tasks at various stages of life; and the degree of success with which tasks are performed, and crises met, spells the difference between good and impaired health" (Bennett, 1970).

Ideally, one should take into account the interconnected arrangement of all parts of the model in order to understand the quality of life of elders. Short of that, understanding is incomplete and, too often, of limited use for life's important decisions. This concept is based on the ecological principle that the determining factors in living nature are irreducible wholes (Bateson, 1979). In other words, the functions and powers of nature as a dynamic, living process are created by the interwoven network of component parts. Although the concept recognizes and accepts the need for studies of parts of a given phenomenon, it stresses the overriding need to understand the organic or functional relationships among the parts or, in other words, to understand what happens when the parts are put together.

To date, scientific approaches to quality of life and quality of care have not been sufficiently holistic. Traditional academia has been prematurely reductionist in dealing with these complex matters and has left out important features of quality of life. For example, the objective–subjective axis is always involved in decision making by or on behalf of elders. Yet, the objective–subjective axis is among the least-understood and least-studied features of the quality of life (d'Iribarne, 1972). Without greater holistic understanding of this phenomenon, information provided by research will continue to be limited and controversial, and progress in understanding the quality of life of elders will be inappropriately slow.

In order to attain holistic insight, science is challenged to begin by developing a common language; that is, a common way of speaking about such generally neglected features of the quality of life of elders as attributes whose definitions currently defy consensus (e.g., life experiences, contexts, beliefs, values, attitudes) and the ways that interconnected components work. Another challenge is to develop the basic concepts, theories, and methods for holistic studies of the quality of life of elders. Building on these fundamental steps, a third challenge is to produce substantive information about the relationship between quality of life and aging, as well as about how the quality of life of elders can be improved. Ideas and works discussed by the other contributors to this book offer substantive and methodological guidance about what is missing and how to meet these challenges.

The present authors have been well aware that these challenges are not trivial; thus, they have been developing practical ways of introducing faculty to holistic research and quality of life. During the fall of 1989, for example, the authors introduced the topic to six junior faculty in professional development seminars at Columbia University. They readily accepted the importance of the challenges. Even as they were adventurous and eager, however, they were appropriately practical-minded and asked questions about how to address complex holistic issues that, at first, appeared overwhelming. Using skeleton graphs and tables, relationships were displayed among selected components of a holistic phenomenon, illustrating the changing likelihood of recovering functional independence over time. We then introduced additional dimensions sequentially (e.g., socioeconomic status and cognitive function) and showed how incremental analysis of interconnected information increases holistic understanding. Through this process, the trainees were able to add new dimensions for analysis, and they experienced the excitement of creative insight.

Summary

This chapter has focused on the need for, and emergence of, a holistically oriented science that will conduct fundamental and applied research into the quality of life of elders. Although philosophers, theologians, and other individual scholars have thought deeply about related matters, a clear, programmatic commitment to the subject has not yet appeared within the contemporary sciences. Investigations of quality of life during the past 10–15 years have generally been the work of isolated explorers whose ability to commit themselves to holistic studies has been limited by reductionist disciplinary policies, priorities, and funding. In fact, one major challenge involves promoting new interdisciplinary approaches to holism by redefining disciplinary missions.

Based on the concept of holism, the authors' underlying premise is that the phenomenon known as "the quality of life of elders" is an irreducible network of interwoven parts, encompassing elders themselves (mind, body, and spirit), their animate and inanimate environment, their life experiences in space and time, and the functions or powers created by the interwoven parts. Progress in understanding this entity is significantly hindered by a lack of information about the foregoing components and their interrelationships. In terms of goals, science is faced with two interdependent challenges: The first is to establish the language, concepts, theories, and methods for a holistically oriented science. The second is to contribute information for use in personal and public activities that transform increasing longevity from years of material and moral dilemmas into years of enhanced, satisfying maturity, in other words, activities that transform the later years from a period that is seen as a time of pain and burden into a period that is a gift of years.

References

Bateson, G. (1979). *Mind and nature: A necessary unity,* pp. 3–22, 98–100. Toronto: Bantam Books.

Bennett, L. L. (1970). Protective services for the aged. In *Working with older people: A guide to practice: 3. The aging person: Needs and services.* (DHEW Publication No. 1459, pp. 52–57). Washington, D.C.: U.S. Government Printing Office.

Callahan, J. J., Jr., & Wallack, S. (1981). Major reforms in long-term care. In J. J. Callahan, Jr., & S. S. Wallack, eds., *Reforming the long-term-care system,* pp. 3–10. Lexington, Mass.: D. C. Heath.

Cath, S. H. (1963). Some dynamics of middle and later years. *Smith College Studies in Social Work, 33,* 97–126.

Collen, M. F. (1985). Information needs for technology assessment. In Institute of Medicine, *Assessing medical technologies,* pp. 502–505. Washington, D.C.: National Academy Press.

Committee for Evaluating Medical Technologies in Clinical Use (1985). Summary and methods of technology assessment. In Institute of Medicine, *Assessing medical technologies,* pp. 25–26, 88–89. Washington, D.C.: National Academy Press.

Committee on Nursing Home Regulation (1986a). Regulatory criteria. In Institute of Medicine, *Improving the quality of care in nursing homes,* p. 79. Washington, D.C.: National Academy Press.

Committee on Nursing Home Regulation (1986b). Introduction and summary: Regulatory criteria. In Institute of Medicine, *Improving the quality of care in nursing homes,* pp. 27, 81–83. Washington, D.C.: National Academy Press.

Committee on Nursing Home Regulation (1986c). Introduction and summary: Concepts of quality: Other factors affecting quality: Key indicators of quality of care. In Institute of Medicine, *Improving the quality of care in nursing homes,* pp. 23, 51–52, 171–189, 382. Washington, D.C.: National Academy Press.

d'Iribarne, P. (1972). The relationship between subjective and objective well-being. In B. Strumpel, ed., *Subjective elements of well-being,* pp. 33–44, (papers at 1972 OECD seminar). Paris: Organization for Economic Cooperation and Development.

Fusfeld, H. I. (1979). Overview of science and technology policy—1979. In H. I. Fusfeld & C. S. Haklisch, eds., *Science and technology policy: Perspectives for the 1980s,* vol. 334, pp. 1–26. New York: New York Academy of Sciences.

Katz, S. (1984). The quality of life. In C. E. Grassley and C. Pell (chairs), *Longevity and the lifestyle of the older individual.* Committee Publication of U.S. Senate. Washington, D.C.: U.S. Government Printing Office.

Katz, S. (1987). Editorial: The science of quality of life. *Journal of Chronic Disease, 40,* 459–463.

Kurowski, B. D., & Shaughnessy, P. W. (1983). The measurement and assurance of quality. In R. J. Vogel & H. C. Palmer, eds., *Long-term care: Perspectives from research and demonstrations,* pp. 103–132. Washington, D.C.: U.S. Government Printing Office.

Lindberg, D. A. B. (1979). The development and diffusion of a medical technology: Medical information systems. In National Research Council, *Medical technology and* the health care system, pp. 201–239. Washington, D.C.: National Academy of Sciences.

Liu, K., Manton, K., & Alliston, W. (1983). Demographic and epidemiologic determinants of expenditures. In R. J. Vogel & H. C. Palmer, eds., *Long-term care: Perspectives from research and demonstrations,* pp. 81–102. Washington, D.C.: U.S. Government Printing Office.

Lohr, K. N. (1989). Conceptual background and issues in quality of life. In F. Mosteller & J. Falotico-Taylor, eds., *Quality of life and technology assessment,* pp. 1–6 (monograph of the Council of Health Care Technology, Institute of Medicine). Washington, D.C.: National Academy Press.

Lovejoy, A. O. (1936). *The great chain of being.* Cambridge: Harvard University Press.

Morris, R., & Youket, P. (1981). The long-term-care issues: Identifying the problems and potential solutions. In J. J. Callahan & S. S. Wallack, eds., *Reforming the long-term-care system,* pp. 11–28. Lexington, Mass.: D. C. Heath.

Nelkin, D. (1979). The social responsibility of scientists. In H. I. Fusfeld & C. S. Haklisch, eds., *Science and technology policy: Perspectives for the 1980s,* vol. 334, pp. 176–182. New York: New York Academy of Sciences.

Pifer, A. (1986). The public policy response. In A. Pifer & L. Bronte, eds., *Our aging society: Paradox and promise,* pp. 391–413. New York: W. W. Norton.

Pirsig, R. M. (1974). *Zen and the art of motorcycle maintenance,* pp. 193–195, 260–269, 335–345. Toronto: Bantam Books.

Rivlin, A. M., & Wiener, J. M. (1988). *Caring for the disabled elderly: Who will pay?,* pp. 3–50. Washington, D.C.: Brookings Institution.

Scanlon, W., Difederico, E., & Stassen, M. (1979). *Long-term care: Current experiences and a framework for analysis* (UI No. 1215–10, pp. 122–123). Washington, D.C.: Urban Institute.

Schumacher, E. F. (1977). *A guide for the perplexed.* New York: Harper & Row.

Somers, A. R. (1981). The geriatric imperative. In A. R. Somers & D. R. Fabian, eds., *The geriatric imperative: An introduction to gerontology and clinical geriatrics,* pp. 3–19. New York: Appleton-Century-Crofts.

Szalai, A. (1980). The meaning of comparative research on the quality of life. In A. Szalai & F. M. Andrews, eds., *The quality of life: Comparative studies,* pp. 7–21. Beverly Hills, Calif.: Sage.

17

Concepts and Content of Quality of Life in the Later Years: An Overview

JAMES E. BIRREN
LISA DIECKMANN

The contributors to this volume deal with quality of life in a variety of ways. Some assume the job of defining, whereas others focus on interventions and measurement issues associated with specific assaults to quality of life in the frail elderly. The purpose of the present chapter is to provide an overview of the volume and an attempt at integration. The difference in approaches makes it difficult to directly compare the content of the preceding chapters. However, it is possible to present a picture of the overlaps, gaps, and controversies associated with the conceptualization of quality of life that emerges from this volume. The present chapter begins with a discussion of the history and current status of the concept of quality of life, followed by a review of methodological issues still to be resolved. The final section provides a chapter summary and some overall conclusions. Although some additional sources are introduced to illustrate points raised by the contributors, this overview is primarily focused on the preceding chapters.

History of the Term

As the chapters of Katz and Gurland (16) and Lawton (1) document, systematic study of quality of life is largely a phenomenon of the last decade. The contributors point out that for many years the concept of quality of life was viewed as abstract, "soft," and difficult to operationalize. Consequently, this concept was overlooked, particularly by psychology and other disciplines intent on achieving "hard science" status. More concrete health measures, such as mortality, morbidity, restricted activity days, and functional status typically have been used to evaluate the cost-effectiveness of interventions or to assess quality of care, and social scientists have relied on related but less complex concepts, such as life satisfaction, to elucidate the subjective aspects of life.

The Concept and Measurement of
Quality of Life in the Frail Elderly

Copyright © 1991 by Academic Press, Inc.
All rights of reproduction in any form reserved.

There is consensus among contributors that the recent interest in the quality of life concept has been stimulated by ethical and financial concerns associated with an aging population and the concomitant increase in chronic illness. Since older adults, particularly those over age 75, are at greater risk for chronic disease and functional disability, the increase in numbers of elderly in the population presents a challenge to the existing health care system that we are ill prepared to meet.

Contributors delineate three distinct issues that have induced social scientists and policymakers to approach, if not embrace, the rather amorphous concept of quality of life: (1) health service resource allocation, (2) intrusive use of medical technologies, and (3) quality of life in institutions.

Underlying the first issue is the fear that unrestricted dispersion of medical services to the old will result in an economic burden that society is unable or unwilling to bear. Technological advances have made it possible to keep people alive longer, but many are afraid that the cost will soon become prohibitive. As the proportion of older adults reaches a new high, so presumably will the number of candidates for life-extending health care.

Policy recommendations such as rationing make us squirm. However, if the premises of high demand and limited fiscal resources are accepted, then medicine will not be able to provide unlimited treatment to everyone who wants it. The next step, it is presumed, is to develop a means to weigh the benefits of treatment to the individual against the costs to society. Some policymakers and clinicians are hoping that quality of life measures can help with this decision making.

The above issues reflects the interest of society at large rather than that of individuals or older adults as a specific group. In fact, it is sometimes framed as an intergenerational equity issue, with the elderly pitted against society in a battle over costly and coveted health services (Caplan, 1990). However, increased attention to quality of life measures also stems from the desire to protect the right of older adults to control the way they live and die.

As we puzzle over how to allocate expensive technologies, we are also wary of inappropriate, intrusive use of life-extending procedures. Since we seem to be more adept at developing technology than devising guidelines for its compassionate, ethical use, questions regarding appropriate practice remain unanswered. How can we ensure that aggressive life-extending medical technology is both wanted and warranted from the perspective of the patient? How can we distinguish between procedures and services that truly increase overall well-being and those that prolong life in a meaningless way, to the point where death may be the better option? Who will make the decisions? Physicians at a prominent university hospital (personal communication) recently described a case in point, that of an 80-year-old women stricken with metastatic cancer whose disinterest in additional assessment and treatment was doggedly challenged by her son and son-in-law. Finally, the female patient wearily agreed to a more thorough, expensive diagnostic workup, although attending physicians acknowledged that little was likely to be gained and that the woman would be put through considerable discomfort. Privately, one physician referred to this as "cover your ass" medicine. Legal considerations prevented him from withholding the additional procedures, but he clearly regarded them as a psychological palliative for the relatives rather than rational treatment for the patient.

In recent years a number of measures have been developed that assess the impact of health conditions on functioning. These address what has been referred to as "health-related quality of life" and have been used in evaluation of intervention strategies and, increasingly, in policy analysis. In fact, the Oregon legislature has included one such measure, the Quality of Well-being Scale (Kaplan, 1988; Kaplan & Bush, 1982) in a recently announced plan to use cost–benefit rankings of medical procedures to determine Medicaid coverage (Egan, 1990). Underlying this plan is a policy that makes a priority of providing basic services to many individuals, rather than expensive procedures to a few. The policymakers report that by eliminating some highly expensive procedures they hope to be able to double the number of people receiving some coverage. In their formula, cost of treatment is weighed against the length of time before the illness would recur and quality of well-being after treatment as defined in terms of severity of symptoms and physical, social, and mobility level.

While this and many other health-related measures have been carefully and creatively developed and are psychometrically sound (see Arnold, Chapter 3), they define quality of life largely in terms of physical and functional status. The contributors to this volume (e.g., Gentile, Chapter 4; Lawton, Chapter 1) argue that, in many situations, it is important to make a distinction between the medical status of the body and the good of the person as a whole. In making this point, many approvingly cite the World Health Organization (1948) definition of health as a complete state of physical, mental, and social well-being, a definition which Lawton notes is specifically rejected by one author of the Quality of Well-being Scale. Lawton also points out that even though some health-related measures assess social as well as physical well-being, the "emphasis is always on whether physical illness or its treatment exerts a decrementing effect on non-health dimensions." The consensus seems to be that quality of life needs to be extricated from a medical context. A multidimensional quality of life concept that weights the emotional, social, and spiritual aspects of life more heavily is seen as the antidote.

Concern for the frail elderly, particularly those in institutions, is a third issue that has prodded social scientists to shape the concept of quality of life into usable form. This is the central focus of many of the contributors to the present volume. It is pointed out that assaults to quality of life are most common in the frail elderly. Whereas healthy older adults do not appear to suffer marked declines in quality of life, the frail elderly are likely to confront an overwhelming accumulation of physical, cognitive, and social losses. For example, Atchley

(Chapter 10) argues that while normal aging has a positive influence on self-concept, this trend is reversed when frailty occurs. Among the threats to self-image he describes are decreased instrumental competence, loss of significant others to affirm one's past self, and service providers who fail to reinforce a positive self-image. Similarly, Abeles (Chapter 14) concludes that sense of control may remain relatively stable in the young old but almost certainly becomes seriously threatened among the frail elderly. Dozens of other threats to quality of life in the frail elderly are described in this volume, and it is safe to say that all authors agreed that there is room for improvement in the way in which these threats are addressed in our society.

The quality of life issues associated with long-term care are as murky as those associated with acute care. Apparently, there is not much consensus as to what constitutes quality of life in institutions, what kind of interventions are the most promising, or whose responsibility it is to decide. In fact, Hofland (1988) suggested that making decisions regarding patient well-being may be more difficult in long-term care than in acute care. He pointed out that in acute care, at least some basic values are likely to be shared by patient and physician (e.g., "health is a paramount good and disease, pain, injury, and death are harms"), whereas "compared to acute care, the choices of diagnostic intervention and treatment are murkier and rely less on the objective assessment of best interests on the part of the physician and more on the subjective preferences and values of the client" (p. 5). One example of conflicting values is given by Wetle (Chapter 13). She describes a nursing home resident who was discouraged by an aide from going outside to make a snowball. The aide was concerned about the risk of falling, whereas the resident was thinking about holding on to one of the small joys in her life. Katz and Gurland (Chapter 16) summarize the problem: "In the final analysis, justification of current actions is based on conflicting judgments and uninformed demand."

Moreover, contributors point out that the search for appropriate interventions and bases for policy-making has been hampered by current approaches to evaluation. The use of both single outcome measures and frameworks derived from the medical model received considerable criticism.

Several authors argue that the use of single outcome measures, medical or otherwise, has made it all too easy to come to the wrong conclusions about the actual impact of long-term care interventions on overall quality of life. For example, an increase in one component of quality of life by an intervention may be offset or negated by a decrement in another. Fernie (Chapter 7) outlines an array of improvements in quality of life that may be afforded by technology. However, noting that many products highlight disability, he reminds us that it is important to keep in mind all the effects of a given product. For example, from one perspective, the increased mobility afforded by a wheelchair seems to constitute an obvious increment in quality of life; however, the physical advantage of using a wheelchair for locomotion must be weighed against the potential stigmatizing effects or perceived indignities. Along the same lines, Wetle (Chapter 13) and Abeles (Chapter 14) point out that autonomy has competing values, such as security and safety; and Cohn and Sugar (Chapter 2) discuss the trade-offs associated with institutionalization (e.g., relief from household responsibilities in exchange for freedom). Measurement of only one of these components can cause serious errors in interpretation and does not provide the kind of information needed to devise interventions that meet diverse sets of needs (e.g., wheelchairs with a less institutional appearance).

Unexpected positive change may also be masked if the focus of evaluation is too narrow. Lieberman (Chapter 6) demonstrates the way in which overreliance on mortality as the single outcome measure for relocation studies has led to methodological and interpretive errors, such as exaggerating the negative impact of change. Expecting the worse, investigators made little effort to assess possible positive effects.

In addition, as Lawton (1983) commented in an earlier article, demonstrating positive effects that extend across several domains is frequently a goal of evaluation research. A program or intervention appears particularly attractive if benefits are multidimensional. Spirduso and Gilliam-MacRae (Chapter 11) describe the multiple beneficial effects—cognitive and emotional as well as physical—that physical exercise may impart.

Some authors (e.g., Gentile, Chapter 4; Lawton, Chapter 1) also argue that health-related quality of life measures and quality of care, both of which fit squarely within the traditional medical model, are also inadequate tools for evaluating quality of life in long-term care. Health-related quality of life may be a particularly inappropriate method for measuring change in recipients of long-term care interventions, since in many cases neither cure nor significant medical improvement is foreseeable. Such measures will be insensitive to psychological and social interventions that may have a negligible impact on life expectancy or functioning but may, nonetheless, deliver significant increases in quality of life.

The concept of quality of care also seems to be too limited to provide a basis for evaluating and improving life in institutions. Although quality of care can be used in a manner implicitly equivalent to quality of life, particularly when access to frail elderlys' opinions is difficult to obtain, the distinction is an important one. Gentile (Chapter 4) distinguishes between the two by stating: "Whereas quality of care is measured by the cleanliness of the environment, compliance with regulations, and the type of nursing and medical care provided, quality of life focuses on the attitudinal and affective atmosphere. . . . " She argues that quality of care guidelines are only one step toward improving the status of the frail elderly and recommends the adoption of a social model that gives more consideration to psychological, social-behavioral, environmental, and spiritual aspects of life.

It appears, then, that the impetus for recent interest in quality of life issues springs in large part from the aging of society. Allocation of medical resources, intrusive use of medical technologies, and quality of life in institutions, although not specific to the old, are issues that have become more pressing because of shifts in the age composition of the population. However, as Katz and Gurland (Chapter 16) point out, quality of life issues are also beginning to arise in the population at large:

> Other contributing forces include continuing social and technological changes that affect people of all ages. For example, new production processes and products lead to concerns about the harmful effects of polluted water, radiation, acid rain, and pesticides. Concerns also prevail about the ultimate effects of such technical processes as organ transplants, genetic manipulation, and artificial methods of life support.

Currently, this is perhaps most evident in the surge of interest in the environment. Considered a fringe cause not too long ago, the environment has moved into the spotlight, with Earth Day 1990 recently celebrated worldwide. Behind all these quality of life issues is a call for a different kind of decision making, one that requires us to think in more complex, integrated ways.

One term for this kind of thinking is *holistic*. Central to Chapter 16 and mentioned in other chapters as well, it is a term frequently associated with nontraditional medicine. Defined in Webster's Third New International Dictionary (1981, 1080) as "emphasizing the functional relations between parts and wholes," the term *holistic* does not sound particularly radical or intellectually suspect. However, a holistic approach runs counter to some of the most well-entrenched (and frequently bemoaned) trends in academic psychology: reductionism/lack of integrating theory, biomedicalization, intellectual fragmentation and "disciplinary territoriality," and the emphasis on the objective at the expense of the subjective.

The study of quality of life, then, can be viewed as a rethinking of these trends. It provides an opportunity for gerontologists to redress the relative neglect of nonmedical aspects of aging that has occurred in the field of gerontology (Estes & Binney, 1989) and to take a leadership role within academia in grappling with complex issues from a multidisciplinary perspective.

Present Status of the Concept of Quality of Life

So far, more has been said about what *is not* quality of life than about what it *is*. As indicated earlier, quality of life is not equivalent to physical health status or quality of care. It has also been pointed out that quality of life is distinct from exclusively subjective constructs such as life satisfaction, morale, and happiness (Gentile, Chapter 4; George & Bearon, 1980). Arriving at a precise, consensual definition of quality of life, however, remains a goal; at its worst, quality of life tends to mean "what investigators mean it to be" (Bergner, 1989, 150) and it "invites being stuffed with anything that suits anyone's fancy" (Callahan, 1987, 178–179).

In the present volume, however, there are several areas of obvious agreement concerning the concept of quality of life among the contributors who address the overall concept. First of all, most authors appear to agree that quality of life is multidimensional—a broader and more complex construct than that suggested by predominant health-related perspectives or by the more subjective concepts such as life satisfaction and subjective well-being.

There is also considerable overlap and no immediately apparent disagreement concerning those elements (domains, aspects, components, qualities of life) that should be included in this broader concept. The contributors to this volume appear to put particular emphasis on the topics of autonomy and choice. Some also make a point of mentioning both subjective and objective elements; but none makes an attempt to derive an exhaustive list. Rather, they list sample elements in introducing the concept of quality of life or emphasize particular components in the context of their chapters. Objective factors include physical health and functional health, cognitive functioning, existence of social network, economic status, and environmental factors. Health perceptions, life satisfaction, self-esteem, and sense of control are frequently described as important subjective criteria.

However, as Lawton (Chapter 1) points out, it is far easier to come up with potential candidates for inclusion in the concept than to derive an exhaustive list or a structure that will contain and organize all possible category members. Criticizing current lists as "a jumble of content and levels of generality," Lawton describes his own efforts to impose some order. Building on his earlier work on "the good life," he puts forth a comprehensive original definition designed to accommodate all possible components of quality of life. Other authors in the present volume present useful recommendations as well. After consideration of these various contributions, this chapter offers the following definition of quality of life: Quality of is a term that refers to an evaluation of the circumstances of life of an individual, group, or population. The concept of quality of life is complex, and it embraces many characteristics of the social and physical environments as well as the health and internal states of individuals. There are two approaches to the measurement of quality of life: One is based upon the subjective or internal self-perceptions of the quality of life; the other approach is objective and based upon external judgments of the quality of life.

As reflected in the above definition, most contributors who address the issue of definition conclude that quality of life is both subjective and objective or normative. Gentile (Chapter 4), for example, cites McDowell and Newell (1987), who "define quality of life in terms of both the adequacy of material circumstances and people's feelings about these circumstances." Lawton (Chapter 1) also combines both types of criteria. Behavioral competence, for example, which is one of four sectors of quality of life Lawton defines, encompasses observable facets such as biological health, functional health, cognition, time use, and social behavior. This is balanced against perceived quality of life, which is the person's subjective evaluation of function in the same areas. In contrast with these authors, Svensson (Chapter 12) primarily emphasizes the subjective in defining quality of life. Taking a more phenomenological perspective, he proposes that the domains that make up quality of life, which he designates "qualities of life," are those areas to which an individual assigns high meaning.

The relationship between subjective and objective or normative viewpoints is a very prominent issue in this book, underscoring the comment by Katz and Gurland (Chapter 16) that the objective–subjective axis is one of the least understood aspects of quality of life. Problems associated with defining quality of life exclusively in terms of objective or normative evaluation is a central topic, the authors citing a number of examples from their own recent works and those of other investigators that reveal discrepancies among viewpoints. Contributors to the present volume also share data and hypotheses about the circumstances under which one gets disparate or close agreement.

Gentile (Chapter 4), for example, describes a study by Pearlman and Uhlmann (1988) that involved the provocative finding that physicians' ratings of quality of life in elderly patients with chronic disease were significantly lower than those made by the patients themselves. In fact, the patients described their status as satisfactory. Clearly, it is fallacious to make the jump from poor health to poor quality of life without reference to the value or meaning assigned to health by the individual and consideration of positive aspects of life that might offset the negative impact of illness. First of all, individuals may have different thresholds of sensitivity to disability, pain, and isolation with resulting different interpretations of the quality of their lives. Furthermore, factors, such as age or illness, in themselves may change the impact of illness on perceived quality of life. For example, Cohn and Sugar (Chapter 2) hypothesize that with age may come an acceptance of disability; and Lawton (Chapter 1) suggests that illness may bring with it a rearrangement of values.

In their study, Cohn and Sugar also found clear differences in the ways in which nursing home residents, staff, and families defined quality of life. Noting that aides rated frequency of baths as more important than other groups and that family members deemphasized the significance of nonfamilial social support, the investigators suggest that groups tended to define quality of life in terms of domains "that validated their roles."

It may be that salience is a factor here as well, with groups highlighting those areas with which they are most familiar or for which they hold responsibility. Along these lines, Pearlman and Uhlmann (1988) hypothesized that physicians may underestimate the quality of life of patients because of their own emphasis on medical factors and because they are exposed to patients primarily during periods of illness. Another study that compared quality of life ratings of elderly patients and those of "proxies" (family member or close friend) found that time spent by the proxy in helping the patient predicted discrepancies in ratings of functional status and social activity (Epstein, Hall, Tognetti, Son, & Conant, 1989). Proxies who spent more time per week in caregiving tended to judge the patient to be more impaired than did the patient. Epstein *et al.* also pointed out that psychologists have documented certain forms of systematic bias (e.g., the tendency of observers to weigh negative information more heavily than positive information) that may influence quality of life judgments.

However, when it comes to program evaluation or understanding quality of life, the limitations of purely subjective assessments also become apparent. Straightforward interpretation of self-report or interview responses may be misleading for a number of reasons. It is probably *not* safe to assume that individuals are aware of the components that contribute most strongly to quality of life and may be the most apt targets for intervention. Moreover, coping strategies or personality style may influence perceived well-being in a manner that renders it impervious to intervention.

Abeles (Chapter 14) and others point out that threats to perceived quality of life may be warded off through the use of coping mechanisms such as shifting standards of comparison, lowering expectations, or denial. Devaluing one aspect of quality of life and upgrading another may also be a common strategy used to maintain a sense of well-being. Moreover, previous studies have suggested that "people's tendency to proclaim themselves satisfied may be accentuated in the elderly" (Lawton, 1983, 352). When faced with reduced capacity to modify the external environment, people may rely on cognitive methods to control affect. Given declines in behavioral competence, the frail elderly may be particularly likely to describe their quality of life in overly positive terms or to pinpoint as problems only those domains over which they have control. Noting that nursing home residents focused on issues of morale and attitude, Cohn and Sugar (Chapter 2) suggest that residents typically make recommendations in areas they view as most amenable to change. They suggest that residents may concentrate "on their own responsibility for creating a good quality of life because they do not feel the institutions can be changed enough to do so." With reference to this hypothesis, Cohn and Sugar also report that residents seldom voiced concerns about fixed elements of the environment and conclude that "recommendations may be constrained by their recognition of institutional practicalities."

Interestingly, precisely the same point is made by Stanford (Chapter 9) in his discussion of quality of life and minority issues. In describing the diverse life patterns concept, he notes that minority elders give feedback based on experiences within their environment and most often are not comparing their life circumstances and experiences with those of other backgrounds. He suggests that minority elders' understanding that "they must live within the constraints of their environment" explains why many minority elders indicate that their quality of life is good when by objective standards it appears to be relatively poor.

Moreover, as Kane comments (Chapter 15), there may be subtle or not-so-subtle pressures within institutions that discourage residents from "making waves." It is difficult to avoid the conclusion that the balance of power within institutions favors the staff. Consequently, residents may be reluctant to voice their views when these differ from staff members upon whom they are dependent.

It is also possible that the difference between the nursing home resident who says, "Life is what you make it," and the one who complains to anyone who will listen lies more in relatively stable personality traits than in relative quality of life. The frail elderly may respond independently or semi-independently of content as a result of lifelong response patterns. This, of course, is the reasoning behind certain types of adjustments made on personality scales for "set" or "response" styles, such as social desirability. Arguably, the life-is-what-you-make-it attitude itself contributes to a better quality of life, but even that is an empirical matter. As Lawton notes in his chapter, hostility has been found to be associated with more positive outcomes in institutionalized elderly (Turner, Tobin, & Lieberman, 1972).

There is another limitation associated with subjective reports that is a particular problem with the frail elderly. As Arnold (Chapter 3) notes, there may be many cases in which cognitive impairment, physical frailty, or acute illness prevent individuals from speaking for themselves. In these cases, objective measures or input from significant others would be the only recourse.

A number of ethical and social policy issues revolve around possible discrepancies in opinion as to what constitutes quality of life, and these have been raised particularly in discussions of autonomy. There appear to be no easy answers. Relying on the input of proxies is problematic, but there are many cases in which the elderly are unable to decide for themselves. The dangers of paternalism are mentioned by several authors (e.g., Kane, Chapter 15; Wetle, Chapter 13). On the other hand, others (e.g., Collopy, 1988) have suggested that there may be cases of neglect that occur in the name of autonomy. In other words, respect for autonomy is not the same as nonintervention. In fact, Kane points out that, given the functional limitations of the frail elderly, their ability to exercise choice may necessitate more, rather than less, involvement on the part of the aides or family.

This issue also extends to the social policy level and may be a particular problem at this political juncture. Rappaport (1981, 14) commented that it is particularly in conservative times that "those we ignore will be described as obtaining their right not to be coerced." An administration not wishing to finance programs for the homeless mentally ill, for example, may interpret their refusal to accept custodial care as evidence that their quality of life is adequate. An example of this is a notorious comment by a former president that, because they resist intervention, homeless mentally ill individuals like living on the street. Expressed satisfaction by minority elderly could similarly be taken as evidence that services are adequate or as justification for cutting back.

Research Recommendations

One cannot avoid the impression that the study of quality of life is in an early stage. While there is evidence of productive research and scholarship, the domain as a whole is not well described. On the basis of frequency with which a topic has been mentioned (with some points for vehemence of argument), some conceptual and methodological topics are apparently considered to be particularly pressing. According to contributors, research should be directed toward the development of a model of quality of life that (1) operationalizes abstract constructs, (2) defines the relationships among specific components and quality of life, (3) weights and integrates components in a meaningful way, (4) incorporates group and individual differences, and (5) incorporates positive and negative change.

The precision and measurement of the overall concept of quality of life will suffer to the extent that the individual components lack clarity. Lawton (Chapter 1) describes operationalization of abstract domains of quality of life such as self-efficacy, agency, and community as the greatest lack in his conceptualization. Similarly, Katz and Gurland (Chapter 16) state that a prerequisite to holistic understanding is the development of a common language, "a common way of speaking about such generally neglected features . . . as attributes whose definitions currently defy consensus (e.g., life experiences, contexts, beliefs, values, attitudes)."

Several chapters in this book aim to clarify the issues related to specific domains and make suggestions for future research. The overall conclusion among those looking at specific components is that much work remains in pinning down the relationship between a given component and quality of life, particularly with the frail elderly. Original assumptions (e.g., relocation has an exclusively negative impact on quality of life; social support always contributes to improved well-being) have broken down and have been replaced with more complex but inchoate models. For example, Chappell (Chapter 8) notes that there may be a nonlinear relationship between some forms of social support and some aspects of quality of life. Some forms of social support may be associated with increased personal control, but too much social support may create decreased sense of control or dependency.

Perhaps some of the most innovative research on quality of life will involve the study of the interrelationships of components. As Katz and Gurland (Chapter 16) argue: "Although the concept recognizes and accepts the need for studies of parts of a given phenomenon, it stresses the overriding need to understand the organic or functional relationships among the parts or, in other words, to understand what happens when the parts are put together." In addition to separate ratings of dimensions of quality of life, individuals also appear to be able to give a general indicator of the overall quality of life (i.e., an answer to the question, "All things considered, how do you rate your quality of life?"). Understanding the ways in which individuals integrate the many aspects of quality of life to arrive at such a pronouncement will be a particular challenge. As Atchley (Chapter 10) and Katz and Gurland (Chapter 16) note, science has been more oriented toward differentiation than integration.

The need for a model that will accommodate individual and group differences is also a recurring theme. Not only do we need to find a way to combine discrete domains, we need to personalize the regression equation. As the earlier discussion on subjectivity suggests, one issue raised again and again by contributors concerns the differences in perception among individuals and groups as to what constitutes quality of life and how it is assessed: "Quality of life means different things to different people" (Cohn & Sugar, Chapter 2); "Different individuals view similar situations in different ways" (Chapell, Chapter 8).

The studies by Kane and Cohn and Sugar (this volume) have revealed differences in the ways in which nursing home residents, staff, and families define quality of life. These and other studies that document group differences have important implications for long-term care policy. Continued work in this area is particularly important given the increasing heterogeneity of the aging population. The ethnic diversity of the aging population is such that the desires, expectations, and perceptions involved in quality of life are likely to vary widely. In Stanford's (Chapter 9) view, this diversity dooms to failure mass-market solutions to the problems of aging. Until differences in the way quality of life is defined among minority groups are spelled out, services may be inappropriate and/or underutilized.

As Wetle (Chapter 13) points out in her discussion of autonomy, there may be considerable diversity *within* groups as well. Autonomy is generally considered to be a highly valued component of quality of life that is limited by institutional constraints or insensitive medical personnel rather than by personal choice. As Kane (Chapter 15) comments, it seems self-evident that personal autonomy is an important human desire. Nonetheless, a survey of residents regarding health care decision making (Wetle, Levkoff, Cwikel, & Rosen, 1988) revealed a wide range of preferences, including a substantial percentage of residents who were satisfied with little or no information or involvement.

In addition to continuing efforts to delineate individual and group differences in the way quality of life is defined, it has been recommended that investigators seek out the mechanisms that account for the diverse patterns of perception. In addition to ethnic background, some possible candidates mentioned included age differences, health status, type of illness, individual coping styles, conditions of entry or duration in long-term care setting, and job or role.

Finally, both Lawton (Chapter 1) and Lieberman (Chapter 6) strongly advise that more attention be paid to positive as well as negative changes in quality of life. Lawton argues that it is important *not* to follow the example of medicine, which has typically gauged health in terms of negative deviations from the usual. He recommends that researchers devote equal time to the study of those factors that elevate quality of life above baseline, and he reminds us that positive and negative affect appear to be at least partially independent. When devising interventions for those in long-term care, the contribution of the positive may be particularly important. Adding the positive may be more feasible than reducing the negative (e.g., symptoms and institutional constraints). Lawton also notes that there may be individual variation in the relative importance of avoidance of negative states versus the proliferation of positive states. Take, for example, the work on individual differences which suggests that introverts may be more sensitive to punishment signals and extroverts more sensitive to reward (Gray, 1971, 1982). Lieberman (Chapter 6) was equally critical of the practice in relocation studies of defining success in terms of absence of change. Noting that the effects of relocation can be beneficial as well as detrimental, he concludes that a more complex model is required.

A Practical Recommendation

The preceding discussion implies that if care is to be humanely as well as efficiently organized, considerable anticipatory research should be initiated. However, one practical strategy that can be put into effect immediately is worth reiterating. Several authors in the present volume recommend eliciting input from nursing home residents and involving them in decision making on quality of life issues. Pynoos and Regnier (Chapter 5) suggest "before and after" resident surveys for the planning and evaluation of design features; Cohn and Sugar (Chapter 2), Gentile (Chapter 4), and Kane (Chapter 15) recommend development of an ongoing dialogue among nursing home residents, families, staff, and administration. Gentile describes one such program that was implemented by Wells and Singer (1988). Nursing home residents and staff were asked to evaluate the social climate of their institution and to describe the way they would like it to be. Results from the survey were then used to form committees and stimulate group discussions on ways to improve quality of life.

Summary and Conclusions

The chapters in this book document the increased interest in quality of life that has resulted from pressing ethical and financial concerns associated with the growing elderly population. The authors, experts in their subject matters, were asked to present their opinions and recommendations about improving the quality of life of the frail elderly.

The resultant chapters of this volume reflect a wide range of approaches to the definition and measurement of quality of life and differences in intervention strategies. Since the authors are senior investigators and scholars, the diversity must be taken as evidence of the early stage of development of the subject matter. One notices little consensus on definition. Evidently, there seems to have been some lack of interest in defining quality of life.

Future research and scholarship on the subject should give more attention to the definition of quality of life lest its boundaries become synonymous with almost all aspects of living. In particular, since measurements flow from concepts and definitions, it is desirable for researchers to state explicitly their meanings of the concept and to bring to the surface of discussion the implicit assumptions as to what constitutes quality of life.

Health, as well as health care, is obviously a component in quality of life, but it does not comprise the necessary and sufficient conditions for high quality of life. The contributors of this book explicitly reject a medical definition of quality of life. Limitations of the medical definition cited were its neglect of psychological, social, environmental, and spiritual factors and lack of attention to positive increments to quality of life. The medical definition is also seen as a contributing factor to the "biomedicalization of aging" and relegation of older adults to "sick-role" status. A few authors define health as total well-being—physical, social, and psychological—which approaches in meaning a broad concept of high quality of life. This leads to the question of how good health (in the WHO sense) is different from high quality of life.

The study of quality of life requires a holistic approach. Not only is multidimensionality called for, but also the study of the relationship among the components. For example, how the various qualities of life are hierarchically organized is an issue to be explored. In weighting individual elements, it may be anticipated that there are marked discontinuities attached to their importance (e.g., if one is in great pain, then the cleanliness of one's room may not enter one's weighted average of quality of life). Similarly, as the environment of the frail person shrinks in space and time, variables may assume a new saliency, some becoming unimportant and others ascending in dominance (such as having the opportunity to spend one's last days and die in a self-defined state of dignity and appropriateness).

One of the important issues in the definition of quality of life and its measurement concerns whose perspective and values form the basis of the evaluation and the dimensions along which the evaluations are made (i.e, that of the observer or that of the observed). This distinction is frequently contrasted by the terms subjective and objective, or normative, quality of life. The subjective, self-perceived quality of life embraces the facets of existence that enter into the awareness of the individual. The individual's personal values and history modify the evaluation or weighting assigned to the elements that enter into a global

quality of life judgment (e.g., answering the question, "How is life for you?").
The objective or normative evaluation of quality of life is made by external
observers. It is based upon estimates of the quality of the physical and social
environments, the physical and mental health of the individual, and the support
systems available to the individual. Also, the objective measurement and concept
of quality of life appears to be equivalent to the World Health Organization
definition of health, which regards total physical, mental, and social well-being.
Obviously, the measurement of quality of life by subjective and objective judgments will not necessarily be in close agreement. For example, in the case of
anxious or depressed persons, there may be wide disagreement between these
two assessments of quality of life.

Professionals tend to assume that their dimensions of judgments about quality
of life are the same as those of the older patients, residents, or clients of service.
The chapters in the present volume lead to the conclusion that we need to study
the structure and weight of the dimensions defined by professionals and observers as well as those of the observed.

Lurking behind the objective stance often lies the assumption of lack of competence of the older person to judge his or her quality of life as well as the latent
parental position of "we who know best." This can lead to protectionism and
medicalization of the aged with overuse of guardianship relationships and social
and physical restraints. The older person may wish to trade some high-quality
care and dependence for more autonomy of action. The opposite extreme is the
exercise of neglect in the name of autonomy.

Obviously, at some point, the institution and its staff become *en loco parentis*
as the individual becomes disabled, of poor mental or physical health, or incompetent. On the other hand, institutions and professionals have to respect the
decisions and desires of the competent elderly who are in good mental health.
The limits of the parental surrogate role will no doubt be explored and defined
more clearly in the future as the forces directed toward the care of the frail elderly
increase in relation to the growing population to be served.

Given the heterogeneity of the aging population, the development and implementation of social policy for the frail elderly will require knowledge about the
norms and values of different ethnic and clinical subgroups. Attention will also
need to be paid to within-group differences that result from personality styles or
life experiences.

Given the early stage of development of quality of life research, many different
kinds of study should and will likely be initiated in the future. Quantification and
the development of indices of quality of life will no doubt increase. However, it
is apparent that there is also a need for naturalistic or case history approaches that
can provide input into designed research. Some investigators will need to saturate
themselves in the "real life" circumstances of frail elderly persons. The complexity of issues necessitates a multidisciplinary approach to defining the land-

scape of quality of life of the frail elderly. Without such an approach and without the additional access to critiques of humanists, our care of the elderly can become industrialized with a bottom-line mentality to guide it.

This chapter puts forth quality of life as a complex concept that needs to be studied in a multivariant manner with different populations. For the competent elderly, there seems little reason to avoid the acceptance of their subjective statements of quality of life as the criterion of significance. However, it is likely that their cognitive assessment, embracing a sweep of time, approaches the concept of a trait rather than an instantaneous evaluation of the state of their present mood or attitude. The psychodynamics of judgments of quality of life remain a wide open territory for exploration. Presumably, not only will the elements of their contemporary milieu enter older persons' evaluations, but their life experiences and cultural backgrounds may lead them to weight differently the environmental opportunities for privacy and autonomy as well as contacts with other persons and the physical features of their environments.

For those elderly persons with limitations in competence and/or with emotional dysfunctions, we will probably have to rely more on external, or perhaps nonverbal, judgments about quality of life. We already know that self-perceptions and the perceptions of others are only modestly related, which suggests caution in moving quickly to define what is good for the frail elderly without considering their opinions.

References

Bergner, M. (1989). Quality of life, health status, and clinical research. *Medical Care, 27* (Suppl.), 148–156.

Callahan, D. (1987). *Setting limits: Medical goals in an aging society.* New York: Simon and Schuster.

Caplan, A. L. (1990). Ethical issues and the care of the elderly. In R. L. Kane, J. G. Evans, & D. McFadyen, eds., *Improving the health of older people,* pp. 667–681. Oxford: Oxford University Press.

Collopy, B. J. (1988). Autonomy in long term care: Some crucial distinctions. *The Gerontologist, 28* (Suppl.), 10–17.

Egan, T. (1990). Oregon lists illnesses by priority to see who gets Medicaid care. *New York Times,* May 3, 1.

Epstein, A. M., Hall, J. A., Tognetti, J. A., Son, L. H., & Conant, L. (1989). Using proxies to evaluate quality of life. *Medical Care, 27* (Suppl.), 91–98.

Estes, C. L., & Binney, E. A. (1989). The biomedicalization of aging: The dangers and dilemmas. *The Gerontologist, 29,* 587–589.

George, L. K., & Bearon, L. B. (1980). *Quality of life in older persons: Meaning and measurement.* New York: Human Sciences Press.

Gray, J. A. (1971). *The psychology of fear and stress.* New York: McGraw-Hill.

Gray, J. A. (1982). *The neuropsychology of anxiety.* New York: Oxford University Press.

Hofland, B. F. (1988). Autonomy in long term care: Background issues and a programmatic response. *The Gerontologist, 28* (Suppl.), 3–9.

Kaplan, R. M. (1988). Health-related quality of life in cardiovascular disease. *Journal of Clinical and Consulting Psychology, 56,* 382–392.

Kaplan, R. M., & Bush, J. W. (1982). Health-related quality of life measurement for evaluation research and policy analysis. *Health Psychology, 1,* 61–80.

Lawton, P. (1983). Environment and other determinants of well-being in older people. *The Gerontologist, 23,* 349–357.

McDowell, I., & Newell, C. (1987). *Measuring health: Guide to rating scales and questionnaires.* New York: Oxford University Press.

Pearlman, R. A., & Uhlmann, R. F. (1988). Quality of life in chronic diseases: Perceptions of elderly people. *Journal of Gerontology, 43,* 25–30.

Rappaport, J. (1981). In praise of paradox: A social policy of empowerment over prevention. *American Journal of Community Psychology, 9,* 1–25.

Turner, B. F., Tobin, S. S., & Lieberman, M. A. (1972). Personality traits as predictors of institutional adaption among the aged. *Journal of Gerontology, 27,* 61–68.

Webster's Third New International Dictionary (1981). Springfield, Mass.: Merriam-Webster, Inc.

Wells, L. M., & Singer, C. (1988). Quality of life in institutions for the elderly: Maximizing well-being. *The Gerontologist, 28,* 266–269.

Wetle, T., Levkoff, S. E., Cwikel, J., & Rosen, A. (1988). Nursing home resident participation in medical decisions: Perceptions and preferences. *The Gerontologist, 28* (Suppl.), 32–38.

World Health Organization (1948). *Constitution of the World Health Organization.* Geneva, Swit.: WHO Basic Documents.

Author Index

Subject Index

Activities of daily living
 assistance with, 173, 175
 autonomy, 321
 competence, 12, 14
 eating, 149
 exercise, 234, 237–239, 248
 housekeeping, 151, 157
 measurement of quality of life, 4, 8,
  18, 62, 81
 toileting, 150
Adaptation (*see also* Coping)
 intelligence, 260
 environments of, 111
 relocation, 130, 133–134
 to institutions, 30
 to life, 20
Affect
 emotional support, 173, 176, 183
 exercise, 242
 measurement, 356
 quality of life, 19
 relocation, 131, 134
 self, 209
 wisdom, 261
Ageism
 definition, 229
 frailty, 230, 249
 sense of control, 303
Aging (*see also* Normal aging, Successful
  aging)
 alteration in perceptions, 46
 control, 297, 304–305, 307–309
 definition, 28, 214
 inactivity, 227
 increase, 345, 249
 influence on self, 215–217, 223
 intellectual function, 266, 270

physical function, 44, 232–235, 249
 trend, 336
Alzheimer's disease
 assistive devices, 156
 autonomy, 323
 dependence, 81
Autonomy (*see also* Control, Independence)
 definition, 279–280, 316, 331
 delegated, 289
 diversity, 355
 environments, 99
 long-term care, 30, 35, 40, 42, 78, 85,
  286, 287–288, 290, 324
 measurement, 325–330
 physical independence, 322
 principle of respect, 316–317
 quality of life, 13, 350, 353
 restriction, 319–320
 values, 315, 348

Blindness
 assistive devices, 159

Cardiovascular function
 exercise, 235–236, 239, 241
Caregivers (*see also* Family, Friends)
 affect, 19
 control, 305
 evaluation, 352
 family, 144, 172–174, 184
 minority, 201
 quality of life, 291
 reciprocity, 180
 technology, 143, 166